Psychiatric and Mental Health Nursing

From
Bill Reynolds

to Ruth Murray
with gratitude for
wonderful hospitality
1st November, 1992

Psychiatric and Mental Health Nursing

Theory and practice

William Reynolds
Senior Tutor, Highland College of Nursing and Midwifery
Raigmore Hospital, Inverness

and

Desmond Cormack
Honorary Reader in Health and Nursing
Queen Margaret College, Edinburgh

CHAPMAN AND HALL
LONDON · NEW YORK · TOKYO · MELBOURNE · MADRAS

1990

UK   Chapman and Hall, 2–6 Boundary Row, London SE1 8HN

USA   Chapman and Hall, 29 West 35th Street, New York
              NY10001

JAPAN   Chapman and Hall Japan, Thomson Publishing Japan,
              Hirakawacho Nemoto Building, 7F, 1–7–11 Hirakawa-cho,
              Chiyoda-ku, Tokyo 102

AUSTRALIA   Chapman and Hall Australia, Thomas Nelson Australia,
              480 La Trobe Street, PO Box 4725, Melbourne 3000

INDIA   Chapman and Hall India, R. Sheshadri, 32 Second Main
              Road, CIT East, Madras 600 035

First edition 1990

© 1990   Chapman and Hall

Typeset in 10/12pt Palatino by
Best-set Typesetter Ltd
Printed in Great Britain by
Page Bros (Norwich) Ltd

ISBN 0 412 31610 2

British Library Cataloguing in Publication Data
Reynolds, William
   Psychiatric and mental health nursing.
   1. Mentally disordered patients. Nursing
   I. Title   II. Cormack, Desmond
   610.7368

   ISBN 0-412-31610-2

Library of Congress Cataloging-in-Publication Data

Psychiatric and mental health nursing: theory and practice / [edited
   by] William Reynolds and Desmond Cormack. – 1st ed.
      p.   cm.
   Includes bibliographical references.
   ISBN 0–412–31610–2
   1. Psychiatric nursing.   I. Reynolds, William, 1945–
II. Cormack, Desmond.
   [DNLM: 1. Models, Psychological.   2. Psychiatric Nursing –
methods.
WY 160   P9715]
RC440.P729   1990
610.73'68—dc20
DNLM/DLC
for Library of Congress   90-1514
                                                           CIP

Contents

Contributors

Philip Barker, RNMH, PhD, Honorary Lecturer, Department of Psychiatry, University of Dundee, Scotland.

Beverly Benfer, RN, MA, FAAN, Consultant in Administrative and Psychiatric Nursing, Marion, IA, USA.

David A. Bertin, RMN, RGN, Cert Behaviour Therapy Nursing, Clinical Nurse Specialist, Argyll and Bute Hospital, Lochgilphead, Argyll, Scotland.

Mary Chambers, RGN, RMN, Dip Nurs (Lond), RNT, BEd (Hons), Senior Lecturer in Psychiatric Nursing, Department of Nursing and Health Visiting, University of Ulster, Coleraine, Londonderry, Northern Ireland.

Desmond F. S. Cormack, RMN, RGN, MPhil, Dip Ed, Dip Nurs, PhD, Honorary Reader in Health and Nursing, Queen Margaret College, Clerwood Terrace, Edinburgh, Scotland.

Bryn Davis, BD, SRN, RMN, RNT, BSc, PhD, Principal Lecturer, Department of Community Studies, Brighton Polytechnic, Brighton, England.

Katherine Dorsey, RN, MS, BSN, Nursing Home Care Unit, Veterans Administration Medical Center, Roseburg, OR, USA.

Anne Hume, RGN, RMN, Cert Behaviour Therapy Nursing, Senior Nurse Therapist, The Montgomery Clinic, Edinburgh, Scotland.

Maxine E. Loomis, RN, CS, PhD, FAAN, Professor and Director (PhD Program), University of South Carolina, College of Nursing, Columbia, SC, USA.

Peggy Martin, RGN, RMN, Dip N (Lond), RCNT, RNT, Senior Tutor, Sussex Downs School of Nursing, Hellingly Hospital, Harlsham, England.

Shelagh Meuser, RN, BS, Lieutenant Commander, The Naval Hospital, Portsmouth, VA, USA.

Anita O'Toole, RN, PhD, CS, Professor and Graduate Program Director (Psychiatric Mental Health Nursing), School of Nursing, Kent State University, Kent, OH, USA.

Hildegard Peplau, RN, EdD, FAAN, Professor Emerita, Rutgers, The State University of New Jersey, New Brunswick, NJ, USA.

Shirley Purcell, RN, MN, Associate Chief, Veterans Administration Medical Center, Roseburg, OR, USA.

William Reynolds, RMN, RNT, RGN, MPhil, Senior Tutor, Highland College of Nursing and Midwifery, Raigmore Hospital, Inverness, Scotland.

Patricia Schroder, RN, MA, CS, Consultant in Psychiatric Nursing, Marion, IA, USA.

Shirley Smoyak, RN, PhD, FAAN, Professor of Doctoral Nursing Studies, Faculty of Planning, Institute of Health Care Policy and Aging Research, Rutgers, The State University of New Jersey, New Brunswick, NJ, USA.

Patricia Underwood, RN, DNSc, FAAN, Professor of Clinical Nursing and Vice Chair, Department of Mental Health, Community and Administrative Nursing, School of Nursing, University of California, San Francisco, CA, USA.

Preface

Psychiatric and Mental Health Nursing: Theory and practice was conceived as a result of three major premises which, in the view of the editors, relate to the practice of psychiatric and mental health nursing. First, that high-quality psychiatric and mental health nursing can be practised only if it is underpinned by appropriate nursing theory. Secondly, that there exists a body of theory which can and should be applied to psychiatric and mental health nursing. Thirdly, that there is a need for a text which will assist teachers, students and clinicians to apply available nursing and borrowed theory to clinical practice.

The general aim of this book is to introduce nursing students to a theory-based approach to caring for people with psychiatric and mental health problems. The phrase psychiatric and mental health problems indicates that the text relates to clients with a psychiatric diagnosis, and also to those who have mental health problems but who do not necessarily have such a diagnosis. The client group to which the material in this text applies will include those who are, or have been, hospitalized and those in the community who have not been, and may never be, hospitalized.

The intended readership is all students of psychiatric and mental health nursing issues, for example basic and post-basic nurses, and their teachers. Established clinicians who are seeking to develop skills in applying psychiatric and mental health nursing theory to practice will, we hope, also find the content of value. While the book is primarily intended for nurses, it should also be of interest to all other groups of psychiatric and mental health workers such as social work, clinical psychology and occupational therapy students.

The special features of this book are that it is essentially a nursing book which seeks to identify problems which nurses can treat, and the means by which that can be done. Selected theoretical models are discussed in relation to general principles and applications, then applied to examples of specific psychiatric and mental health problems. It is intended to rectify the relative weakness of many texts on nursing theory which do not fully address nursing practice, and many relating to nursing practice which do not fully address nursing theory. By addressing both nursing theory and practice via the application of theory, the text will introduce readers to the rationale underpinning a variety of nursing treatment strategies.

Part One of the text (Chapters 1 and 2) introduces the role of nurse in terms of using theory-based strategies in order to personally influence the mental health of clients. Chapter 1 traces the development of the nurse's role from that of providing custodial care, to the identification and treatment of human responses to psychiatric and mental health problems, via the application of nursing theory. The application of theory to practice is dependent on making one or more nursing diagnoses as a means of focusing nursing care on one or more specific patient needs/problems. Chapter 2 gives a classification of human responses which, we believe, provides an appropriate framework from which to make nursing diagnoses. Many of these responses are dealt with in practical terms in the subsequent two parts of the text (Chapters 3 to 18) and provide demonstrations of how diagnoses were made, and the application of theory to practice in order to effect desired change through appropriate nursing intervention.

Part Two (Chapters 3 to 10) provides insight into the rationale, content and general principles of a number of selected major nursing and borrowed theories, and demonstrates the general application of these in relation to psychiatric and mental health nursing. Readers may wish to use Part Two in one of two ways. First, Chapters 3 to 10 might be read independently of the remainder of the text in order to study the principles and general applications of a number of major theories. Alternatively, readers may wish to study an individual chapter on principles and general applications, then move on to the corresponding chapter in Part Three which deals with clinical applications. Because of the common origins of some of the theories presented in this book, and because of similarities in the way in which some are interpreted and applied, there is inevitably a degree of overlap in the chapters in this and the subsequent part of the text. We make no apology for this overlap and view it as a demonstration of the need for nurses to be familiar with and, when appropriate, make use of more than one theory. This approach to nursing is reflected in our decision to include Chapters 10 and 18 which view psychiatric and mental health nursing from an eclectic perspective.

Part Three (Chapters 11 to 18) demonstrates how each of the selected theories can be applied in particular clinical situations. Authors present a brief case-study of a client with specific needs/problems and describe how nursing care based on relevant theory can be delivered. These chapters enable readers to consider why clients behave in a certain way, guide them to an appropriate nursing diagnosis and intervention, and assist in the prediction and assessment of outcome.

Part Four (Chapters 19 to 21) focuses on issues relating to teaching and learning psychiatric and mental health nursing, and on the nature and scope of psychiatric nursing research. The first two chapters in this part (Chapters 19 and 20) indicate our belief that teaching and learning this subject requires special insights, innovative and special teaching/learning approaches, and the development of a teacher–learner relationship which is not unlike the client–patient relationship. Finally, Chapter 21 reviews the contributions to, and limitations of, existing psychiatric and mental health nursing research.

As with any textbook, *Psychiatric and Mental Health Nursing: Theory and practice* has its limitations. It does not deal with the pathology or aetiology of mental illness, with the contributions of other professionals, or with the structure and organization of psychiatric and mental health care generally, or nursing in particular, for example. However, these limitations are deliberate in that the general aim of the text is to demonstrate how nursing theory can be applied to clinical practice, and to place that application in the context of how the subject is being, and can be, taught, learned and researched.

W. J. Reynolds (Inverness) and D. F. S. Cormack (Edinburgh), 1990

Part One

THE ROLE OF THE PSYCHIATRIC NURSE

This section sets the scene for the rest of the book. Chapter 1 by Reynolds and Cormack is essentially a summary of the aims of the text, examining such fundamental issues as the focus for psychiatric nursing practice and the need for it to be theoretically based. Loomis and O'Toole provide an excellent nursing diagnostic classification system. It is our contention that the content of Chapter 2, nursing diagnosis, will be at the forefront of future debate about the role and function of psychiatric nurses. Indeed, an understanding of such a diagnostic framework is essential to the application of theory to practice.

The relevance of nursing diagnosis to nursing practice was emphasized by Peplau (1988) when she stated that '...over the years, nurses have called public attention to their duties, obligations, activities and roles. These items tell what nurses do, but not what nurses set out to fix, change, correct, relieve, remedy or prevent.' In other words, Peplau is suggesting that nurses have found it difficult to identify the focus for their work. They have hinted at, but not named, nursing's domain. A classification system, such as the one presented in Chapter 2, is intended to help psychiatric and mental health nurses to organize their functions and define their scope. We also believe that such a classification system will expedite nursing research and assist communication between nurses, consumers and other health care providers.

Readers are invited to reflect upon the stated motives for the development of a diagnostic or classification system for psychiatric and mental health nursing.

References

Peplau, H. (1988) Substance and scope of psychiatric nursing. Paper presented at the 3rd. National Conference on Psychiatric Nursing. Montreal, Canada.

Chapter 1

Psychiatric and mental health nursing: theory and practice

W. REYNOLDS and D. CORMACK

Contemporary psychiatric nursing has its recent history in the custodial model of care which caused the mentally ill to be isolated, frequently under lock and key, from the rest of the population. Such people were housed in psychiatric institutions, and provided with clothing, heat, food and other physical requirements. The main purpose of medical intervention was to separate patients from the rest of the community, to keep them in reasonably good physical health, and to provide physically based psychiatric treatment. Medical intervention was, for the most part, confined to making psychiatric diagnoses, the prescription of a small range of tranquillizers, and to other forms of physical treatment. For the most part, psychiatric nurses functioned in support of this isolate and tranquillize philosophy. Up until the 1940s and 1950s, one of the main attributes of a psychiatric nurse was adequate physical stature and strength. The main purpose of psychiatric nursing was to contain patients, keep them in reasonable physical health, and prevent patients from harming themselves, other patients, and staff. The custodial role of the nurse in these areas was of paramount importance, with the psychiatrist being the sole source of decision making, determining the type and focus of nursing care, and generally being responsible for all aspects of patient treatment. This relationship between doctor and nurse, with the former being responsible for and directing the activities of nursing staff, was little changed from that existing 100 years earlier when Connelly (1856, p. 37) wrote: '. . . all his [the physician's] plans, all his care, all his personal labour, must be counteracted, if he has attendants [nurses] who will not observe his rules, when he is not in the ward, as conscientiously as when he is present.'

Thus, the period which emphasized custodial care began and ended with a psychiatric nursing role which included little more than a caretaking custodial function. The primary function of the nurse, therefore, was to maintain the safety and physical health of patients under the close direction and supervision of medical staff, and to carry out the treatments prescribed by them. That view contrasts with that of Reynolds (1988a) who stated that the primary function of the psychiatric nurse is to formulate and deliver his or her own treatment strategies, rather than to focus exclusively on giving assistance to other professionals. During the 1950s, when an array of psychopharmacological treatments became available, the custodial approach began to be extended to include a range of more sophisticated and selective treatments. At that stage, the role of the psychiatric nurse was extended to include the administration of a much wider range of medical prescriptions, and to monitoring the effects and side-effects of these. As a consequence of the use of these pharmacological agents, many patients became considerably more accessible to nursing staff, leading to the formation of a variety of nurse–patient relationships. Although these nurse–patient relationships were relatively unsophisticated, frequently unplanned, and not designed to fulfil any specific goals, they undoubtedly had the potential for enabling nursing staff to positively influence the health status of patients. Indeed, there followed some debate regarding the extent to which psychopharmacology influenced patient behaviour, and the extent to which nurse–patient interactions and relationships produced change. McGhie (1957, p. xiii), in a discussion of the role of the psychiatric nurse, stated: '...psychiatrists, while not doubting the efficacy of these [medical] treatments to many psychiatric conditions, have referred to the difficulty in differentiating between the therapeutic value of the treatment itself and the interpersonal influences which are an integral part of any treatment situation'.

Increased nurse–patient contact, frequently resulting in the formation of informal relationships, added a new dimension to the role of the psychiatric nurse. Nursing staff were now able to influence the mental health status of patients, although this was almost certainly done in an unstructured, unsystematic and random way which had no theoretical underpinning. Indeed, it might be argued that nurses used their new access to patients in order to encourage/motivate patients to continue to accept that which was offered in terms of the custodial model of care, and to accept those specific (medical) treatments which were provided by psychiatrists. Nurses were perceived as being those who facilitated the work of others, primarily that of medical staff. Johnson and Martin (1958), in a sociological comment on the psychiatric nurses' role suggested that they might have a specialist function in terms of maintaining the equilibrium of the patient/ carer sphere, and in facilitating success of patient care within the medical model. In discussing these aspects of the psychiatric nurses' role Johnson and Martin (1958, p. 373) stated: 'We call actions which are directly related to moving the system towards its goal instrumental, and actions which are related to maintaining motivational equilibrium in the individuals composing the group expressive'.

In the previous year Belknap (1956) placed nurses in the role of mediators between patients and doctors, preventing the latter from being over-whelmed by large numbers of patients who may have wished to see the doctor.

Thus, the increased ability of nurses to relate to, and interact with, patients enabled them to give additional support to the care of the patient within the context of the medical model. It was to be some considerable time before psychiatric nurses generally began to see opportunities for development of a role which would enable them to make a personal con-tribution to achieving positive changes in the mental health status of patients. During the 1970s a number of research studies were undertaken to try to identify those areas of psychiatric nursing which constituted a special and unique contribution by psychiatric nurses. For example, the study by Towell (1975, p. 13) attempted to: '...discover how nurses understand the behaviour of patients in these various ward settings and with what consequences for their action in relation to patients'. Towell (1975) concluded, as did Cormack (1976), that nurses were not making use of potentially therapeutic relationships in the manner which was described in much of the contemporary psychiatric nursing literature. Although the reasons for nurses' inability or reluctance to encompass a personal thera-peutic role may be difficult to establish, evidence of that position continued to exist in the early 1980s. Cormack (1983, p. 12) reported the following anecdotal information which was derived from his meetings with trained nursing staff in a Scottish psychiatric hospital. A staff nurse said: 'I can see how it is possible to identify patients' specific non-physical problems, disorientation for example. However, our role does not involve influencing these problems, that is the job of the psychiatrist.' On being asked how the psychiatrist would influence the above problem, and others such as trust, anxiety and hostility the staff nurse replied: 'The psychiatrist prescribes medication, that is how the problems are treated. The nurse assists in the treatment by giving the medications, feeding patients and making sure they are safe and so on'.

In trying to understand the continued dependence of psychiatric nurses on the medical model of care, one must look closely at psychiatric nurse education and (more importantly) on the published materials which are available upon which to underpin the notion of a personal therapeutic role. The purpose of this text is to provide nurse clinicians and educators with a clinically applicable theoretical basic upon which psychiatric nurses can develop personalized therapeutic skills. It is hoped that the content of this text will go some way towards answering questions raised in the seminal text by Altschul (1972). These questions were: 'What is the theoretical basis on which sound nursing practice is to be based?' and 'What criteria can be used to evaluate the effect of nursing care?' Central to the philosophy of this text is acceptance of the notion that a central part of the role of the nurse is 'the diagnosis and treatment of human responses to an actual and potential health problem' (American Nurses' Association, 1980).

The role of the psychiatric nurse

The role of the psychiatric nurse has three important elements: that relating to custodial care, that which is supportive to the medical model of care, and that which requires psychiatric nurses to personally influence the mental health status of patients. Whilst we regard all three elements as important, we submit that the latter element (that which requires psychiatric nurses to personally influence the mental health status of patients) is the primary role of the psychiatric nurse, and that which makes psychiatric nursing unique.

The custodial role

The biological maintenance of all human beings is essential and of immediate importance. In psychiatric institutions this (immediate) responsibility has, for historical reasons, become part of the psychiatric nurse's role. This responsibility, which will remain for the foreseeable future, is one which relates to and interacts with the personal therapeutic function of the psychiatric nurse. That this function has extended into the therapeutic domain can be demonstrated by the fact that a nurse who encounters a patient who is undernourished by his/her refusal to eat, will regard this as a problem which can be influenced by the use of a range of therapeutic techniques. In other words, the nurse would no longer focus on nutrition as being the primary problem; rather, she would attempt to understand and influence the psychodynamics of this phenomenon.

Custodial care, therefore, remains an important part of the psychiatric nurse's role. Patients who cannot eat will continue to require to be fed, patients who are incontinent will require to be changed and cleaned, and patients who cannot walk will need to be assisted with mobility. For some patients, these deficits present no additional problems which require additional therapeutic interventions. For others, however, these deficits may cause the patient to have superimposed problems which do require such intervention. For example, patients may have difficulty in coming to terms with an inability to eat unaided, being incontinent, or having to be moved with assistance. Where these superimposed difficulties occur, they require to be understood and treated by the use of a range of therapeutic techniques.

The role of the psychiatric nurse, therefore, encompasses a range of biological/physiological patient needs. In particular, it addresses patients' psychological responses to experiencing those particular needs. Chapter 2, which provides a classification of human response patterns for psychiatric mental health nursing practice, includes a range of human response patterns in physiological processes. The psychiatric nurse will diagnose and treat these items in the context of the patient's mental health status rather than as isolated physiological needs and responses.

The medical model

Clark (1981, p. 21) suggests that: '. . . the traditional medical model views the client as a passive host of disease processes, tended by experts who always know best, and who believe that the client's conceptualization of his predicament has little relevance to his condition'. According to Clark, the client's stay in hospital consists of treatment sessions, for example, drugs and/or electro-convulsive therapy, or brief chats with his doctors and nurses. The time spent between the sessions are merely waiting periods to be filled in as best as possible. A psychiatric admission ward operating on the medical model makes a (superficially) reassuring impression on those who view it. Clients may be seen in bed waiting for a physical examination, or wandering around in casual clothes, watching TV or engaged in some other social activity. Some patients may be playing table tennis, billiards, or otherwise engaged in one of a range of activities. Nursing staff, who may be actively engaged in this activity, see their major role as maintaining and occupying patients, with the main thrust of treatment being provided by medical colleagues. They regard medical treatment as being the main focus of cure. People who have been patients in such a setting frequently speak well of the medical treatment, and of the support which nursing staff provided to achieve this. In large part, the causes of mental health problems are externalized, with help being available only in the form of that provided by medical staff. However, many patients will speak of the tedium generated by the hospital stay with time essentially being used by waiting for the medical treatment to take effect. Clearly, some psychiatric wards have a more dynamic approach to treatment and care, one which emphasizes the treatment potential of all forms of social interaction. However, there are still large elements of the medical model existing in contemporary psychiatric institutions. Clark (1981, p. 7) provides the following description of the medical model in the long-term ward: 'Most of the patients are sitting in quiet submissive rows or pacing to and fro, or standing motionless and muttering in corners. They sit for long periods waiting for basic routine to intervene such as meals or medication. On fine days they will sit in the sun, walk to and fro, or occasionally kick a ball about'. These are examples of the medical model of care. However, there are variations to this pattern. Some long-term wards have included other treatment modalities with this model, such as the best aspects of milieu (social) therapy and interventions borrowed from behaviour modification therapy. Examples include the behavioural treatment of semimute schizophrenic patients (Fraser *et al.*, 1981).

Figure 1.1   Secondary sub-roles of the nurse (traditional medical model)

Work role	Role action (purpose)
1. Mother (parent) surrogate	Bathing, feeding, dressing, toileting, warning, disciplining, etc
2. Technical	Medicating and monitoring the effects of others' treatment, etc
3. Socializing agent	Social chitchat, playing cards, games, and walks with patients, etc
4. Environmental safety	Prevention of self-harm, wandering, hostility, starvation, etc

The role of the nurse within the traditional medical model tends to consist of activities which Peplau (1986a) has described as secondary sub-roles. Some examples are given in Fig. 1.1.

The secondary sub-roles (custodial – medical model)

Many would agree that these interventions, described as secondary sub-roles, are legitimate functions of the psychiatric nurse. Few would dispute that there is a need for nurses to assist, and work in collaboration with, other professionals. Similarly, many would agree that a legitimate function of the psychiatric nurse is to provide care which meets patients' basic physiological needs. It is not our intention to devalue these sub-roles by suggesting that they are not necessary, or that they are not a legitimate part of the role of the psychiatric nurse. However, there is a need for nurses to be consciously aware of the circumstances which have caused them to take on, and give high profile to, these sub-roles. Questions which need to be asked are: 1. Should these sub-roles continue to take precedence over one in which a therapeutic personal contribution is made by the psychiatric nurse? 2. Do these sub-roles meet a need which cannot be met in any other way? 3. What is the client's perception of these sub-roles? 4. Do these psychiatric nursing sub-roles make anyone sick? Questions (1) and (2) are necessary due to the cloning nature of large institutions, particularly within the traditional custodial/medical models of care. Within such care systems, even though good interpersonal relationships may be taught, the goal of such a relationship is often that of getting the client to conform. Jourard (1964) expressed it thus: 'Much of the contemporary interpersonal competence seems to entail success in getting patients to conform to roles they are supposed to play in the social system of the hospital, so that the system will work smoothly.'

Peplau (personal communication to W.R., 1988a) suggested that we should ask whether the client is accurately perceiving the role adopted by the nurse. The nurse may believe that she (the nurse) is teaching, and the client may think that she (the nurse) is mothering. Peplau (1960) had earlier stated that nurses were often unaware of, or did not make explicit to the client, the purpose of the nurse/client relationship. In more recent times, Reynolds (1986) noted (with alarm) that some Scottish nurse-teachers appeared to be unaware of the purpose of one-to-one talks with patients. This suggests that nurses and clients may be confused about the purpose of the nurse's role. This role confusion can, on occasions, cause the nurse to become unconsciously involved in a pathological behavioural pattern which may have been familiar to the client, but not made known to the nurse. Smoyak (1984) alluded to this when she described a concept taken from general systems theory called coalition across generations. In Smoyak's example she described a child approaching his father for a favour such as ice-cream before a meal, and being turned down. However, children tend to test out the systems, rules and norms. In this case the child next asked his mother for an ice-cream. The mother agreed to the child's demands, then compounded the violation of the rules by saying 'Don't tell father.' According to Smoyak, the main sufferer in this triad tends to be the mother who subsequently develops migraine or feels self-conscious. The dynamic can be replicated in a hospital situation between doctor, nurse and client. Nurses often acquiesce to clients' demands. Unfortunately, not only may the nurse become sick but the client may be labelled manipulative by the social system.

Relevance of the custodial/medical model

Adams and Macione (1983) suggested that much of the current research supports the usefulness of the medical model. They point out that there have been extensive recent advances in neurochemistry, psychopharmacology, and systematic diagnosis. Research and adoption studies have suggested the presence of genetic factors in major psychiatric illness. In addition, the increasing number of pharmacological preparations capable of helping people with emotional disorders has led to major revisions in thought about the causation of such disorders. Further support comes from the notion that the medical model approach has, for many years, been used by nurses and others to gain access to patients/clients in order to use psychotherapeutic techniques.

However, as nursing evolves as a field of scientific enquiry, there is an increasing effort among nurses to dissociate themselves from the medical paradigm, and to define the boundaries and goals of their discipline as being essentially different from those of medicine. This has been particularly true of psychiatric nursing with its distinct psychosocial emphasis. That psychiatric nurses have a distinct function which is different from that of medical colleagues has come from several sources.

First, numerous contributors to the literature have suggested that the bias in medicine towards predominantly chemical interventions restricts the role of the psychiatric nurse. Peplau (1986a, pp. 5–6) stated that: '. . . the nature of psychiatric work, how it is defined by both society and nurses, is central to the development of nursing skills. If, for example, mental illness is defined solely as a medical problem, primarily pathophysiological and biochemical in origin and nature, then nurses are likely to envision skills related to medical prescriptions – carrying them out and monitoring their effects'. Peplau goes on to say that if, on the other hand, mental illness is viewed as primarily an interpersonally derived adaptation to traumatic life experiences, then the nursing skills required will be of a very different and more complex nature.

Secondly, it has been suggested that nurses and doctors within the traditional medical system may sometimes damage their clients' health. Peplau (1964, p. 1), a strong advocate of that view, suggested that: 'The very place to which tormented people turn for help, often provides a scene for the day-to-day, week-by-week, year-by-year re-inforcement of a client's illness until he is virtually incurable.' Some support for that view can be found in the literature. Of particular interest is a study by Cohen and Struening (1963). They compared the discharge rates of hospitals which provided a fairly rigid medical model, with less traditional care facilities which emphasized interpersonal experience and the ability of staff to empathize with their clients' distress. Clients treated by the traditional model spent far fewer days in the community than did those treated by the less traditional model. Twenty years later Rippere and Williams (1985, p. 18), in a book entitled *Wounded Healers: Mental health workers experiences of depression*, provide graphic case studies taken from the personal experiences of professionals who were being treated for depression. An account taken from a psychiatrist who was admitted to hospital following a suicide attempt emphasizes the potential of the mental hospital for creating learned helplessness. He said: 'I was now one of them. The whole business was about being a helpless patient – a passive, inert lump of problems, some intractable. The days were endless. We waited around, sitting and lounging, for drugs, ECT and doctors' visits. We suffered from a kind of stimulus deprivation in that all normal events had been removed from our lives. I must have displayed the same child-like dependence of the others for doctors' rounds and amateurish interviews with nurses.' This description suggests that the goal of independent living may not always be achieved through hospitalization.

Thirdly, Wilson and Kneisl (1983) suggest that people's actions in a situation are based on the unique meaning that a situation has for them. Consequently, the psychiatric nurse should be wary of interventions that convey an invalidation of the meaning that an experience has for the client. Peplau (1988b) provided cautionary tales for nurses when she suggested that it was common practice in the 1950s to label as schizophrenic housewives who expressed dissatisfaction about their emotional and economic dependence upon their husbands, and their social isolation from the rest of the world outside of the home. Peplau quotes Warren (1987, p. 153): 'In hospitals they were given electroshock as treatment, and when they finally verbalised acceptance of the housewife role, they were given conditional discharge [which] continued the coalition of psychiatric and marital authority over their lives.'

Many conventional situations in psychiatric nursing account for meanings such as normal and mentally ill by regarding them as intrinsic to the nature of behaviour. Wilson and Kneisl (1983, p. 4) believe that meanings arise in the process of interaction with others. They state that: 'Meanings are social products formed in and through interpersonal processes.' It is therefore essential that nurses take into account the social and cultural environment of each client. A holistic assessment (one that considers both biological and psychosocial needs) accounts for social norms and interaction patterns in that person's social world. A shaved head or a Mohawk haircut may appear bizarre in a milieu of middle-class professionals, but represents social norms amongst the punk-rock sub-culture.

All of this suggests that nurses should develop the skills of building an empathic therapeutic relationship with their clients. Empathy, the ability to put yourself in another person's place, has been said to be the most important facilitator of the therapeutic (helping) relationship (Reynolds, 1987; Reynolds and Presly, 1988). Clearly, there is little point in knowing that the client feels down or tense unless one understands the personal meaning that those terms have for the individual. Understanding by the nurse requires a more dynamically oriented investigative approach than that prescribed within the medical model. In order to understand accurately it is also necessary to study the client's culture and social system by moving out of the institutional frame of reference into the family and world in which the client lives.

The primary function of the psychiatric nurse

We propose that the primary function of the psychiatric nurse is a psychotherapeutic one. By psychotherapeutic we mean those strategies which are used by psychiatric nurses to diagnose and personally influence patients' responses to, alterations of or threats to their mental health status. Peplau (1962) proposed that the manner in which the nurse personally influenced the mental health status of a client (the psychotherapeutic role) was the primary function of the psychiatric nurse. Later, Peplau (personal communication to W.R., 1983) suggested that: 'Most psychiatric illness is reflected in the language of the client; if it is a thought disorder, the only way that this can be corrected or helped is by the language of the nurse interacting with the language of the client.'

The psychotherapeutic role has been variously described by nursing theorists as relationship therapy (Kalkman, 1967), counselling and psycho-therapy (Reynolds and Cormack, 1987), and interpersonal relations (Peplau, 1987). This role includes several treatment modalities such as individual psychotherapy, group psychotherapy, psychodrama and family therapy. This function of the nurse has expanded in recent decades, particularly as a consequence of the Masters degree programmes for psychiatric nurses in the USA, and the availability of a number of post-registration specialist courses in the United Kingdom and elsewhere.

The primary focus of psychiatric nursing

The focus of psychiatric nursing is different from the function of psychiatric nurses. Focus determines function; it is concerned with the patient's prob-lems and needs. The question which needs to be asked is: what is it that psychiatric nurses focus on in terms of correcting, ameliorating, changing or preventing? Peplau (1988b, p. 3) argues that psychiatric nurses have a responsibility to define the substance (the focus) of psychiatric nursing. She defines substance as the essential part, and goes on to say that it is less concerned with what nurses do, than with what they set out to focus on. She stated that: 'This issue is important: it is the named focus of the work that determines what theories practices require, the major content of the curriculum, the most relevant foci for nursing research, and the major information which the public needs and wants from nurses for purposes of self-maintenance of health.' This change suggests that instead of asking what nurses do, we should be asking what do nurses treat? In other words, what are the phenomena to which the skills of the psychiatric nurses are addressed so as to achieve outcomes for clients? Thus, instead of asking the question 'What shall we do?' we should ask 'What does the client need?'

Reynolds and Cormack (1982, p. 233) had earlier alluded to this issue when they suggested that psychiatric nursing was different from psychiatry due to the fact that nurses were concerned with the problems that psy-chiatrists did not normally treat. They stated that: 'Clearly there is a wide range of variation in the nursing needs of individuals who share the same psychiatric diagnosis.' Reynolds (1985) expanded this theme when he suggested that if nurses were not aware of specific nursing needs they would not know whether their responses towards clients were appropriate or not, and would not be aware of the existence of problems which were within the scope of nurses to treat. Those problems, which may include a tendency for a client to isolate himself, or to be hostile towards others, require nursing diagnosis and intervention.

Peplau (Chapter 5) proposes that the phenomena commonly observed by nurses during their relationships with psychiatric clients should be the focus for nursing intervention. She refers to the definition of nursing of the American Nurses' Association (1980) which pinpoints the work of nurses as being: '...the diagnosis and treatment of human responses to actual and potential health problems'. Thus, the emphasis is on the problematic, psychosocial, behavioural human responses of clients, rather than upon medical diagnostic categories of mental illness which are diagnosed and treated by psychiatrists. Peplau (1988b) suggests that the substance (focus) of psychiatric nursing includes a considerable array of problems classified under the heading of 'human response patterns'. Examples of such human response patterns include anxiety, disorientation, hallucinations, negative self-concept, loneliness, envy, and passive aggression. Peplau (1988b, p. 5) also states that hallucinations, anxiety, loneliness, grief and other such phenomena are often dysfunctional human responses to gravely distressing human conditions. She goes on to suggest that: '...psychiatric nurses have an unparalleled opportunity – beginning today – to make themselves experts in a humanistic alternative approach to such problems of psychiatric clients and to speak out on the prevention of such problems'.

It has been suggested that the focus for nursing practice arises from concerns of clients, which nurses observe during nurse–client interactions. These clinical data yield theoretical constructs which set in logical order our ideas about clinical phenomena such as self-concept and dependency. These constructs, derived from our observations of human responses, have explanatory power and provide the basis for the development and testing of nursing theory.

Theory-based approaches to nursing practice

Hage (1972) identified six elements of a theory, specifying the contribution which each element makes to the whole. These elements were: concepts, theoretical statements, definitions, linkages, ordering of concepts and definitions, and ordering of statements and linkages.

Concepts, which may be described as the building blocks of theories, classify the phenomena with which psychiatric nursing is concerned. The concepts are not considered in isolation from the theoretical system of which they form a part, and from which they derive their meaning. The development of concepts, and a conceptual framework, enable the description and classification of the phenomena with which psychiatric nursing is concerned. Examples of concepts which are the concern of psychiatric nurses are anxiety, dependence, hostility and disordered orientation.

Theoretical statements, which utilize concepts which are the building blocks of theory, are connected and integrated into a meaningful whole. As the theory develops, the linkages and relationships between the previously identified concepts will become possible (Mullins, 1971; Reynolds, 1971; Walker and Avant, 1983).

Definitions of concepts enable clear and unambiguous descriptions of the concepts to be made. Hage (1972) recommended that the concept label and definition were necessary for subsequent identification of the concept.

Linkages between concepts is an important part of the development of theory. In addition to identifying connections between concepts, these linkages also describe the rationale for identifying connections between specific concepts. Theoretical linkages are a means by which connections between concepts are described and explained. They provide a means by which the relationships between concepts are understood.

Ordering of concepts offers the means by which to establish the logical arrangement of concepts, and of bringing some conceptual order into the elements of the theory. Hage (1972) suggested that concepts (and definitions) be ordered if the theory contains more than ten concepts.

Ordering of statements and linkages becomes necessary if the theory contains a greater (rather than smaller) number of theoretical statements (Hage, 1972). Thus, a theory is a set of specifically defined and interrelated concepts such as self-esteem, affect, and hostility, which present a systematic view of a phenomenon. The theories utilized in this text relate specifically to psychiatric and mental health nursing. Such theories propose, explain and predict specific cause and effect relationships between concepts (components of the theories) and the general phenomenon to which they apply.

Flaskerud and Halloran (1980) suggested that whilst nurses were reluctant to describe nursing models or conceptual frameworks as theories, they were relatively more willing to label frameworks from other fields such as sociology and psychology as theories. They argued that this had resulted in difficulty in the development of nursing theories. However, if nursing is to be an applied science, it desperately needs theoretical constructs which explain the problems which constitute the focus of nursing practice. Peplau (1988b, p. 9), one of the strongest advocates of the notion of nursing theory development, stated that: '...nurses have a gold-mine opportunity to collect data about any one problem that comes up repeatedly in their practice as seen in several clients and from that, the case history and interview data, to formulate a theoretical construct of the origins, nature and variations of that problem'.

Reynolds and Cormack (1987) proposed that if the nurse did not have a theory, she would be forced to rely upon trial and error, precedent, or the authority of others. The problem with this approach is that solutions are often accepted without question or rationale, and even if the nurse finds a solution, she cannot be certain that it is the best one, or one that will enable the client to achieve the optimal amount of health. It also means that she must rely upon the biases and belief systems of physicians and others in authority to decide what the nursing role is. The focus of human responses may be lost in favour of psychiatry and a medical disease model of illness.

The usefulness of theory

Theory provides focus and direction to psychiatric nursing practice. Essentially a theory should provide answers to the following questions:

1. What is the range of human responses to actual or potential mental health problems? At this stage, the nurse requires a full understanding of the manner in which individuals may respond to actual or potential mental health problems. This phase is guided by reference to a diagnostic or conceptual framework which will enable the understanding and labelling of potential individual responses.

   A conceptual framework specifies the discipline's focus of enquiry, it identifies those responses which are of special interest to nursing, and it focuses attention on those concepts which are treatable by nurses. In the early days of the formation of conceptual frameworks, they tended to be relatively limited and unsophisticated. A natural development of this approach to making nursing diagnoses has been the formation of a formal nursing diagnostic classification system. This topic is addressed in Chapter 2.

2. How can a nursing diagnosis be made, and what is the basis of that diagnosis? With reference to a diagnostic categorization system, the nurse then makes a diagnosis of specific needs (human responses) and labels these in a way which can be understood by others. The nursing diagnosis has a basis in, and relates to, nursing theory. The diagnosis is accompanied by written evidence of the existence of a particular problem. As with other aspects of nursing intervention, nursing diagnoses are subject to change as new data are generated via interactions with patients.

3. Why do individuals respond in the way they do? Human responses to actual or potential mental health problems are relatively independent of medical diagnoses. Use of a nursing theory will enable the nurse to interpret and understand individual responses and, subsequently, inform her of the individual needs of that particular patient in these particular circumstances.

4. What form of nursing intervention is required? Making use of a nursing theory will enable the nurse to select and implement nursing interventions which are appropriate in this particular circumstance. Unless nursing interventions have a theoretical underpinning, they may, at best, be inappropriate. At worst, they can harm the patient.

5. What is the desired outcome of the intervention? Reference to an appropriate theory will enable the nurse to identify the specific goals of the intervention. It will enable the nurse to determine whether success has been achieved, and will inform her of alternative nursing strategies which may be used. Thus, nursing becomes a structured and less haphazard activity, eliminating trial and error. Currently, nursing tends

to borrow from theories (explanation systems) which originate from other disciplines. Examples include: Client-Centred Therapy (Rogers, 1957), Operant Learning Theory (Allyon and Michael, 1965), Cognitive Therapy (Barker, 1983) and General Systems Theory (Smoyak, 1975). Such borrowed theories can be reshaped into a form that renders them applicable to nursing. Several nurse theorists have contributed towards the development of an array of theoretical models which are now available to nursing. These include: the interpersonal model (Peplau, 1952), the self-care model (Orem, 1980), and the adaptation model (Roy, 1976).

According to Peplau (1986b, 1987) theories which explain recurring health problems are the major tools of a professional nurse. She suggests that practising nurses are expected to have a full understanding of, and have readily available for recall and application, a range of theories.

In order to demonstrate how a theory can be applied to clinical practice, Rogers' Client-Centred Therapy will be briefly described. Application of Rogers' theory requires that the following questions be answered:

1. What is the range of human responses to actual or potential mental health problems? Rogers' (1957) theory suggests that the goal of the therapist is to understand the client. Clinical data are collected during interaction with the client when the therapist achieves accurate empathy (the ability to understand the client as if you were he). Those clinical data reveal a variety of human responses such as anger, anxiety, depression, memory impairment and so on.
2. How can a nursing diagnosis be made, and what is the basis of that diagnosis? Classification of the human responses that may be observed during empathic linkages poses a challenge for nursing. Reynolds and Cormack (1982) evaluated a limited taxonomy of human responses developed earlier by Cormack (1980). Elements of that taxonomy included needs/problems relating to broad areas such as self-esteem, affect, hostility, social skills, trust and dependence. That global taxonomy was limited in that it failed to describe discrete behaviours which may be typical of the problems which it identified. O'Toole and Loomis (in Chapter 2) present a considerably more detailed (and linked) taxonomy of nursing diagnoses. For example, low self-esteem (negative self-concept) has been categorized in several ways including hopelessness, loneliness and powerlessness. Full operational definitions, which include descriptions of the patterns, variations and circumstances of clinical phenomena, can only emerge from clinical data. Categorizing phenomena by using a panel of experienced clinicians (Chapter 2) forms the basis of establishing the content validity of a diagnostic taxonomy.
3. Why do individuals respond in the way they do? The client-centred point of view sees human beings as being basically rational, socialized, forward moving and realistic. Furthermore, human beings are said to be

basically co-operative, constructive and trustworthy when they are free of defensiveness. As individuals, human beings possess the capacity to move from a state of maladjustment towards a state of psychological adjustment. These capacities and tendencies will be realized in a relationship that is perceived as non-threatening by the client.

4. What form of nursing intervention is required? Rogers (1957) suggests that the non-threatening relationship occurs when the helper displays certain attitudes and behaviours. He described those attitudes and behaviours as 'the facilitative conditions for therapeutic change'. The facilitative conditions which have received most attention are empathy, warmth and genuineness. These facilitative conditions are delivered within a counselling relationship with the client.

5. What is the desired outcome of the interventions? When the client experiences those conditions in abundance, he is enabled to feel non-defensive and to be able to consider and experiment with alternative coping strategies. Outcome will be measured against realistic and measurable goals.

Nursing research

The application of theory to named phenomena, such as low self-esteem, hallucinations and disorientation, provides a focus for nursing research. We need research evidence to support assumptions that nursing interventions, which are separate from medicine, make a difference. Nursing research is approximately 50 years old, but the available studies are beginning to support the assumptions that nursing can become an applied science. The following studies support that view.

First, Field (1985) conducted a study in Texas with hallucinating clients. Nurses were trained to use a counselling approach which originated from Peplau's Theory of Interpersonal Relations (Field, 1979). Interventions occurred during the accepting/supporting and derogatory phases of the auditory hallucinatory process, and were designed to help the client dismiss the voices. The results of the study revealed that clients did express relief from hallucinations and developed the ability to dismiss voices when nursing prescriptions directed at dismissal were followed. Clients' self-esteem was enhanced and greater control was achieved over their thoughts, feelings and actions. It was also found that the dismissal method reported by Field (1985) was of greater benefit than neuroleptic drugs.

Second, Barker (1988) studied nursing interventions with clients suffering from major affective disorders in Dundee, Scotland. That study was the first experimental examination of the role of the nurse in caring for such a population, mounted anywhere in the world. A structured care system based on the conceptual framework of cognitive/behavioural theory has been developed as a result of that study. That treatment approach gained significantly better results than did more traditional nursing approaches with depressed women in respect of locus of control (beliefs about being in control of personal circumstances) and vulnerability to stressors as measured on a dysfunctional attitude scale.

The third study, although not using experimental design, provides questions for further nursing outcome studies. Reynolds (1986) found a significant increase between client ratings of student nurses' empathy among measures during a series of counselling interviews. The students were trained in the Rogerian client-centred approach. Despite some methodological weaknesses associated with client ratings, unsolicited comments made to the researcher during the completion of an empathy instrument tended to support the assumption that clients found it easier to relate to the students by the fifth counselling interview. Typical of the comments made by patients were: 'We didn't really talk about my illness' (second interview); 'We talked about my current difficulties. Today I cried. She [the student] understands my point of view and feels how upset I am' (fifth interview). The specific nature of these comments suggested that clients experienced sensitive understanding by the student and became less defensive. These data suggested that a trust relationship was developing. Trust is another example of phenomena which psychiatric nurses can treat.

Earlier it was suggested that the psychotherapeutic role was the primary function of the psychiatric nurse. The rationale is based upon the view that the focus for psychiatric nursing (human responses) is different from that role in which a psychiatric nurse functions as a supporter of the psychiatrist. Peplau (1988b, p. 6) proposed that '...the decision psychiatric nurses face is this: whether assisting psychiatrists is their primary function, or whether they will make that function secondary, and, instead, develop their own primary function by taking the option of elaborating a different viewpoint and treatment approach.'

If psychiatric nurses accept the medical view of mental health (primarily brain dysfunction), then, possibly, assisting psychiatrists is their primary function. If they view mental health in terms of human responses to stresses (a psychodynamic process), then activities such as pouring medicine, or being a mother to the client, are clearly a secondary role. The primary role then becomes any response on the part of the nurse which assists the client to achieve the most adaptive response possible to a traumatic life event. That role requires a nursing diagnosis of the client's level of adaptation to stressors, and interventions which are guided by theory. That role is primarily a psychotherapeutic one.

The responsibilities of nurse education

Peplau (1986a) suggested that it was during educative clinical experience, followed by supervisory review of interaction data, that skill in theory application and in the use of theory-derived interventions was learned, refined and evaluated. This is the labour-intensive and costly part of nurse education; it takes much time for well-qualified nurse teachers to supervise the collection of, and review of, clinical data. Unfortunately, at present, not all societies are willing to provide the resources for such in-depth skilled training of nurses.

Reynolds (1988b) proposed that it was important for teachers of psychiatric nurses to practise psychiatric nursing with their students; otherwise, it may become a case of 'those who have never done leading those who cannot do'. Reynolds' approach to psychiatric nurse education stems largely from professional experience of past limitations of traditional approaches to nurse education, and has been influenced by theories of learning. Examples of learning theories which influenced Reynolds' approach to supervised clinical practice include:

Rogers' student-centred model
The principles of Rogers' conceptualization include the view that learning is retained when it is experiential and meaningful, that telling slows down learning, and that teachers should create learning environments within clinical settings. All of this, however, is difficult to achieve if teachers are classroom-based practitioners (see Reynolds, 1984).

Bandura's social learning theory
Bandura's theory (1977) states that self-efficacy, the degree of confidence in our ability to achieve, controls our efforts and persistence. Self-efficacy is achieved by graded exposure to a skill, observing a competent role model, and receiving positive feedback from an experienced supervisor. Again, this is difficult to achieve unless teachers are prepared to accept the risks of clinical practice with their students.

Festinger's theory of cognitive dissonance
Festinger (1957) stated that anxiety is created when learners are pressurized during clinical practice to act in a way that is incompatible with their values. The resultant conflict blocks innovation and results in theory not being practised. Reynolds (1988) proposed that consistency between theory and practice could only be achieved when theory and practice are taught by the same individual.

Conclusion

In conclusion, it has been argued that the primary task facing psychiatric nurses is to identify and address problems related to the substance of psychiatric nursing. It has been argued that psychiatric nursing diagnosis and treatment differ from medical diagnosis and treatment. For example, psychiatrists diagnose diseases such as schizophrenia and then prescribe drugs for symptoms such as hallucinations. These drugs mask the symptoms. Psychiatric nurses, on the other hand, recognize hallucinations as a human response to pervasive anxiety and loneliness. Consequently, there is a need for nurses to formulate and apply theories of intervention and to test these theories via subsequent research.

References

Adams, C. and Macione, A. (1983) *Handbook of Psychiatric Mental Health Nursing*, Wiley, New York.

Allyon, T. and Michael, J. (1965) The psychiatric nurse as a behavioural engineer, in *Case Studies in Behaviour Modification* (eds V. Ullman and A. Krosner), Rinehart, Orlando, FL.

Altschul, A. (1972) *Patient–Nurse Interaction. A study of interaction patterns in acute psychiatric wards*, Churchill Livingstone, Edinburgh.

American Nurses' Association (1980) *Nursing: A social policy statement*, American Nurses Association, Kansas City, MO.

Bandura, A. (1977) Self-efficacy: Toward a unifying theory of behaviour change. *Psych. Rev.*, **84**, 191–215.

Barker, P. (1983) *Understanding Your Feelings and Solving Your Problems*, Behaviour Nurse Therapy Department, Royal Dundee Liff Hospital, Liff by Dundee, Scotland.

Barker, P. (1988) 'Nursing the Patient with Major Affective Disorder', Unpublished PhD thesis, Dundee College of Technology, Dundee, Scotland.

Belknap, I. (1956) *Human Relations in a State Mental Hospital*, McGraw-Hill, New York.

Clark, D. (1981) *Social Therapy in Psychiatry*, Churchill Livingstone, Edinburgh.

Cohen, J. and Struening, E. (1963) Opinions about mental illness: mental hospital occupational profile and profile cluster. *Psych. Rep.*, **12**, 111–24.

Connolly, J. (1856) *The Treatment of the Insane Without Mechanical Restraint*, Smith, Elder and Co., London.

Cormack, D. (1976) *Psychiatric Nursing Observed*, Royal College of Nursing, London.

Cormack, D. (1980) The nursing process: an application of the SOAPE model. *Nurs. Times*, **76**, 37–40.

Cormack, D. (1983) *Psychiatric Nursing Described*, Churchill Livingstone, Edinburgh.

Festinger, L. (1957) *A Theory of Cognitive Dissonance*, Row-Peterson, New York and London.

Field, W. (1979) *The Psychotherapy of Hildegard Peplau*, PSF Productions, New Braunels, TX.

Field, W. (1985) Hearing voices. *J. Psych. Nurs.*, **23**, 9–14.

Flaskerud, J. and Halloran, E. (1980) Area of agreement in nursing theory development. *Adv. Nurs. Sci.*, **3**, 1–7.

Fraser, D., Anderson, J. and Grimes, J. (1981) An analysis of the progressive development of vocal responses in a mute schizophrenic patient. *Behav. Psychother.*, **9**, 2–12.

Hage, J. (1972) *Techniques and Problems in Theory Construction in Sociology*, John Wiley, New York.

Johnson, M. M. and Martin, H. W. (1958) A sociological analysis of the nurse's role. *Am. J. Nurs.*, **58**, 373–7.

Jourard, S. (1964) *Transparent Self*, 1st edn, Van Nostrand Reinhold, New York.

Kalkman, M. (1967) *Psychiatric Nursing*, McGraw-Hill, New York.

McGhie, A. (1957) The role of the mental nurse 1. Historical development. *Nurs. Mirror*, **105**, xii–xiii.

Mullins, N. (1971) *The Art of Theory Construction and Use*, Harper and Row, New York.

Orem, D. (1980) *Nursing Concepts of Practice*, 2nd edn, McGraw-Hill, New York.

Peplau, H. (1952) *Interpersonal Relations in Nursing: A Conceptual Frame of Reference for Psychodynamic Nursing*, Putnam, New York.

Peplau, H. (1960) Talking with patients. *Am. J. Nurs.*, **60**, 946–66.

Peplau, H. (1962) Interpersonal techniques: the crux of psychiatric nursing. *Am. J. Nurs.*, **62**, 50–4.

Peplau, H. (1964) *Basic Principles of Patient Counselling*. Report of Smith, Kline and French Seminars.

Peplau, H. (1983) Personal communication to W.R.

Peplau, H. (1986a) Psychiatric nursing skills: today and tomorrow – a world overview. Paper presented at 'A Celebration of Skills', Third International Congress of Psychiatric Nursing, Imperial College, London.

Peplau, H. (1986b) Interpersonal constructs for nursing practice. Paper presented at The First Hildegard Peplau Seminar, Highland College of Nursing, Inverness, Scotland.

Peplau, H. (1987) Interpersonal constructs for nursing practice. *Nurs. Ed. Today*, **7**, 201–8.

Peplau, H. (1988a) Personal communication to W.R.

Peplau, H. (1988b) Substance and scope of psychiatric nursing. Paper presented at The Third Conference on Psychiatric Nursing, Montreal.

Reynolds, P. (1971) *A Primer in Theory Construction*, Bobbs-Merrill, Indianapolis, IN.

Reynolds, W. (1982) Patient-Centred teaching: A future role for the psychiatric nurse teacher? *J. Adv. Nurs.*, **7**, 469–75.

Reynolds, W. (1984) Psychiatric nursing in the USA. *Nurs. Mirror*, **158**, 25–7.

Reynolds, R. (1985) Issues arising from interpersonal skills in psychiatric nurse training, in *Interpersonal Skills in Nursing: Research and applications* (ed. C. Kagan), Croom Helm, London.

Reynolds, W. (1986) *A Study of Empathy in Student Nurses*, MPhil thesis, Dundee College of Technology, Scotland.

Reynolds, W. (1987) Empathy: We know what we mean, but what do we teach? *Nurs. Edu. Today*, **7**, 265–9.

Reynolds, W. (1988a) The primary and secondary role of the psychiatric nurse. Keynote Speech, National Conference on Psychiatric Nursing, Wellington, New Zealand.

Reynolds, W. (1988b) Nurse teachers should practise nursing? Debate (chaired by A. Altschul) PNA Conference, University of Stirling, 21st June, 1988.

Reynolds, W. and Cormack, D. (1982) Clinical teaching: An evaluation of a problem-oriented approach to psychiatric nurse education. *J. Adv. Nurs.*, **7**, 231–7.

Reynolds, W. and Cormack, D. (1987) Teaching psychiatric nursing: interpersonal skills, in *Nursing Education: Research and Developments* (ed. B. Davis), Croom Helm, London.

Reynolds, W. and Presly, A. (1988) A study of empathy in student nurses. *Nurs. Ed. Today*, **8**, 123–30.

Rippere, V. and Williams, R. (1985) *Wounded Healers: Mental Health Workers' Experiences of Depression*, John Wiley, New York.

Rogers, C. (1957) The necessary and sufficient conditions of therapeutic personality change. *J. Consult. Psycho.*, **21**, 95–103.

Roy, C. (ed.) (1976) *Introduction to Nursing: An adaptation model*, Prentice Hall, New York.

Smoyak, S. (1975) *The Psychiatric Nurse as a Family Therapist*, John Wiley, New York.
Smoyak, S. (1984) Family Therapy: the evolution of theoretical perspectives used in treatment. Videotaped lecture to Module 8 students, Highland College of Nursing, Inverness, Scotland.
Towell, D. (1975) *Understanding Psychiatric Nursing*, Royal College of Nursing Research Series, RCN, London.
Walker, L. O. and Avant, K. C. (1983) *Strategies for Theory Construction in Nursing*, Appleton-Century-Crofts, Norwalk, CT.
Warren, C. A. B. (1987) Madwives: schizophrenic women (unpublished report), Rutgers University, New Brunswick, NJ.
Wilson, H. and Kneisl, C. (1983) *Psychiatric Nursing*, 2nd edn, Addison-Wesley, Menlo Park, CA.

Chapter 2

Classifying human responses in psychiatric and mental health nursing*

A. W. O'TOOLE and M. E. LOOMIS

This chapter discusses the work of the American Nurses' Association (ANA) in developing a classification system for psychiatric and mental health nursing practice. The forces that gave impetus to the establishment of the ANA task force on the classification system are described, and the various stages of the task force's work are explained. Appendices provide two draft lists of the phenomena of concern for psychiatric and mental health nurses.

History and background

Impetus for the development of a classification system for psychiatric and mental health (PMH) nursing practice was provided by *Nursing: A social policy statement* (American Nurses' Association, 1980). This landmark document defined nursing as 'the diagnosis and treatment of human responses to actual or potential health problems', and identified the 'four defining characteristics of nursing: phenomena, theory application, nursing action, and evaluation of effects of action in relation to phenomena' (American Nurses' Association, 1980, p. 9).

In 1984, the Executive Committee of the ANA Division on Psychiatric and Mental Health Nursing Practice responded to the ANA priority to implement *Nursing: A social policy statement* with a proposal to develop a comprehensive list of the phenomena of concern to their speciality practice. A task force composed of a panel of specialists, selected for their expertise in psychiatric nursing care of patients in each developmental age group, was authorized to develop the phenomena of concern. Members of the

*Presented in part at Northeast Regional Conference, 'Classifying Nursing Diagnoses: State-of-the-Art', Andover, Massachusetts, October 24, 1987. Published with permission of American Nurses' Association, 2420 Pershing Road, Kansas City, MO 64108, USA.

task force are Maxine Loomis, PhD, RN, CS, FAAN (South Carolina) and Anita O'Toole, PhD, RN (Ohio), co-chairpersons, both representing psychiatric nurses who work with the adult population; Marie Scott Brown, PhD, RN (Oregon), an expert on the mental health of infants; Patricia Pothier, MS, RN, FAAN (California), whose field is children's mental health; Patricia West, MSN, RN, CS (Michigan), an expert on adolescent mental health; and Holly Skodol Wilson, PhD, RN, FAAN (California), a geropsychiatric nurse. The members of the task force held meetings over a period of several years and have continued working on the classification project on an individual basis.

The revision of the *Standards of Psychiatric and Mental Health Nursing Practice* (American Nurses' Association, 1982) also gave impetus to the development of a list of phenomena of concern. The third standard addresses diagnosis: 'The nurse utilizes nursing diagnoses and/or standard classification of mental disorders to express conclusions supported by recorded assessment data and current scientific premises' (p. 4). The 'standard classification of mental disorders' referred to in the above statement is, of course, the *Diagnostic and Statistical Manual of Mental Disorders*, third edition (DSM-III), published by the American Psychiatric Association. In 1981, when the standards committee was revising the ANA standards, the committee conducted a lengthy discussion about whether or not to include nursing diagnosis in the above statement. It was the belief of some committee members that the DSM-III would facilitate interdisciplinary communication in mental health settings. Others recommended abandoning DSM-III and relying exclusively on nursing diagnosis as a way to identify the autonomous contributions of nursing to the psychiatric team. A compromise was to endorse both systems of diagnosis, as the committee described in the following:

> Since the primary objective of the Task Force to Develop a Classification System of Phenomena of Concern for PMH Nursing was to extend *Nursing: A social policy statement* (ANA, 1980), the task force began its work without a bias for either the DSM-III or the North American Nursing Diagnosis Association (NANDA) diagnostic systems, yet with an awareness that any PMH nursing specialty classification system must eventually interface with DSM-III and the NANDA nursing diagnoses...
> The task force concluded that identifying the scope of nursing practice by classifying the phenomena of concern for nursing diagnosis is necessary in order to develop adequate criteria to operationalize standards. An important aspect of standards implementation is the development of outcome criteria sets for specific nursing diagnoses. This activity requires an established list of nursing diagnoses and some consensus about the identifying assessment criteria for each diagnosis (Loomis *et al.*, 1987).

Assumptions

A classification system of the phenomena of concern to PMH nursing practice provides a means whereby consensus within the speciality and within the discipline of nursing may be achieved. We need to be able to identify or diagnose the specific phenomenon that we are trying to treat. 'Educators, researchers, and theoreticians must be able to systematically address the objects of their conceptual and practical pursuits if the speciality area is to flourish as a scientific and academic endeavour' (Loomis *et al.*, 1987).

According to Loomis *et al.* (1987), the development of a classification system for PMH nursing involves two major issues:

> The first is political: the need to identify the domain of PMH nursing practice and claim a rightful share of scarce resources for the delivery of PMH nursing care. The second is a conceptual issue: the need to label or name the phenomena of concern for the speciality in order to develop and test theories that will lead to explanations of the phenomena and guide clinical interventions... Ultimately the phenomena must be grouped or classed in a conceptually logical manner so the interrelationships between categories and between specific phenomena can be understood and explained.
>
> Any diagnostic classification is flexible. It must be tested continuously and be subjected to refinement and revision. It will never be exhaustive, since members of the discipline will always be in the process of discovering new knowledge and classifying previously unidentified phenomena. Utility of the classification system is pragmatic. That is, it must be useful in the clinical setting and serve to guide interventions. Without clinical or pragmatic utility a classification system will serve neither the political nor the conceptual purposes for which it was intended.

Methods

The work of the task force was conceptualized in a three-stage process. Stage one was the development of a conceptual classification system for categorizing the phenomena of concern for PMH nursing practice. Stage two involves validity testing with input from content experts and structured feedback from certified generalists and specialists in PMH nursing, as well as reliability testing in selected clinical settings. Stage three is the development and implementation of a plan for dissemination and utilization of the classification system. The task force is currently completing stage one and some aspects of the validity testing of stage two. Formal reliability testing and implementation will require extramural funding, so we are currently exploring sources for such support.

We will elaborate upon stage one, development of a conceptual classification system, by presenting the definitions of key concepts that were agreed upon, discussing the conceptual focus of the task force members, and describing the sources we used to develop the system.

Definitions   It became apparent early in our work that we would need to arrive at some conceptual agreement about the definition of two key concepts: phenomena and human response. *Nursing: A social policy statement* offers clues to the intended meaning of phenomena within the context of the definition of nursing: 'the phenomena of concern to nurses are human responses to actual or potential health problems. Any observable manifestation, need, condition, concern, event, dilemma, difficulty, occurrence, or fact that can be described or scientifically explained and is within the target area of nursing practice is of interest to nurses' (American Nurses' Association, 1980, p. 9).

Dictionary definitions of phenomenon range from 1. a fact, occurrence, or circumstance observed or observable; to 2. something that impresses the observer as extraordinary; and 3. a thing as it appears to or is constructed by the mind; as distinguished from neumenon, or thing-in-itself. This definitional range from objective to subjective reality mirrors the range of phenomena of concern to nurses. The task force concluded that phenomena are human responses, and that phenomena can represent either subjective or objective reality.

Nursing: A social policy statement identifies two kinds of human responses that are the objects of nursing action: '1. reactions of individuals and groups to actual health problems (health-restoring responses), such as the impact of illness effects upon the self and family, and related self-care needs; and 2. concerns of individuals and groups about potential health problems (health-supporting responses), such as monitoring and teaching in populations or communities at risk in which educative needs for information, skill development, health-oriented attitudes, and related behaviour changes arise' (American Nurses' Association, 1980, pp. 9–10).

The use of the term response caused some difficulty because of the cause-and-effect nature of its definition. In common usage, a response is a reaction or any behaviour resulting from the application of a stimulus. Yet in most mental health situations, the nature of cause-and-effect relationships is highly speculative. The task force finally concluded that human responses are human behaviours. These behaviours may or may not be responses to identifiable stimulation. The human responses of concern for nurses are health-related. In most cases aggregates, clusters or patterns of human responses are used to group behaviours and formulate diagnostic categories. For example, the defining characteristics of the NANDA nursing diagnoses and the diagnostic criteria of the DSM-III psychiatric diagnoses are actually human responses. In DSM-III a predictable configuration of human responses is a diagnostic category. The task force was then faced with the difficulty of defining the level of generalization or specificity at which a human response became a nursing diagnosis.

Conceptual focus   We had decided to approach the task of developing the classification system from an atheoretical stance. PMH nursing has traditionally supported an eclectic approach to the use of psychiatric theories. Nursing theories did not appear to be developed in sufficient enough detail to provide guidance for our work. We were, of course, biased by our own personal theoretical positions about human behaviour, but such biases were divergent enough among the committee members to allow for representation of a variety of points of view. Selection of committee members by their expertise in a developmental age group introduced a conceptual perspective, that of a developmental model, and supported the view that a classification system for PMH nursing should have relevance to age-related subspecialities within the field: child psychiatric and mental health nursing, adolescent, adult, and geropsychiatric nursing.

The initial intent of the committee was to develop a classification system that addressed three major response classes: individual, family, and community. These three response classes may be viewed as a secondary conceptual focus. Individual, family, and community represent target populations for which interventions in PMH nursing are designed. As such, they can be found as a basis for graduate curriculum development in the speciality. Research and other publications are often directed toward explication of methods of interventions in each of these three categories. After the task force had worked extensively on the individual response class, however, it became apparent that it was almost impossible to separate responses into these three classes. It was particularly problematic to separate individual from family responses in the infant, child, and adolescent populations and seemed artificial to do so. As a consequence we abandoned our effort to develop three separate classes and included aspects of all three in the final draft.

Sources   The process by which the task force selected the phenomena to be included in the classification system involved review of a number of sources. First, as mentioned earlier, panel members were selected for their knowledge and expertise in the nursing care of clients in a selected developmental era. All of the members of the task force had extensive clinical experience in the area of their expertise and had conducted research and published. So it was possible to use the accumulated knowledge of the group in formulating a beginning list of phenomena.

In addition, the group reviewed psychiatric and psychiatric–mental health nursing assessment tools to abstract the broad categories, which became level one in the classification system. Behavioural criteria in DSM-III were assumed to represent our definition of a human response and were therefore abstracted for review as phenomena. We reviewed the psychiatric–mental health nursing literature. O'Toole (O'Toole, 1981; O'Toole, Jones and Wilson, in press) did an extensive review of published research articles between 1970 and 1986. From this review key concepts or variables were abstracted and reviewed for inclusion in the final classification system. Loomis (1985) summarized major concepts from nursing dissertation abstracts. Psychiatric nursing textbooks provided key sources of information for the classification system. We looked at how these texts were organized to get ideas on the major categories in level one and then reviewed the content for examples of phenomena.

Finally, we talked to other psychiatric–mental health nurses. We reviewed nursing care plans written for patients in psychiatric units and nursing process studies written by students in graduate and undergraduate psychiatric–mental health nursing courses. We elicited specific review of several different drafts of the classification from members of the ANA Council on Psychiatric and Mental Health Nursing. Their feedback was invaluable in formulation of the current draft.

We found that the concepts or phenomena abstracted from the various sources were remarkably similar. It was then a matter of intuitively deriving the level one categories. That was not a very difficult task. The difficulty came later when we tried to fit the phenomena under each major category. The task of classifying or categorizing phenomena under each major heading led to considerable disagreement about what belonged where and in some instances whether a major heading was appropriate for inclusion. Categories were renamed and phenomena reclassified until we reached consensus within the group.

Results

The first draft of the classification system, completed in July 1986, included six level one categories within the individual response class. (This draft was prepared during the time we still thought we could divide response classes into individual, family and community.) The level one categories within the individual response class comprised:

1. biological response patterns
2. socio/behavioural response patterns
3. emotional response patterns
4. defensive response patterns
5. perceptual/cognitive response patterns
6. value/belief response patterns.

The completion and dissemination of the first draft of the classification system for PMH nursing created considerable interest and controversy within the profession. The controversy was related to concerns about the extent to which ANA should be involved in the development of diagnostic classification systems. After all, diagnosis was considered to be the primary mission of the North American Nursing Diagnosis Association (NANDA).

Both ANA and NANDA supported the need for the development of a uniform classification system for nursing practice, although there was some disagreement as to how that would be implemented. To express that support and discuss ways to achieve consensus about a uniform system, representatives of our task force and NANDA met in July and December of 1986. These meetings were held at the request of the ANA Cabinet on Nursing Practice '...to advise on the process for synthesis and inter-petation of information on the state of the art of nursing classification systems and on the development of a strategic plan for the adoption of classifications for nursing practice for the profession by 1992'. This group of consultants, chaired by Norma M. Lang, PhD, RN, FAAN, recommended to the Cabinet on Nursing Practice that ANA facilitate the classification of nursing practice within the categories of assessment, diagnosis, interventions, and outcomes. They also recommended that ANA make a commitment to the development of a single, comprehensive system for classifying nursing practice and that the professional association collaborate with intradisciplinary and interdisciplinary groups in the development of classification systems for nursing and health care. These recommendations with strategies for achievement were accepted by the ANA Board of Directors.

The commitment to a single, comprehensive system for classifying nursing practice and the opportunity to submit a diagnostic classification system for inclusion in the International Classification of Diseases, 10th edition (ICD-10), led to the initiation of work on an integration of the NANDA taxonomy and the PMH nursing classification system. Members of the joint task force on nursing classifications, composed of representatives from the PMH task force and NANDA, met to draft a document which combined the then current PMH classification system (draft 1) and the NANDA taxonomy. A copy of that draft, which we refer to here as draft 2 (see Appendix A), was forwarded to the World Health Organization for inclusion in the revision of the International Classification of Diseases (ICD-10).

The second and third drafts of the PMH nursing classification system of human responses are organized according to human response patterns in:

1. physiological processes
2. interpersonal processes
3. emotional processes
4. decision processes
5. perception processes
6. cognition processes
7. valuation processes
8. activity processes
9. ecological processes.

Draft 1 and draft 2 differ in the following ways: biological became physiological; sociobehavioural became two categories, interpersonal and activity;
emotional remained the same; defensive was deleted in draft 2; perceptual/
cognitive became two categories, perceptual and cognitive; value/belief
was changed to valuation; and ecological was added to draft 2. The task
force also decided at this point to give up the effort to identify three separate
systems – individual, family and community – and instead to combine
them into one system.

The task force met again in March 1987 to revise draft 2. Draft 3 (Appendix
B), the current draft, differed from draft 2 in the following ways: the
categories at each level were alphabetized, the category of decision processes was dropped; and the categories undeveloped and potential for
were added. Decision processes in the second draft included the NANDA
diagnoses of ineffective individual and family coping. Both of these diagnoses seemed too broad to be of value to PMH nursing. Ineffective coping
did not distinguish between patients. The undeveloped designation was
added to be used when the person (adult or child) has not yet reached the
stage of development represented by the response pattern. The designation of potential for alterations is to be used when there is reason to believe
that a person is at an increased risk for a specific alteration. For example,
depressed persons are often at risk for aggressive/violent behaviours
toward themselves and require special observation and precautions in the
environment. The designation NOS (not otherwise specified) used in draft
1 was retained. It allows for the recording of processes not yet classified,
and will provide data for further refinement of the classification system.

Recent efforts of the task force have been focused on developing PMH
speciality diagnoses that would fit within a generic classification system of
nursing diagnoses. Thus PMH speciality diagnoses would be a subset of
general nursing diagnoses in somewhat the same way that the DSM-III-R
psychiatric diagnoses fit into the ICD-9 medical diagnostic system.

We have proposed that, in our classification system, generic nursing
diagnoses would appear at the four-digit level and PMH speciality nursing
diagnoses would be presented at the six- and eight-digit levels.

Our working definition of **diagnosis** is a name for a cluster or pattern of
human responses which may include a statement specifying related to or
associated with when data are available. Thus a nursing diagnosis can be
made at varying levels of abstraction depending on the amount and type of
information available about the client and the level of sophistication of the
nurse. Nursing diagnoses are important in so far as they provide direction
for nursing interventions. The more specialized or specific the nursing
diagnosis, the greater the level of sophistication required for nursing interventions. For example, a nurse generalist would be expected to diagnose a
client with altered thought content, but would rely on a PMH specialist to
diagnose and treat the difference between delusions, ideas of reference,

magical thinking, and obsessions. Our task force is continuing to refine and revise the classification system. A current priority for our work is to submit as many of the new diagnoses as possible to NANDA for review. The opportunity for NANDA and ANA to develop a truly collaborative relationship in relation to the formation of classification systems is unprecedented. Our future efforts will be directed toward supporting that collaboration, while, at the same time, encouraging individuals and groups to continue to work on the development of classification systems for generic and speciality practice.

References

American Nurses' Association (1980) *Nursing: A social policy statement*, Kansas City, MO.

American Nurses' Association (1982) *Standards of Psychiatric and Mental Health Nursing Practice*, Kansas City, MO.

American Psychiatric Association (1980) *Diagnostic and Statistical Manual of Mental Disorders*, 3rd edn, Washington, DC.

Loomis, M. E. (1985) Emerging content in nursing: an analysis of dissertation abstracts and titles 1976–1982. *Nurs. Res.*, **34**, 113–9.

Loomis, M. E., O'Toole, A. W., Brown, M. S. *et al.* (1987) Development of a classification system for psychiatric/mental health nursing: Individual response class. *Arch. Psych. Nurs.*, **1**, 16–24.

O'Toole, A. W. (1981) When the practical becomes theoretical. *J. Psychosoc. Nurs. Mental Health Serv.*, **19**, 11–19.

O'Toole, A. W., Jones, S. L. and Wilson, H. S. Research in psychiatric nursing, in *Psychiatric Nursing*, 3rd edn, (eds C. R. Kneisel and H. S. Wilson), Addison Wesley, Menlo Park, CA (in press).

Appendix A: working classification schemata of nursing diagnoses, December, 1986 (Draft 2)

```
01.   Human response patterns in physiological processes
      01.01   Altered circulation processes
              01.01.01   Altered vascular circulation
                         01.01.01.01   Tissue perfusion
                         01.01.01.02   Altered fluid volume
              01.01.01   Altered cardiac circulation
      01.02   Altered elimination processes
              01.02.01   Altered bowel elimination
                         01.02.01.01   Constipation
                         01.02.01.02   Diarrhea
                         01.02.01.03   Incontinence
                         01.02.01.04   Encopresis
              01.02.02   Altered urinary elimination
                         01.02.02.01   Incontinence
                         01.02.02.02   Retention
                         01.02.02.03   Enuresis
              01.02.03   Altered skin elimination
```

01.03 Altered endocrine/metabolic processes
    01.03.01 Altered growth and development
    01.03.02 Altered hormone regulation
        01.03.02.0.1 premenstrual stress syndrome
01.04 Altered gastrointestinal processes
    01.04.01 Altered absorption
    01.04.02 Altered digestion
01.05 Altered neuro/sensory processes
    01.05.01 Altered levels of consciousness
    01.05.02 Altered sensory capacity
    01.05.03 Altered sensory processing
    01.05.04 Altered sensory integration
        01.05.04.01 Learning disabilities
01.06 Altered oxygenation processes
    01.06.01 Altered respiration
        01.06.01.01 Impaired gas exchange
        01.06.01.02 Ineffective airway clearance
        01.06.01.03 Ineffective breathing pattern
01.07 Altered reproductive/sexual processes
    01.07.01 Altered menstrual processes
        01.07.01.01 Amenorrhea
        01.07.01.02 Dysmenorrhea
    01.07.02 Altered sexual functioning
        01.07.02.01 Dyspareunia
        01.07.02.02 Infertility
01.08 Altered nutrition processes
    01.08.01 Altered cellular processes
    01.08.02 Altered systemic processes
        01.08.02.01 More than body requirements
        01.08.02.02 Less than body requirements
        01.08.02.03 Potential for more than body requirements
    01.08.03 Altered eating processes
        01.08.03.01 Bulemia
        01.08.03.02 Anorexia
01.09 Altered physical integrity processes
    01.09.01 Potential for injury
        01.09.01.01 Potential for suffocating
        01.09.01.02 Potential for poisoning
        01.09.01.03 Potential for trauma
    01.09.02 Altered physical integrity
        01.09.02.01 Altered skin integrity
        01.09.02.02 Altered tissue integrity
01.10 Altered physical regulation processes
    01.10.01 Altered immune responses
        01.10.01.01 Potential for infection
    01.10.02 Altered body temperature
        01.10.02.01 Potential altered body temperature
        01.10.02.02 Hypothermia
        01.10.02.03 Hyperthermia
        01.10.02.04 Ineffective thermoregulation
01.99 Altered physiological processes not otherwise specified

02. Human response patterns in interpersonal processes
  02.01 Altered communication processes

02.01.01 Altered verbal communication
02.01.02 Altered nonverbal communication
02.02 Altered role performance processes
    02.02.01 Altered parenting roles
    02.02.02 Altered sexual roles
    02.02.03 Altered work roles
    02.02.04 Altered family roles
    02.02.05 Altered social/leisure roles
02.03 Altered socialization processes
    02.03.01 Impaired social interaction
    02.03.02 Social isolation/withdrawal
02.04 Altered conduct/impulse processes
    02.04.01 Aggressive/violent behaviors
        02.04.01.01 Aggressive/violent behaviors toward self
        02.04.01.02 Aggressive/violent behaviors toward others
        02.04.01.03 Aggressive/violent behaviors toward environment
        02.04.01.04 Potential for violence
    02.04.02 Dysfunctional behaviors
        02.04.02.01 Bizarre behaviors
        02.04.02.02 Compulsive behaviors
        02.04.02.03 Disorganized behaviors
        02.04.02.04 Age-inappropriate behaviors
        02.04.02.05 Unpredictable behaviors
02.05 Altered sexuality processes
02.99 Altered interpersonal processes not otherwise specified

03. Human response patterns in emotional processes
  03.01 Altered feeling patterns
    03.01.01 Anxiety
    03.01.02 Fear
    03.01.03 Anger
    03.01.04 Envy
    03.01.05 Guilt
    03.01.06 Shame
    03.01.07 Sadness
    03.01.08 Grieving
  03.02 Post-trauma response patterns
    03.02.01 Rape trauma syndrome
  03.99 Altered emotional processes not otherwise specified

04. Human response patterns in decision processes
  04.01 Altered coping
    04.01.01 Ineffective coping patterns
        04.01.01.01 Individual ineffective coping
        04.01.01.02 Family ineffective coping
        04.01.01.03 Community ineffective coping
  04.02 Altered participation
    04.02.01 Ineffective participation patterns
        04.02.01.01 Individual ineffective participation
        04.02.01.02 Family ineffective participation
        04.02.01.03 Community ineffective participation
  04.03 Altered judgment
    04.03.01 Ineffective judgment patterns
        04.03.01.01 Indecisiveness

04.99 Altered decision processes not otherwise specified

05. Human response patterns in perception processes
05.01 Altered self-concept
05.01.01 Altered body image
05.01.02 Altered self-esteem
05.01.03 Altered personal identity
05.01.04 Altered gender identity
05.01.05 Altered social identity
05.02 Altered attention
05.02.01 Distractibility
05.02.02 Hyperalertness
05.02.03 Inattention
05.02.04 Selective attention
05.03 Altered sensory perception
05.03.01 Visual
05.03.02 Auditory
05.03.03 Kinesthetic
05.03.04 Gustatory
05.03.05 Tactile
05.03.06 Olfactory
05.03.07 Hallucinations
05.03.08 Illusions
05.04 Altered comfort patterns
05.04.01 Pain
05.04.02 Discomfort
05.04.03 Distress
05.99 Altered perception processes not otherwise specified

06. Human response patterns in cognition processes
06.01 Altered memory
06.01.01 Amnesia
06.01.02 Distorted memory
06.01.03 Impaired long-term memory
06.01.04 Impaired short-term memory
06.02 Altered orientation
06.02.01 Confusion
06.02.02 Delirium
06.02.03 Disorientation
06.03 Altered thought content
06.03.01 Delusions
06.03.02 Illusions
06.03.03 Magical thinking
06.03.04 Obsessions
06.04 Altered thought processes
06.04.01 Impaired abstract thinking
06.04.02 Impaired concentration
06.04.03 Impaired problem solving
06.05 Altered knowledge processes
06.05.01 Knowledge deficit
06.05.02 Impaired intellectual functioning
06.06 Altered learning processes
06.99 Altered cognition processes not otherwise specified

07. Human response patterns in valuation processes
    07.01   Altered meaningfulness
            07.01.01   Hopelessness
            07.01.02   Helplessness
            07.01.03   Loneliness
            07.01.04   Powerlessness
    07.02   Altered spirituality
            07.02.01   Spiritual distress
            07.02.02   Spiritual despair
    07.03   Altered values
            07.03.01   Conflict with social order
            07.03.02   Inability to internalize values
            07.03.03   Unclarified values
    07.99   Altered valuation processes not otherwise specified

08. Human response patterns in activity processes
    08.01   Altered motor behavior
            08.01.01   Catatonia
            08.01.02   Impaired coordination
            08.01.03   Hyperactivity
            08.01.04   Hypoactivity
            08.01.05   Muscular rigidity
            08.01.06   Psychomotor retardation
    08.02   Altered self-care
            08.02.01   Feeding
            08.02.02   Bathing/hygiene
            08.02.03   Dressing/grooming
            08.02.04   Toileting
            08.02.05   Health maintenance
    08.03   Altered sleep/arousal patterns
            08.03.01   Hypersomnia
            08.03.02   Insomnia
            08.03.03   Somnolence
            08.03.04   Nightmares
    08.04   Altered recreation patterns
            08.04.01   Inadequate diversional activity
    08.05   Altered growth and development
            08.05.01   Developmental lag
    08.99   Altered activity processes not otherwise specified

09. Human response patterns in ecological processes
    09.01   Altered home maintenance
            09.01.01   Home sanitation hazards
            09.01.02   Home safety hazards
    09.02   Altered community maintenance
            09.02.01   Community sanitation hazards
            09.02.02   Community safety hazards
    09.03   Altered environmental integrity
    09.99   Altered ecological processes not otherwise specified

ILH:pm:001
01/02/87
01/05/87

Appendix B: working draft of the classification of human responses of concern for psychiatric mental health nursing practice, March 6, 1987 (Draft 3)[†]

01   Human response patterns in activity processes
    01.01   Altered motor behavior
        01.01.01   Bizarre motor behavior
        01.01.02   Catatonia
        01.01.03   Impaired coordination
        01.01.04   Hyperactivity
        01.01.05   Hypoactivity
        01.01.06   Muscular rigidity
        01.01.07   Psychomotor retardation
    01.02   Altered recreation patterns
        01.02.01   Inadequate diversional activity
    01.03   Altered self-care
        01.03.01   Altered eating
      *01.03.02   Altered grooming
        01.03.03   Altered health maintenance
      *01.03.04   Altered hygiene
        01.03.05   Altered participation in health care
      *01.03.06   Altered toileting
    01.04   Altered sleep/arousal patterns
        01.04.01   Difficult transition to and from sleep
        01.04.02   Hypersomnia
        01.04.03   Insomnia
        01.04.04   Nightmares
        01.04.05   Somnolence
    01.97   Undeveloped activity processes
    01.98   Altered activity processes not otherwise specified
    01.99   Potential for altered activity processes

02   Human response patterns in cognition processes
    02.01   Altered decision making
    02.02   Altered judgment
  *02.03   Altered knowledge processes
        02.03.01   Agnosia
        02.03.02   Altered intellectual functioning
      *02.03.03   Knowledge deficit
    02.04   Altered learning processes
    02.05   Altered memory
        02.05.01   Amnesia
        02.05.02   Distorted memory
        02.05.03   Long-term memory loss
        02.05.04   Short-term memory loss
    02.06   Altered orientation
        02.06.01   Confusion
        02.06.02   Delirium
        02.06.03   Disorientation

[†]M. Loomis, A. O'Toole, P. Pothier, P. West, H. Wilson, American Nurses' Association, Phenomenon Task Force, 1987. This classification is based on previous work of the Phenomenon Task Force and the Advisory Panel on Classifications for Nursing Practice of the American Nurses' Association.

02.07 Altered thought content
    02.07.01 Delusions
    02.07.02 Ideas of reference
    02.07.03 Magical thinking
    02.07.04 Obsessions
*02.08 Altered thought processes
    02.08.01 Altered abstract thinking
    02.08.02 Altered concentration
    02.08.03 Altered problem solving
    02.08.04 Thought insertion
02.97 Undeveloped cognition processes
02.98 Altered cognition processes not otherwise specified
02.99 Potential for altered cognition processes

03 Human response patterns in ecological processes
03.01 Altered community maintenance
    03.01.01 Community safety hazards
    03.01.02 Community sanitation hazards
03.02 Altered environmental integrity
*03.03 Altered home maintenance
    03.03.01 Home safety hazards
    03.03.02 Home sanitation hazards

04 Human response patterns in emotional processes
04.01 Abuse response patterns
    *04.01.01 Rape trauma syndrome
04.02 Altered feeling patterns
    04.02.01 Anger
    *04.02.02 Anxiety
    04.02.03 Elation
    04.02.04 Envy
    *04.02.05 Fear
    *04.02.06 Grief
    04.02.07 Guilt
    04.02.08 Sadness
    04.02.09 Shame
04.03 Undifferentiated feeling pattern
04.97 Undeveloped emotional responses
04.98 Altered emotional processes not otherwise specified
04.99 Potential for altered emotional processes

05 Human response patterns in interpersonal processes
*05.01 Altered communication processes
    05.01.01 Altered nonverbal communication
    *05.01.02 Altered verbal communication
05.02 Altered conduct/impulse processes
    05.02.01 Aggressive/violent behaviors
        05.02.01.01 Aggressive/violent behaviors toward environment
        05.02.01.02 Aggressive/violent behaviors toward others
        05.02.01.03 Aggressive/violent behaviors toward self
    05.02.02 Dysfunctional behaviors
        05.02.02.01 Age-inappropriate behaviors
        05.02.02.02 Bizarre behaviors

          05.02.02.03   Compulsive behaviors
          05.02.02.04   Disorganized behaviors
          05.02.02.05   Unpredictable behaviors
   05.03   Altered role performance
       05.03.01   Altered family role
       05.03.02   Altered leisure role
    *05.03.03   Altered parenting role
       05.03.04   Altered play role
       05.03.05   Altered student role
       05.03.06   Altered work role
   05.04   Altered sexuality processes
   05.05   Altered social interaction
       05.05.01   Social intrusiveness
    *05.05.02   Social isolation/withdrawal
   05.97   Undeveloped interpersonal processes
   05.98   Altered interpersonal processes not otherwise specified
   05.99   Potential for altered interpersonal processes
    *05.99.01   Potential for violence

06   Human response patterns in perception processes
   06.01   Altered Attention
       06.01.01   Distractibility
       06.01.02   Hyperalertness
       06.01.03   Inattention
       06.01.04   Selective attention
  *06.02   Altered comfort patterns
       06.02.01   Discomfort
       06.02.02   Distress
    *06.02.03   Pain
   06.03   Altered self-concept
    *06.03.01   Altered body image
       06.03.02   Altered gender identity
    *06.03.03   Altered personal identity
    *06.03.04   Altered self-esteem
       06.03.05   Altered social identity
       06.03.06   Undeveloped self-concept
   06.04   Altered sensory perception
    *06.04.01   Auditory
    *06.04.02   Gustatory
       06.04.03   Hallucinations
       06.04.04   Illusions
    *06.04.05   Kinesthetic
    *06.04.06   Olfactory
    *06.04.07   Tactile
    *06.04.08   Visual
   06.97   Undeveloped perception processes
   06.98   Altered perception processes not otherwise specified
   06.99   Potential for altered perception processes

07   Human response patterns in physiological processes
   07.01   Altered Circulation Processes
       07.01.01   Altered Vascular circulation
          *07.01.01.01   Tissue perfusion
          *07.01.01.02   Altered fluid volume
       07.01.02   Altered cardiac circulation

07.02 Altered elimination processes
    07.02.01 *Altered bowel elimination
        *07.02.01.01   Constipation
        *07.02.01.02   Diarrhea
        *07.02.01.03   Incontinence
        07.02.01.04   Encopresis
   *07.02.02 Altered urinary elimination
        *07.02.02.01   Incontinence
        *07.02.02.02   Retention
        07.02.02.03   Ensuresis
    07.02.03 Altered skin elimination
07.03 Altered endocrine/metabolic processes
    07.03.01 Altered growth
    07.03.02 Altered hormone regulation
        07.03.02.01   Premenstrual stress syndrome
07.04 Altered gastrointestinal processes
    07.04.01 Altered absorption
    07.04.02 Altered digestion
07.05 Altered neuro/sensory processes
    07.05.01 Altered levels of consciousness
    07.05.02 Altered sensory acuity
    07.05.03 Altered sensory processing
    07.05.04 Altered sensory integration
        07.05.04.01   Learning disabilities
07.06 Altered nutrition processes
    07.06.01 Altered cellular processes
    07.06.02 Altered systemic processes
        *07.06.02.01   More than body requirements
        *07.06.02.02   Less than body requirements
    07.06.03 Altered eating processes
        07.06.03.01   Anorexia
        07.06.03.02   Pica
07.07 Altered oxygenation processes
    07.07.01 Altered respiration
        07.07.01.01   Altered gas exchange
        *07.07.01.02   Ineffective airway clearance
        *07.07.01.03   Ineffective breathing pattern
07.08 Altered physical integrity processes
   *07.08.01 Altered skin integrity
   *07.08.02 Altered tissue integrity
07.09 Altered physical regulation processes
    07.09.01 Altered immune responses
        07.09.01.01   Infection
07.10 Altered body temperature
   *07.10.01 Hypothermia
   *07.10.02 Hyperthermia
   *07.10.03 Ineffective thermoregulation
07.97 Undeveloped physiological processes
07.98 Altered physiological processes not otherwise specified
07.99 Potential for altered physiological processes

08 Human response patterns in valuation processes
   *08.01 Altered meaningfulness
       *08.01.01 Hopelessness

08.01.02   Helplessness
08.01.03   Loneliness
*08.01.04   Powerlessness
08.02   Altered spirituality
*08.02.01   Spiritual distress
08.02.02   Spiritual despair
08.03   Altered values
08.03.01   Conflict with social order
08.03.02   Inability to internalize values
08.03.03   Unclarified values
08.97   Undeveloped valuation processes
08.98   Altered valuation processes not otherwise specified
08.99   Potential for altered valuation processes

*NANDA diagnosis.

Part Two

THEORETICAL MODELS: PRINCIPLES AND GENERAL APPLICATIONS

This section examines the key principles and general applications of several different, and occasionally related, theoretical approaches to psychiatric nursing. Some readers may feel that there is a considerable difference between models and theories; particularly nursing models (such as Adaptation or Self-Care) and models of therapy such as Cognitive, or Client-centred therapies. However, because the extent to which theories and models differ or overlap is often unclear, all means of understanding and treating the client using approaches which have a clear theoretical underpinning have, for the purposes of this text, been referred to as theoretical models.

The differing writing styles in this section reflect the multicultural backgrounds and professional experiences of the writers. Also, the balance of treatment models, often borrowed from other disciplines, and nursing models highlights a debate which is current within the profession. That debate is largely concerned with the applicability and usefulness of nursing models, and the extent to which nursing theory can be said to exist.

It is possible that readers of this section might avoid what may essentially be a semantic debate about the ownership of theory and make their own assessment of the usefulness of the theory based approaches described here. Questions which the readers might apply to each theoretical model include:

1. To what extent does the theoretical model help me to identify the range of human responses to actual or potential health problems?
2. How can a nursing diagnosis be made and what is the basis for that diagnosis?
3. Does the model explain why individuals respond to health problems in the way that they do?
4. What does it say about the form of nursing intervention that is required to enable the client to move towards optimum health?

5. Does the model help me to understand the desired outcome of nursing intervention?

References

Fox, D. (1983) *Fundamentals of Research in Nursing.* Appleton-Century-Crofts, Norwalk, CT.

Mowinski-Jennings, B. (1987) Nursing theory development: successes and challenges. *J. Adv. Nurs.*, **12** (1), pp. 68–9.

Smoyak, S. (1988) *Strategies for Theory Development.* Proceedings: Fifth Nursing Science Colloquium. Boston University School of Nursing, Boston, MA.

Chapter 3

Cognitive therapy model: principles and general applications

P. BARKER

Much psychological distress has to do with being happy. People who might be described as depressed clearly are unhappy, to say the least. However, many other life-problems are described, however circularly, from a happiness perspective. People who have relationship difficulties, for instance, might not be happy about the way their husbands/wives/children/relatives/friends behave. Such unhappiness can be expressed as anger, frustration or fear, rather than sadness. At its most fundamental, however, people interpret such experiences as distressing or disturbing. The way the world is, as opposed to the way they would like it to be, upsets their emotional equilibrium. As a result they are unhappy.

The philosophy of living which underpins this chapter could be called hedonistic. Aristippus is credited with establishing the doctrine of hedonism: the idea that pleasure or happiness is the chief good or chief end of man. A crude analysis of the philosophical basis of the therapies covered in this text would suggest that they are all, basically, concerned with the pursuit of happiness. It should become apparent also that many contributors to the development of these therapies have also asserted their belief in the intrinsic value of man. Therapy often means the means by which people loosen the shackles which restrict their awareness of their basic human worth. A precedent for such psychotherapeutic assumptions might be found in Goethe's dictum that the man who is happy as well as great needs neither to obey nor command in order to be something.

This chapter should be read with a number of potential clinical problems in mind. People who devalue themselves, feel depressed, are hostile, are overly dependent or find it difficult to trust people, or who experience severe anxiety, might all be considered suitable for cognitive therapy. To this list could be added, arguably, those with distorted perceptions of reality, such as people experiencing hallucinations and delusions. The therapeutic model addressed here would view such groups as experiencing life-problems which are rooted in their perception and interpretation of themselves and their world. It will be argued here that cognition is primary to the generation or maintenance of such problems. To avoid the implication that cognitive therapy is appropriate for some, but not all, of such problems, I shall address the model in more general terms, identifying the content and its relationship to various psychological or psychiatric problems of living. I shall try to illustrate how a cognitive therapy approach might help people to live less restricted, happier lives, by revising their conceptual model of themselves and their world. Such a revision, of necessity, deals with phenomena such as low self-esteem, affect, hostility, trust, dependency and so on, all of which are secondary to cognition.

Cogito ergo sum

The next chapter gives the reader an introduction to the traditional behaviourist perspective on problems of living (see Chapter 4). The analysis of psychological problems from a contemporary behavioural perspective emphasizes their acquired nature. Some develop through a process of social learning, whereas others exist largely because of the absence of essential social, survival or problem-solving skills. The contribution made by modern behaviourism to the explanation of psychological difficulties and psychiatric distress cannot be underestimated. Within the past quarter-century, however, increasing concern has been expressed, within behavioural psychotherapy itself, that extrapolations from Pavlovian and Skinnerian conditioning theories are inadequate to explain the genesis of many patterns of behaviour (Mahoney, 1974). Such critiques led to the development of cognitive behaviour modification and/or therapy which paid more attention to the role of the mediational processes of thought described by Bandura (1969). This identity crisis within the behavioural camp closely reflected anxieties expressed, almost contemporaneously, by dissident thinkers within the psychoanalytic movement (Ellis, 1962). The review of the development of the cognitive therapy model within this chapter will attempt to acknowledge influences from both the behavioural and the psychoanalytic viewpoint.

Although all counselling aims to influence the ways in which people think, differences exist in the methodology involved. The term cognitive therapy commonly refers to a group of psychological interventions which share the aim of tackling specific psychological problems through teaching clients how to modify maladaptive thinking through using the skills of effective thinking. The approach represents a middle-ground dissatisfaction with, at one extreme, behavioural approaches which de-emphasize affect and cognition, and at the other, psychoanalytic psychotherapy which emphasizes unconscious processes and distal life-events to the exclusion of contemporary concerns and problems.

The term cognition means the faculty of knowing (Watson, 1976) but is probably related to gnomon, the pin of a sundial. The gnomon measures the heavens from shadows. This serves as an apposite metaphor for the role of cognitions, which translate experiences into shadows cast in human memory (Gregory, 1987). In this latter sense cognition represents attending, perceiving, thinking and remembering. In the cognitive therapy literature reviewed here, however, the term is commonly used to refer to thinking only. It will become apparent, however, that the cognitions manipulated within the therapeutic model do not deal solely with active thinking in the here-and-now. Instead, the patient's recollections of events, the immediate (or automatic) thoughts, or judgements associated with such events, how certain events are selected and others rejected, as well as a host of fantasies, imaginings, and other manipulations of imagery, will all be considered. All such phenomena are mediated by cognitive processes and are, therefore, cognitions. It is clear that mental health nurses devote a great deal of their time to the assessment and analysis of the patient's cognitions: how he sees himself, his view of past, present and future, and the overall relationship of self, world and future to the everyday business of living. The overwhelming importance of cognition as a focus for nursing activity represents the underlying rationale for the writing of this chapter.

Cognitive behaviour modification and cognitive therapy

The cognitive model of therapy described in this chapter and illustrated in Chapter 11 is based largely upon an integration of the therapeutic methods of Beck and Ellis. The importance of the former lies in his articulation and description of specific therapeutic strategies and outcome evaluation. Ellis' contribution lies primarily in his description of rational emotive therapy (RET), which served as the genuine progenitor of cognitive therapy. Ellis suggests that RET is a comprehensive psychotherapy, since it embraces not only specific methods but also a guiding philosophy. It would appear that such a philosophy is largely missing from Beck and his colleagues' therapeutic model.

Classification of cognitive therapies

Before addressing the cognitive therapy (CT) model which has emerged from the influences of Beck and Ellis, it may be worthwhile to consider the four main groups of cognitive therapy techniques. Most, if not all, are to be found in some form or another in the CT model described later.

1. Dealing with intrusive thoughts. Where persistent patterns of negative thinking which disrupt the fulfillment of everyday living are reported, it may be essential to establish control over such phenomena as part of the overall therapeutic intervention. Usually the procedure is combined with

other cognitive techniques, and behavioural methods such as relaxation, in a treatment package (Wisocki, 1976). Thought stopping is a popular procedure for eliminating perseverative thinking which, characteristically, is unrealistic, unproductive, anxiety-provoking or otherwise disruptive. The procedure described here could equally be used with a person experiencing ruminative negative thoughts or auditory hallucinations. The procedure involves the following stages:

(a) The person is asked to relax, close his eyes and allow himself to think a typically negative thought.
(b) As soon as the thought is produced the person signals to the therapist by raising his forefinger.
(c) The therapist shouts STOP loudly, asks the person to open his eyes and reports his response. Typically, the person will report a startle response and the loss of the negative thought.
(d) A second trial is set up preceded by the provision of the simple rationale that interruption, if practised regularly enough, can establish control over negative thinking, leading to its elimination.
(e) In the second trial the therapist waits a second or two before introducing the startle response.
(f) The person is instructed further in the use of stop as a self-control strategy. Initially, the person is told to imagine himself shouting STOP very loudly. If problems are encountered the person is advised to practise shouting STOP aloud several times before returning to the imaginal practice. If difficulty is met in manipulating the imaginal STOP the person is advised to imagine seeing the word depicted in neon, or graffiti or in symbolic form such as a road STOP sign. This image or symbol is matched with the imagination of the word STOP shouted aloud.
(g) Approximately 10 minutes are then spent practising thought stopping, alternating between therapist and person-induced interruption. This usually represents about 20 distinct trials, ten apiece.
(h) At the end of the session the person is instructed to practise the procedure at specified times during the day, usually two or three sessions of approximately 20 trials. In addition, the person is asked to invoke the procedure whenever negative thoughts occur spontaneously. The value of the procedure in reducing, and ultimately bringing negative thoughts under the person's control, is further emphasized. Although used mainly as a strategy for dealing with obsessional ruminations (Taylor, 1963) the procedure has been reported as having wider applications (see Cautela and Wisocki, 1977; and Wisocki, 1976).

2. Manipulating self-statements. Self-statements are thoughts which a person has about specific events and their meaning for the person concerned. Most authorities regard self-statements as lower-order cognitive phenomena which are situation-specific and conceptually limited. Usually

these statements represent the internalization of statements which originally were declared overtly: for instance 'I am going to make a mess of this test...I'll never manage to go to the shops'. The manipulation of such negative self-statements involves the following stages:

1. The person is helped to recognize the occurrence of such thoughts through use of self-monitoring.
2. The person is helped to generate challenges to the negative thoughts, as well as the production of alternative self-statements.
3. The person is helped to assess his reaction to the manipulation of self-statements, in terms of his eventual behaviour and concomitant emotions.

This approach is fundamental to a number of different cognitive therapies, such as rational emotive therapy (Ellis, 1962), self-instructional training (Meichenbaum, 1977) and some forms of assertiveness training (Alberti, 1977). Meichenbaum was influenced greatly by Luria (1961) in developing his ideas of the relationship between language, thought and behaviour. His view of self-talk differs significantly from that of Ellis in that the internal dialogue is not seen as equivalent to thought. Rather, the process is seen as one of both listening and talking to oneself. The concept of this dialogue provides the underpinnings of problem-solving training described below. In addition to its popular application to stress management (Meichenbaum, 1983) the approach has been used most successfully in anger-management with adults (Novaco, 1977) and impulse-control in children (Meichenbaum and Genest, 1981).

3. Challenging beliefs and assumptions. Beliefs and assumptions represent either conscious or unconscious (implicit) evaluations of life experiences. In cognitive therapy the focus is almost exclusively upon dysfunctional or absolutistic evaluations. Within Ellis' rational emotive therapy (RET) model such beliefs are viewed as predominantly embodying unconditional shoulds, musts, demands and commands (Ellis, 1962). These beliefs co-exist with the negative cognitions noted in (2) above, but in practice appear to follow in a logical process of negative evaluation. For example, the person who is faced with a demanding task may self-state, 'I'll never manage this'. When asked to explain what this situation might MEAN for him, 'what would be so bad about that anyway', the person might conclude that this would mean that 'I'm hopeless (or useless, a failure, all washed up)'. Both RET and Beck's cognitive therapy (CT) involve direct challenging of beliefs and assumptions. In the Ellis model, the therapist actively and forcefully disputes the person's belief systems with him. A typically confrontative disputation might be as follows:

OK, so you find it difficult to make friends. Sometimes people you like reject you. Where is it written on tablets of stone that you are incompetent or worthless if you find it difficult to make friends or get rejected by some people? The answer is NOWHERE, except maybe in your head. The facts are that you are just another person who has had a hard time with people recently. You are just someone who has had better experiences with some people in the past, and who can keep on trying to improve your relationships with people until you get it right!

In the Beck model the focus upon dysfunctional beliefs not only is less confrontational, but is located within a therapeutic time-scale: in CT the person is helped to identify, challenge and subsequently classify specific forms of thinking errors, in the form of specific self-statements, before moving on to tackle dysfunctional belief systems *per se*. When such dysfunctional beliefs are tackled, differences in the therapist's method, rather than overall aim, would become apparent. Beck's approach would involve a more sensitive invitation to the patient to identify the evidence for thinking that (for example) 'you are worthless'. Ellis has asserted that a wide range of people can benefit from this approach, including those diagnosed as personality disorder, schizophrenic, manic depressive and even mildly mentally handicapped (Ellis and Whiteley, 1979). The more severe the person's problems, the more likely that this intervention would be linked to adjunct drug therapy and hospitalization. More research is needed to determine the efficacy of this approach with different populations. For nurses, however, this approach offers a structured basis for responding to people who display overtly dysfunctional belief systems.

4. Developing problem-solving. A range of strategies are encompassed by the generic title problem-solving training. These focus upon the importance of cognitions in understanding, mediating and resolving intrapersonal and interpersonal problems. Problem-solving abilities are directly related to adjustment in children, adolescents and adults. Where such skills are not in evidence, life problems are expressed through depression, anxiety, substance abuse, marital discord or parenting difficulties. The approach emphasizes five main stages:

1. The person is helped to recognize and understand the nature of his interpersonal problems and to be aware of their origin. This is generally construed as a problem sensitivity and orientation stage.
2. The person is then helped to assess his main problems, identifying targets in the form of realistic and specific goals. This stage involves problem definition and formulation.
3. The person is then helped to generate a range of possible solutions, usually through use of brainstorming. Where this approach is used in a group, other members take turns in proposing options. Where solution generation is undertaken on an individual basis the person is encouraged to view the problem from the perspective of other people,

using the experience of others or expectations of how they might respond to the situation.

4. The fourth stage involves decision-making. The person selects the option which, in his view, looks most likely to effect the change necessary to resolve the problem or reach the target. This is achieved by thinking through the short- and long-term effect of each optional solution, considering the personal and social effects of the action. In addition to considering how the option might work, obstacles are considered along with possible strategies for circumventing them. Usually a rating is given for each optional solution, based upon an evaluation of the possible advantages and disadvantages.

5. The final stage involves the implementation and evaluation of the selection solution.

This approach has been applied to a broad spectrum of problems: those involving children of pre-school and school age, considered normal, as well as disturbed children (Urbain and Kendall, 1980); parents with child-rearing difficulties (Spivack and Shure, 1978); a range of psychiatric problems (Spivack, Platt and Shure, 1976). A specific form of problem-solving training is contained within so-called behavioral marital therapy (Jacobsen and Margolin, 1979). A sizeable literature exists which demonstrates the benefits of facilitating problem-solving, rather than merely offering advice or unconditional support. For nurses, who often are engineered into providing solutions to maintain their helpful image, problem-solving offers a viable alternative.

These four categories of cognitive intervention are no more than a crude summary of specific technical methods, taken largely out of context. All the authors referred to above would emphasize the location of such technical interventions within a broader therapeutic system involving careful assessment, cognitive-behavioural analysis, establishment of a positive therapeutic relationship (in some cases emphasizing a collaborative relationship), homework assignments and the development of personal discovery through self-monitoring and testing thinking and belief systems through experimental action. Most if not all of these aspects of the therapeutic programme will be discussed later under the Beck and Ellis cognitive models. For this reason no further discussion of these therapeutic variables will be included here.

An integrated cognitive therapy model

The contribution of Ellis: rational emotive roots
While practising psychoanalytic psychotherapy in the late 1940s Ellis became disillusioned with its unscientific nature and the passivity required of the therapist (Ellis, 1949). Experience of employing active–directive home-

work assignments in sex therapy, coupled with a long-standing interest in the philosophy of human happiness, led Ellis to develop rational emotive therapy (RET). In RET, Ellis developed a model of therapy based upon the idea of using reason in the pursuit of short-term and longer-term hedonism. In his view people have a strong innate (biological) tendency to think irrationally, which is supported (reinforced), especially in childhood development, by the irrational ideas of parents and society expressed through mass media. People's failure to think rationally and face reality, in Ellis' view, leads to the development of emotional disorder and its concurrent behavioural disturbances.

In RET, Ellis proposed that human thinking and emotion were not two different processes but, for all practical purposes, overlapped. The view that thought and feeling were essentially the same thing was, indeed still is, a provocative concept. The relationship between the four basic life processes, sensing, moving, thinking and feeling were described by Ellis (1962, p. 39) thus: 'If an individual senses something...he also tends, at the very same time, to do something about it...to have some feeling about it...and to think about it... Similarly, if he acts, emotes or thinks, he also consciously or unconsciously involves himself in the other behaviour processes.' In this sense Ellis described RET as a comprehensive system of psychotherapy, based upon a range of theories of human behaviour and behaviour change. Ellis has acknowledged Watson and Dunlap, of the early behaviourists, as influential figures in overcoming his own social anxiety (Ellis, 1972) as well as philosophical activists such as Epicurus, Epictetus, Schopenhauer and Santayana, in shaping the philosophy which underpins RET. Ellis saw these writers as encouraging people to do something to challenge their 'misery-creating thinking'. It should be noted that RET is one of the few schools of therapy which does not espouse self-esteem. Instead, in the basic spirit of hedonism, people are encouraged to enjoy themselves, rather than prove themselves. Rather than encourage people to develop themselves through a process of working towards goals accompanied by self-rating, Ellis emphasizes self-acceptance. For nurses who have, traditionally, paid a lot of attention to trying to develop the patient's sense of self-worth, this represents a significant conceptual shift. Philosophically, RET argues that people have a right to individuality, freedom, self-interest and self-control. At the same time as people are helped to access such rights they are encouraged to live in an involved, committed and selectively loving manner. The approach thereby facilitates both individual and social interest (Ellis, 1973), and is undoubtedly a genuine humanistic psychotherapy.

Ellis has identified several irrational (dysfunctional) beliefs. These include demandingness where the person mistakes preferences or choices for demands or commands. Such beliefs inevitably include reference to words like must, should, ought. Ellis has also referred to this belief in terms of perfectionism or intolerance (Ellis, 1973). Although he has identified as many as 11 or 12 irrational beliefs (Ellis, 1962), in his view every disturbed feeling is closely linked to one or other of the following irrational, or self-defeating, beliefs (iBs):

1. I must do well and must win approval for everything I do, otherwise I am a rotten person.
2. You must act kindly, considerately and justly towards me or else you are a louse.
3. The conditions under which I live must remain good and easy, so that I get practically everything I want without too much effort or discomfort, or else the world turns damnable, and life hardly seems worth living (Ellis, 1977).

These three core beliefs are examples of what Ellis has called musturbation. In Ellis' view there is no escape from individual responsibility. People are responsible for the rational fashioning of their existence, no matter how unfairly other people or the world may be treating them (Ellis and Grieger, 1977). Ellis' approach aims to minimize the person's self-defeating outlooks, and to attain a more realistic, tolerant philosophy of life, by mercilessly attacking his methods of responsibility avoidance which are reflected in his belief systems. His therapeutic tactics emphasize disarming the patient on a conceptual level, often using punchy, direct language. One of his favourite dictums, often used to illustrate his model to patients, is 'Freud was wrong, masturbation isn't the source of psychological distress, it's MUSTURBATION.' RET aims to help the client semi-automatically think about himself, others and the world in a more sensible way in future (Ellis, 1977). Ellis was one of the people responsible for popularizing the use of role-play in sessions, use of homework assignments, using imaginal techniques and self-reward, as well as directed reading and replaying of recordings of therapy sessions by clients (Ellis, 1972).

Beck's cognitive model

The conceptual model upon which Beck's cognitive therapy is based represents a synthesis of five distinct theoretical elements, each of which has been used to explain the genesis and maintenance of specific problems of behaviour. Four functions within the individual (cognition, behaviour, mood and biology/biochemistry) interact with each other, all four interacting with the person's environment. Such reciprocal interactions can lead, from the perspective of this model, to the genesis of problems such as anxiety and depression. In Beck's view, this conceptual framework could be used to explain a much wider range of emotional problems (Beck, 1976).

Predisposing and precipitating factors The model acknowledges the role of predisposing and precipitating factors. Hereditary characteristics are accepted as potential predisposing factors, as are physical illnesses which might generate neurochemical abnormalities. From a developmental perspective, inadequate exposure to experiences essential for the formation of adequate coping mechanisms, would constitute a learning deficit which might predispose the person to psychological problems in later life. Equally, the acquisition of rigid, dysfunctional belief systems, such as values and assumptions, would represent further predispositions toward psychological problems in later life.

The model accepts that such predisposing factors are not sufficient to generate psychological problems. Physical illness, or exposure to toxic substances might represent a precipitating trigger for the onset of a psychological crisis. Whereas such an influence would be felt within the person, external stresses might also precipitate psychological breakdown: single major losses, such as bereavement or a series of more minor losses being further examples of external stress. Finally, the model emphasizes that where a stressful event impinges upon a specific vulnerability of the person, its effects will be considerably more traumatic than even major losses such as bereavement.

The cognitive triad   Beck proposed that three specific thinking patterns were common in emotional disorders. These involved a negative view of self; a negative interpretation of life experiences (the world); and a tendency to take a negative view of future events. These parallel closely the views of Ellis, noted above. In the case of people who are experiencing depression, for example, these thinking patterns appear to revolve around ideas of loss and deprivation. They tend to report a view of themselves which describes them as deficient in important qualities, unworthy or generally inadequate. Such a view is based upon their presumed mental, physical or moral defects. When problems are encountered in everyday life, these are attributed to such personal defects: deficiencies within the self.

The patient also tends to misinterpret past and present life experiences, viewing the world as making unacceptable demands, or presenting insurmountable obstacles, which prevent the fulfillment of life's ambitions. Failure to overcome such obstacles is interpreted as evidence and symbols of defeat and deprivation.

The patient is also likely to believe that present life problems will continue indefinitely. Projected outcomes for any undertaking are invariably construed in negative terms, and standards may well be set so high as to almost guarantee the failure expected.

Thinking errors   The patient's negative view of life events is expressed through specific dysfunctional cognitive distortions. The patient may predict failure: 'I'll never make it, so why bother,' or attribute negative evaluations of himself to others: 'they must be tired of me being like this.

I'm a burden on everyone.' The theme of the cognitive distortions is likely to reflect the nature of the problem experienced: depressed people think depressing, self-critical thoughts; anxious people think threatening or doom-laden thoughts. However, much common ground exists in terms of a general set of self-defeating thoughts which co-vary with a range of life problems (Hallon and Kendall, 1980).

Such dysfunctional thoughts intertwine with a range of fairly discrete thinking errors which involve faulty information processing. Among the errors identified are: dichotomous reasoning (black-and-white thinking): 'if I don't succeed at everything I do then I am a total failure'; arbitrary inference (jumping to conclusions); 'we had a row, this means he doesn't love me any more'; selective attention (discounting the positive); 'but I always do that anyway, that's not important'; magnification/minimization' (catastrophizing); 'this is awful and there is nothing I can do about it'; personalization; 'why does this always happen to me?'

Underlying schemas The term schema designates relatively stable cognitive patterns. These form the basis of the person's interpretation or organization of experience. Schemata represent the person's beliefs about himself. They are commonly construed as unspoken premises, rather than conscious thoughts, such as those noted above. The person who fears specific situations (such as rejection) may think 'I couldn't bear that.' This negative prediction (jumping to conclusions or crystal-ball gazing) might arise from the silent assumption that 'If I am left all alone, I will die.'

Burns (1980) has classified seven discrete 'silent assumptions', expressed in terms of needs. The need for:

1. approval
2. love
3. achievement
4. perfectionism
5. entitlement
6. omnipotence
7. autonomy

The practice of cognitive therapy

The practice of cognitive therapy involves five main goals. The person learns to:

1. Identify, evaluate and examine his thoughts in relation to specific life events.
2. Judge the validity of such thoughts using objective evidence as a guide.
3. Identify the silent assumptions (unspoken schemata) which underpin his negative thoughts.

4. Practise a range of behavioural and cognitive strategies which can be applied *in vivo* when confronted by new or unexpected stresses.
5. Develop alternative, more adaptive, thoughts about himself, the world and the future, as well as less dysfunctional schemata.

Beck's explanation of dysfunctional behaviour can be summarized thus:

1. Certain psychopathological states are either caused and/or maintained by negative automatic thoughts.
2. Cognitive distortions (negative automatic thoughts) reflect unrealistic views of self, world and future (the cognitive triad).
3. Although appearing illogical to others, dysfunctional cognitions are consistent with the patient's view of reality.
4. Life events may trigger cognitive distortions, but these are maintained by fixed dysfunctional schemata.
5. Such schemata serve as the basis for all evaluation and categorization of experience, past and present.
6. These schemata are shaped by relevant life experiences, usually in childhood.

The process of cognitive therapy

The process of therapy emphasizes a number of elements, not all of which are exclusive to the cognitive model, but which are essential to the practice of effective cognitive therapy. As noted earlier in the discussion of the four main classes of cognitive intervention, the following elements represent the framework which supports the various techniques. Although described here in terms of the practice of psychotherapy, I find it difficult to distinguish these elements from the framework of an effective nurse–patient relationship.

The assessment

Assessment aims in cognitive therapy differ little from those in behavioural psychotherapy in general (Barker, 1982; 1985). The problems which the patient wished to focus upon within the therapy would, first of all, be defined explicitly. Priorities would be set for tackling problems in order of importance, and an important target would be identified for early intervention, to demonstrate that such problems were not insoluble.

The patient's life-problems would be summarized in a coherent and meaningful way, making connections between the presenting problems and life experiences, past and present. An assessment of significant stressors would be made. These might represent debts, domestic difficulties, and interpersonal problems involving children, spouse, colleagues etc. Some of these might need referral on to another agency, such as social worker or educational psychologist. Significant assets would be identified:

personal qualities, or significant others willing to help. The overall severity of the presenting problems would be measured using questionnaires, rating scales and structured interview schedules. These would be used to evaluate progress as well as to identify difficulties which might, otherwise, have been overlooked. Finally, the effect of resolving these problems would be considered. The possibility that some problems, such as dependency for example, might offer a positive pay-off to family members or some other significant other, would need to be considered. The potential effect of the patient changing his behaviour radically would need to be considered in terms of both himself and those most important to him.

Emphasis upon the here-and-now

Emphasis is given to the problems presently experienced by the patient. The specific life-problems encountered by the patient, as well as the thoughts, feelings and interpersonal issues involved, would be focused upon. Although past events, both recent and distant, might form the focus of a specific session, these would be related unequivocally to the here-and-now. For instance, the patient who reports feeling terrible at the beginning of a session, would be asked 'what are you thinking about?' Although this might result in information about a past or anticipated future event, the importance of the primacy of the patient's thoughts in the generation, or maintenance, of the negative affect would be emphasized. In this sense, the past is past. The question is, what can the person do NOW. How can he learn from such past experience?

Problem-orientation

The initial assessment aims to identify the person's life-problems. These might involve specific troublesome thoughts and feelings, but might also involve relationship difficulties such as with spouse children, or other problems involving finance, housing conditions, career development and examinations for example. The therapist aims to encourage the person to explore these problem areas, identifying his thoughts about past or future events, relating these to concomitant emotions. In later stages the role of underlying silent assumptions is stressed, in an attempt to increase awareness of why such dilemmas or difficulties emerged or are maintained.

Time-limited interaction

Consonant with contemporary interest in brief psychotherapy, cognitive therapy often tries to limit therapeutic contact to a prescribed number of sessions. This would be fixed early in the contact, as part of a general therapeutic contract. Typically, this would entail at least 16 one-hour sessions, which would be necessary for accomplishing symptom relief and the modification of key dysfunctional assumptions. However, some flexibility is indicated and the time scale would be negotiated with the patient, with extensions added as required. In the case of in-patients a different time-structure is indicated. The need to frame all contacts with the patient within a projected timetable would, however, still be indicated.

Collaborative relationship

The process of cognitive therapy relies heavily upon an active interchange between therapist and patient. This is true for both Ellis- and Beck-influenced models. The basic tenets of cognitive therapy are introduced along with an outline of the goals of treatment. This provides a basis for the subsequent explanation of the rationale of assignments and homework. This also provides a rational and coherent context within which the therapy can operate. Beck considers all traditional therapeutic qualities (such as warmth, empathy, genuineness, support) to be important. The therapist functions, however, primarily as a guide or teacher. An objective, non-judgemental, stance is vital (unconditional positive regard). The therapist aims always to convey the idea that the person's problems are not to be judged negatively, but are understandable within the context of cognitive theory. Ellis emphasizes empathy and unconditional positive regard, with active listening and revolving discussion (Crawford, 1982). He places more importance on the therapist serving as an authoritative (not authoritarian) teacher, who is not unduly warm or reinforcing to the person who might, inadvertently, have his dire need for approval met (Ellis, 1984a).

Through collecting information about the outcome of specific cognitions or silent assumptions, in everyday life, the therapist and patient can explore the value or otherwise of specific cognitions and schemata. Within this process the therapist encourages the patient to challenge patterns of distorted or dysfunctional thinking. For Beck, this challenging needs to be done indirectly, encouraging the patient to identify the fallacy of his own argument, through the therapist's careful use of Socratic irony (Beck *et al.*, 1979). For Ellis, it is more important to engage in active disputation, in an effort to encourage the person to accept responsibility for his own happiness. Ellis would opt for quite radical strategies to encourage people to confront difficulties met in negotiating change: for example, by contracting with patients to pay stiff penalties, such as burning amounts of money, if they fail to achieve set goals. He emphasizes that the use of self-punishment must always exclude self-damnation in any form.

In both models the therapeutic relationship involves collaborative empiricism. Bordin (1976) has referred to this as the 'working alliance:...the complex of understandings and attachments that are formed when a person in a state of personal crisis...turns to another for his or her expert help and a contract is made. This contract or alliance is a subtle mixture of explicit and implicit understandings and acknowledged and unacknowledged attachments.'

Didactic

Emphasis upon learning is a vital part of the overall therapeutic process. In general, the therapist's role is primarily that of guide or teacher. This is made explicit in the initial stages when some reading material may be offered as a homework assignment (e.g., the booklet *Coping with Depression* (Beck and Greenberg, 1974) or the tape recording *Twenty-one Ways to Stop Worrying* (Ellis, 1971). Within the context of such bibliotherapy (Watson and Tharp, 1981) the person is encouraged to read, and subsequently review with the therapist, information which might simply describe the process of therapy or might be applied successfully to the modification of some life-problem. Later the outcome of conversations within the sessions are reviewed in an effort to define more clearly the mechanism of general problem-solving and coping strategies. Homework assignments, where the patient confronts specific situations, are used to explore alternative ways of responding to difficulty. Here again, the therapist helps the patient actively towards identifying what needs to be done and how the situation might be handled, later reviewing the whole process in the spirit of potential discovery.

Structure

As noted above, emphasis is given to active collaboration between patient and therapist. Clear indications are given of the possible time-scale of the contact, length of sessions and content. Specific goals are negotiated with the patient, and sessions are usually structured to allow adequate time for addressing the important issues. The typical structure of a therapeutic session might be as follows:

Review of assignment The patient reviews briefly events since the last session; is invited to comment upon his recall of the content of the last session; reviews what took place in his planned assignment, identifying as clearly as possible the results; and finally summarizes briefly what needs to be done next.

Agenda setting Patient and therapist then set the focus for the session, drawing this, perhaps, from a list of possibilities provided by the patient.

Target(s) The focus of the session is then defined as explicitly as possible. The patient is asked to identify associated automatic thoughts, which are then investigated using relevant techniques, and evaluated in terms of the effect upon original thoughts and feelings.

Homework Therapist and patient then negotiate specific tasks to be undertaken as preparation for the next session. The rationale for undertaking each task is emphasized. Any doubts, predictions about outcome and anticipated difficulties are discussed. The patient is encouraged to make his own *aide-mémoire* for the assignment and to report back at the next session.

Feedback   Finally the patient is invited to review what has been learned from this session and is asked also to comment upon the therapist's behaviour during the session. Any other comments or questions are considered briefly before fixing the next session.

Preparation of the patient

A series of tasks is tackled in preparing the patient for cognitive therapy. The patient's expectations of treatment are addressed. People seeking help can have feelings and expectations which are either inappropriate or unrealistic, either in terms of what they expect can be achieved or involving their possible role in the therapeutic process. Such expectations are discussed right from the start, the therapist gently correcting any misconceptions concerning the content, method or general aims of the therapy.

Practical aspects of the treatment process are discussed next: the approximate expected length of the therapy, the frequency of sessions and their duration. It is appropriate here to negotiate the timing of sessions and any other practical considerations involving the patient's attendance.

Finally, the specific demands which the therapist expects to make on the patient are discussed. In cognitive therapy these are quite explicit. The need for a strong collaborative relationship would be discussed, emphasizing the requirement for the active participation of the patient and his role in commenting directly on the work of the therapist and the progress of his treatment. Other issues might also be discussed, such as homework assignments, keeping a daily journal and the use of hand-outs and other forms of bibliotherapy. Such explanations are not only necessary to the establishment of the therapeutic alliance but also extend the rationale of the therapy to cover events planned for future sessions.

Who can cognitive therapy help?

I have noted at points during this chapter examples of problems, both general and specific, which research evidence suggests are responsive to cognitive therapy intervention. More elaborate research studies have shown cognitive therapy to be at least as effective as drug therapy in the treatment of severe depression. When both interventions are combined the results are significantly better than for either intervention alone (Blackburn *et al.*, 1981). More recently the supremacy of cognitive therapy over behaviour therapy in the treatment of generalized anxiety has also been demonstrated within a controlled clinical study (Durham and Turvey,

1987). These studies suggest the considerable potential of cognitive therapy, especially where drug dependence or abuse is a risk factor. The potential of cognitive therapy interventions has also been demonstrated in slightly different formats with a wide range of clinical phenomena. Klerman and Weissman (1980) reported significant results using a problem-solving format with severely depressed patients. Similar results, using much the same problem-solving approach, have been reported by McGuire and Sifneos (1970) with bereavement, divorce and redundancy, and by Marlatt (1978) in the management of alcohol abuse. Further research support for specific interventions in relation to different clinical problems, will be noted in Chapter 11. Here, I would like to address the question of who might be helped by a cognitive therapy approach, in more general terms.

Contemporary research in mental health care tends to emphasize the usefulness of different therapeutic processes for different psychiatric disorders or illnesses. The treatment of such problems of living by traditional verbal psychotherapy has shown variable if not wholly negative results. Eysenck (1986) challenged the traditional psychoanalytic approach to psychological disorder, noting the virtual absence of any controlled research data to support its efficacy. Rachman and Wilson (1980) earlier noted that of the alternatives, Rogerian psychotherapy, which they praised in an earlier review, had given rise to 'widespread disappointment... specific claims made by or on behalf of Rogers can call on little empirical support' (p. 259). Alternatively, Kazdin and Wilson (1980) noted that, in general, behavioural methods were at least as effective as – and often more effective than – alternative approaches, particularly the verbal psycho-therapies, the term behavioural being used to denote both strictly be-havioural and cognitive–behavioural methods. One problem with such observations is the assumption that all psychotherapies tackle the same thing. Clearly this is not the case. Rogerian psychotherapy appears to address the subtle manipulation of the person: an approach which is essentially developmental in nature. Psychoanalytic-based psychotherapy addresses the manipulation of dysfunctional processes which, hypo-thetically, give rise to certain disorders of living or experience. Behaviour therapy tries to change behaviour, pure and simple. Given the diversity of processes and objectives it is not surprising that comparison of one therapy with another is difficult.

This chapter has focused upon one aspect of psychological functioning, albeit an exceptionally complex one. It has been suggested that cognition underpins a range of life-problems. Dysfunctional cognitions, therefore, are the primary problems which cast secondary shadows in the form of discrete behavioural disturbance. The person for whom a cognitive–behavioural approach is appropriate employs dysfunctional cognitive processes: these either generate or maintain the life problem. For some problems, such as habit disorders, specific phobias or obsessional rituals, the deeper cognitive processes expressed in automatic thoughts and belief systems, *do not* play a significant part. Contemporary research would suggest that cognitive interventions might be, at least, ineffective in such areas. One task of the nursing assessment is to evaluate the role played by the patient's thinking in the generation of life problems. If cognitive processes are not significantly linked to the problem, then the selection of a cognitive therapy approach is not indicated.

Conclusion

This chapter has summarized the general principles underlying the cognitive therapy model and has outlined some of the main strategies used to manipulate cognitive processes which underpin problems of living. Although sharing the characteristics of many other psychotherapies, especially behaviour therapy and humanistic therapy and counselling, the approach of figures like Beck and Ellis is distinctive. The model emphasizes the use of a collaborative relationship to promote awareness and problem-solving through a structured examination of the person's life style and alternatives. The emphasis upon empiricism demonstrates links with the behavioural sciences. The emphasis upon relationship factors and the therapeutic process reflects many of the considerations of the humanistic therapies. The idea that cognition plays a significant part in the generation of affective disturbance is of ancient pedigree. The cognitive therapy model has grafted such timeless, philosophical considerations into a therapeutic structure geared to meet the needs of late 20th-century psychiatric services. Although as yet largely untested as a conceptual framework for nursing practice, the limitations seem few, whereas the potential seems to be great. Traditionally, nurses have viewed problems such as anxiety, depression, anger, dependency, overprotectiveness, as primary problems. Their response has often been to try to remedy these through advice or counselling, or to provide generalized support to those who are unwilling or unable to confront change. The cognitive therapy model proposes a radical alternative. Firstly, it suggests that disturbances of affect and behaviour are secondary phenomena: a function of dysfunctional cognitions. Although the therapeutic system is multifaceted, focusing upon the manipulation of mood and behaviour, ultimately the emphasis is upon awareness, understanding and manipulating the various processes of thought. The face validity of the approach for a wide range of nursing situations seems self-evident. The clear definition of the processes and strategies involved offers nurses an ideal opportunity for experimental research before adding yet another model to their already bulging conceptual suitcase.

References

Alberti, R. E. (1977) *Assertiveness: Innovations, Applications and Issues*, Impact Publishing, San Luis Obispo, CA.

Bandura, A. (1969) *Principles of Behaviour Modification*, Holt, Rinehart and Winston, New York.

Barker, P. J. (1982) *Behaviour Therapy Nursing*, Croom Helm, London.

Barker, P. J. (1985) *Patient Assessment in Psychiatric Nursing*, Croom Helm, London.

Beck, A. T. (1976) *Cognitive Therapy and the Emotional Disorders*, International Universities Press, New York.

Beck, A. T. and Greenberg, R. L. (1974) *Coping with Depression*, Institute for Rational Living, New York.

Beck, A. T., Rush, A. J., Shaw, B. F. and Emery, G. (1979) *Cognitive Therapy of Depression*, Guildford Press, New York.

Blackburn, I. M., Bishop, S., Glen, A. I. M. *et al.* (1981) The efficacy of cognitive therapy in depression. A treatment trial using cognitive therapy and pharmacotherapy, each alone and in combination. *Bri. J. Psych.*, **139**, 181–9.

Bordin, E. S. (1976) The working alliance: basis for a general theory of psychotherapy. Paper presented at the meeting of the American Psychological Association, Washington, DC, September, 1976.

Burns, D. (1980) *Feeling Good: The New Mood Therapy*, William Morrow, New York.

Cautela, J. and Wisocki, P. A. (1977) The thought stopping procedure: description, application and learning theory interpretations. *Psych. Rec.*, **1**, 255–64.

Crawford, T. (1982) Communication and relational–emotive therapy. Paper presented in Los Angeles, October (cited by Ellis, 1984b).

Durham, R. C. and Turvey, A. T. (1987) Cognitive therapy versus behaviour therapy in the treatment of chronic generalized anxiety. *Behav. Res. Ther.*, **25**, 229–34.

Ellis, A. (1949) Towards the improvement of psychoanalytic research. *Psychoan. Rev.*, **36**, 123–43.

Ellis, A. (1962) *Reason and Emotion in Psychotherapy*, Lyle Stuart, New York.

Ellis, A. (1971) *Twenty-one Ways to Stop Worrying* (cassette recording), Institute for Rational–Emotive Therapy, New York.

Ellis, A. (1972) Psychotherapy without tears, in *Twelve Therapists* (ed. A. Burton), Jossey-Bass, San Francisco.

Ellis, A. (1973) *Humanistic Psychotherapy: The Rational–Emotive Approach*, Julian Press, New York.

Ellis, A. (1977) Irrational ideas (hand-out), Institute for Rational Living, New York.

Ellis, A. (1984a) *Rational–Emotive Therapy and Cognitive Behaviour Therapy*, Springer, New York.

Ellis, A. (1984b) Foreword in *Rational–Emotive Therapy: Fundamentals and Innovations* (W. Dryden), Croom Helm, London.

Ellis, A. and Grieger, R. (eds) (1977) *Handbook of Rational–Emotive Therapy*, Springer, New York.

Ellis, A. and Whiteley, J. M. (eds) (1979) *Theoretical and Empirical Foundations of Rational–Emotive Therapy*, Brooks/Cole, Monterey, CA.

Eysenck, H. J. (1986) *The Decline and Fall of the Freudian Empire*, Pelican, Harmondsworth.

Gregory, R. L. (ed.) (1987) *The Oxford Companion to the Mind*, Oxford University Press, Oxford.

Hollon, S. D. and Kendall, P. C. (1980) Cognitive self-statements in depression: development of an automatic thoughts questionnaire. *Cognit. Ther. Res.*, **4**, 383–98.

Jacobsen, N. S. and Margolin, G. (1979) *Marital Therapy: Strategies Based Upon Social Learning and Behaviour Exchange Principles*, Brunner/Mazel, New York.

Kazdin, A. E. and Wilson, G. T. (1980) *Evaluation of Behaviour Therapy: Issues, Evidence and Research Strategies*, University of Nebraska Press, Lincoln, NB.

Klerman, G. and Weissman, M. (1980) Depression among women, in *The Mental Health of Women* (eds M. Gutemag and D. Belle), Academic Press, New York.

Luria, A. (1961) *The Role of Speech in the Regulation of Normal and Abnormal Behaviours*, Liveright, New York.

Mahoney, M. J. (1974) *Cognition and Behaviour Modification*, Ballinger, Boston, MA.

Marlatt, G. A. (1978) Craving for alcohol, loss of control and relapse: a cognitive behavioural analysis, in *Alcoholism: New Directions in Behavioural Research* (eds P. E. Nathan, G. E. Marlant and T. Loberg), Plenum Press, New York.

McGuire, M. and Sifneos, P. E. (1970) Problem-solving in psychotherapy. *Psych. Quart.*, **44**, 667–73.

Meichenbaum, D. (1977) *Cognitive Behaviour Modification: An Integrative Approach*, Plenum Press, New York.

Meichenbaum, D. (1983) *Coping with Stress*, Century, London.

Meichenbaum, D. and Genest, M. (1981) Cognitive behaviour modification: An integration of cognitive and behavioural methods, in *Helping People Change* (eds F. H. Kanfer and A. P. Goldstein), Pergamon Press, New York.

Novaco, R. W. (1977) Stress inoculation: a cognitive therapy for anger and its application to a case of depression. *J. Consult. Clin. Psych.*, **45**, 600–8.

Rachman, S. J. and Wilson, G. T. (1980) *The Effects of Psychological Therapy*, 2nd edn, Pergamon Press, Oxford.

Spivack, G. and Shure, M. (1978) *Problem-Solving Techniques in Child-Rearing*, Jossey-Bass, San Francisco.

Spivack, G., Platt, J. and Shure, M. (1976) *A Problem-Solving Approach to Adjustment*, Jossey-Bass, San Francisco.

Taylor, J. (1963) A behavioural interpretation of obsessive–compulsive neurosis. *Behav. Res. Ther.*, **1**, 237–44.

Urban, E. S. and Kendall, P. C. (1980) Review of social-cognitive problem-solving interventions with children. *Psych. Bull.*, **88**, 109–43.

Watson, O. (1976) *Longman Modern English Dictionary*, Longman, London.

Watson, D. L. and Tharp, R. G. (1981) *Self-Directed Behaviour: Self-Modification for Personal Adjustment*, 3rd edn, Brooks/Cole, Monterey, CA.

Wiscoki, P. A. (1976) A behavioural treatment programme for social inadequacy: multiple methods for a complex problem, in *Counselling Methods* (eds J. Krumboltz and C. Thoresen), Holt, Rinehart and Winston, New York.

Chapter 4

Behaviour therapy model: principles and general applications

A. HUME

Introduction

In the Therapy Family, Behaviour is often the most maligned and misunderstood of the offspring. Behaviour is criticized as being cold, mechanical or simplistic; he is accused of having a malevolent desire to control his fellow man and he has to bear the brunt of endless jokes about clipboards, forms and stop-watches. Behaviour's accusers have one thing in common – they do not really know him. This chapter is an introduction to Behaviour, who he is, his growth and development, and how he promotes a greater quality of life by helping others to learn more adaptive ways of living.

Behaviour therapy is the application of various learning theories to problems of living. Frequently these problems occur within the context of a clinical disorder. Behaviour therapy is not, however, limited to the clinical field. It can just as appropriately be the means whereby individuals achieve personal growth by expanding their skills repertoire. The ambitious junior executive, for example, may improve his promotional prospects by increasing his social effectiveness or by developing additional assertion skills. Conversely, personal growth may involve the reduction or elimination of a particular behaviour, decreasing for example, the amount of work taken home to improve the quality of life, of promoting physical health by learning how to stop smoking.

The historical roots of behaviour therapy are based in the two fundamental learning theories of classical and operant conditioning. Modern behaviourism however, has developed beyond these two traditional constructs. The social learning theory of Bandura (1969), which significantly contributed to the recognition of the role of cognitions on overt patterns of behaviour, was followed by the introduction of various therapeutic techniques which effected a change in observable behaviour by focusing on the mental processes or hidden behaviours referred to by Bandura. The role of the mediational processes and the subsequent development of covert treatment strategies are viewed by many practitioners as a complementary extension of traditional behavioural concepts. Others however, contest the inclusion of covert techniques under the umbrella of behaviourism. Generally speaking, the controversy over what is, or is not, behaviour therapy, is of greater academic than clinical significance. The adoption of a purist or more radical behavioural model does, nevertheless, influence the clinician's use of terminology and perception of applicability. The conventionally orientated tend to use the term behaviour modification, which is usually associated with clinical practices arising primarily from operant learning theory. Others who stress the resolution of problem behaviours by the development of incompatible responses to stimuli which previously elicited maladaptive reactions (counter-conditioning procedures), tend to favour behaviour therapy rather than behaviour modification (Masters *et al.*, 1987). More recently, a third label has been devised to reflect additional therapeutic advances in Bandura's original model (Mahoney, 1974; Meichenbaum, 1977; Rosenthal, 1982) – that of cognitive-behavioural psychotherapy, the exponents of which embrace behavioural as well as cognitive therapies, articulated for example by Ellis (1962) and Beck (1976). To add to the confusion, there is little consistency in the use of the three terms. In this, and in the subsequent Chapter on the clinical application of the behavioural model, the author will use the term behaviour therapy to include all the conceptual models previously mentioned which, despite their differences, do share two common themes. As postulated by Kazdin and Wilson (1978), first they all represent 'a psychological model of human behaviour that differs fundamentally from the traditional intrapsychic, psychodynamic or quasi-disease model of mental illness'. Secondly, they reflect 'a commitment to scientific method, measurement and evaluation'. Furthermore, the author's stance on the applicability of behaviour therapy reflects the philosophy of Kazdin and Wilson (1978), who argue that a broad range of problems of living are amenable to behavioural-cognitive intervention.

In recent years, adopting a behavioural perspective to problems of living has grown in popularity. The recognition by parents, teachers, social workers and relatives, as well as nurses, of the effectiveness of behavioural intervention has resulted in an increased demand for short introductory courses (Matthews, Gelder and Johnston, 1981; Sheldon, 1982; Jones and Robson, 1983; Hall, 1984). For nurses, courses which offer a qualification in behaviour therapy are now an established part of the national post-basic education curriculum.

Modern behaviour therapy has a rich ancestral pedigree. Historical precursors of present-day clinical practices are illustrated in the literature of Greek and Roman antiquity, as well as in the principles of early Buddhism and its descendant, Zen Buddhism. A number of the similarities between early Buddhism and behaviour therapy are striking. There is the focus, for example, on the here-and-now, on observable phenomena, the avoidance of metaphysical theories, and the emphasis given to objectivity and testability (Mikulas, 1978). There is a delightful account in early Buddhist literature of the treatment of obesity, which contains unequivocal behavioural elements. The story describes how the King of Kosala's eating problem was resolved by a multi-component intervention programme comprising the techniques of modelling and response cost, a systematic approach to reduce the quantity of food eaten and the use of a co-therapist (Dhammapada Commentary Translation, 1921). Equally illuminating is the tale of Aggidata, a farmer whose son devised a social skills training programme which equipped his father with the social competence to appropriately address members of the King's Court. While the training package included behavioural rehearsal, modelling and role play, it unfortunately omitted specific anxiety management strategies. When Aggidata was eventually brought before the King, in his excitement he offered, rather than requested, an additional ox. However, the story does have a happy ending: the King, sympathetic to the poor farmer's confusion, presented him with not one, but sixteen oxen to plough his fields!

Japanese Zen Buddhism of 12th-century Chinese origin should not be minimized as just one of the later variants of early Buddhism. According to Humphrey (1967), Zen is uniquely different from other Buddhist schools with its intrinsic philosophy of self-effort. The emphasis in Zen Buddhism on behaviour (action) which is a central characteristic of the Zen-like Morita psychotherapy, allows further parallels to be drawn with behaviour therapy (Shapiro and Zifferblatt, 1976; Shapiro, 1978; Reynolds, 1981).

The literature of Western antiquity also documents prehistorical precursors of behavioural methods. One example described by Franks (1969) involved the use of aversive conditioning by the Roman writer, Pliny the Elder (AD 23–79), in the treatment of alcoholism. Similarly, illustrations can also be found in the more recent past of the 19th century. In the 1800s, a Royal Navy officer, Captain Alexander Maconochie employed, in a South Pacific penal colony, a method of controlling the prisoners which echoed the later development of token economy systems (Pitts, 1976). An early ancestor of Joseph Wolpe's theory of reciprocal inhibition (Wolpe, 1958) may be recognized in the case study reported by a French physician who, in 1845, described the successful use of competing responses and contingency management in the treatment of a 30-year-old wine merchant with a 10-year history of obsessional ruminations (Stewart, 1961).

While all these examples are early approximations of later behavioural practices, they are not primary antecedents. They were without theoretical structure and any potential theoretical significance went unrecognized.

They are, however, valuable and fascinating contributions to the pre-historical development of behaviour therapy, valuable in the sense that they demonstrate unstructured observations of human behaviour and methods of behavioural change thousands of years before Pavlov's dogs or Skinner's rats. Perhaps greater familiarity with the literature of antiquity would undermine the pejoratively viewed association between animal experimentation and behaviour therapy.

Behaviourism is essentially a 20th-century phenomenon. In 1914, an American psychologist, John B. Watson, in response to the variance of opinion on the definition and study of the mind, proposed a radical alternative. Rather than becoming immersed in conceptual and functional controversies about consciousness and mind, Watson suggested that the dominant focus of attention should be on what was definable, measurable and observable; overt behaviour, he argued, was a substantive which could be studied scientifically. Watson further believed that the origins of behaviour lay in the environment (Watson, 1924). The mechanics of environmental manipulation and behavioural response were to be found, according to Watson, in the work of Ivan Pavlov, a Russian physiologist who, in 1904, had won the Nobel Prize for medicine. In his Nobel Laureate address, Pavlov described the principles of classical conditioning which evolved into one of the fundamental learning theories upon which the behavioural model is based (Pavlov, 1927). Classical learning theory is solely concerned with the process by which involuntary behaviour is learned. The aroma of freshly baked bread will produce salivation, a particle of dust settling on the surface of the eye will result in a blink response, the leg will automatically jerk if the patellar tendon is struck, and a sudden loud noise will elicit a startled response. All are examples of reflex or involuntary behaviours, elicited by events (stimuli) which precede them. The responses to these stimuli are inbred: we do not for example have to learn how to salivate in response to food; it is an innate mechanism. Pavlov, however, noticed that salivation occurred in some of his dogs in the absence of food, in much the same way as fear can be experienced without the presence of a naturally fear-provoking stimulus. Pavlov's studies demonstrated how such responses occur. In a series of experiments, a selection of neutral stimuli (the ringing of a bell, the sounding of a buzzer) repeatedly accompanied the presentation of food. A neutral stimulus is regarded as such because it has no innate ability to elicit the response. Eventually, the reflex behaviour of salivation occurred to the ringing of a bell without the food accompaniment. The neutral stimulus, the bell, seemed to have acquired the power of food, an unconditioned stimulus. Associative learning had occurred, a process which Pavlov termed conditioning. Classical conditioning therefore involves the pairing of a neutral stimulus with an unconditioned stimulus, the result being an unconditioned response. When the neutral stimulus acquires the power of the unconditioned stimulus, it is termed a *conditioned* stimulus, and the resultant reflex behaviour now becomes a *conditioned* response. At the time, Pavlov was critical of, in his view, Watson's precipitous application of theories derived from animal studies to the complexities of human behaviour. Some two years earlier, however, a little-known American psychologist, Edwin Twitmyer (Twitmyer, 1902), had accidentally demonstrated classical conditioning while investigating muscle tension in relation to the knee-jerk reflex. Twitmyer's report received little attention from his peers. Similarly, historical accounts of behaviour therapy rarely acknowledge the significance of his findings. One can only assume that the status of a Nobel Laureate inadvertently obscured the contribution of a lesser-known mortal.

The early application of classical learning principles to human behaviour was demonstrated in Watson's highly unethical experiment with little Albert. Watson and his co-worker, Rosalie Raynor (Watson and Raynor, 1920), successfully conditioned a fear response in an eleven-month-old toddler to a white rabbit. It was observed that little Albert reacted in a startled manner (unconditioned response) when a loud sudden noise occurred (unconditioned stimulus). After allowing little Albert to play quite happily with a white rabbit (neutral stimulus), Watson and Raynor arranged for a steel bar to be struck (unconditioned stimulus) each time little Albert reached for the rabbit. After several pairings of the neutral stimulus with the unconditioned stimulus, Albert became intensely frightened every time he saw the rabbit, even though the loud crash produced by the striking of the steel bar no longer occurred. The white rabbit had become a conditioned stimulus, and little Albert's reaction a conditioned response. Regrettably, little Albert was removed from hospital before attempts could be made to extinguish the manufactured response. While such experimentation would now be regarded as disgraceful, it is important to remember that in the infancy of any movement, events can occur which are later judged to be unacceptable. Four years later, Watson did assist another female colleague, Mary Cover-Jones (Jones, 1924) to develop a procedure which resolved a young boy's phobic response to small animals and other fluffy objects – on this occasion the fear had not been experimentally generated.

Conditioning experimentation with animals continued during the following decades. The early work of Liddell (1938) and Masserman (1943) provided in later years the solution to a variety of practical problems. Laboratory research into classical learning theory allowed, for example, Gustavson and Garcia (1974) to control effectively the killing of lambs by coyotes on sheep ranches in the western United States.

The clinical significance, however, of the pioneering work of Watson, Raynor and Jones went largely unrecognized until after the Second World War. It was not until the 1950s that behaviour therapy truly emerged. In Britain, Eysenck (1952) published his famous critique of psychoanalytical therapy. Eysenck, in this highly influential paper, challenged the therapeutic effectiveness of psychoanalytical intervention. On the basis of his study there were no significant differences in outcome between those who had received analytical therapy and those who had received no treatment. Although Eysenck's data was not derived from a controlled experiment, later studies have reflected his findings (Appel, Amper and Schefler, 1961; Levitt, 1963), although his conclusions have been questioned (Paul, 1967; Smith and Glass, 1977). Eysenck's report most certainly gave impetus to the exploration of alternative psychotherapeutic strategies. Eysenck additionally contributed to the development of behavioural psychotherapy by the publication of *Behaviour Therapy and the Neuroses* (1960), and by the establishment of the first professional journal, *Behaviour Research and Therapy*.

At the same time that Eysenck was questioning the validity of psychodynamic therapy, a South African doctor, now living in America, Joseph Wolpe, was similarly dissatisfied with the current state of the art. Wolpe's subsequent contribution in the translation of classical learning theory to clinical practice is, to say the least, substantial. His area of particular interest lay in the acquisition of the neuroses. Wolpe's original Pavlovian animal experiments culminated in his conceptualization of reciprocal inhibition which resulted in the development of systematic desensitization, a treatment technique designed to resolve avoidance behaviour such as phobias. Systematic desensitization is based on the premise that anxiety and relaxation are mutually exclusive: relaxation will inhibit an anxiety response. Wolpe taught his patients to imaginally create a series of anxiety provoking scenes and then to inhibit their anxiety by the introduction of progressive relaxation. The construction of a hierarchy allowed for a graded approach to this desensitizing procedure. Each step of the hierarchy is representative of an increasing level of anxiety arousal. His book *Psychotherapy by Reciprocal Inhibition* (1958), describing the integration of anxiety-provoking imagery, inhibiting relaxation and graded hierarchical construction, is acknowledged as a classic text in behavioural literature.

The second fundamental learning theory of the behaviour model, operant conditioning, has its origins in the work of Edward Thorndike who, in the later 1800s, focused not on reflex behaviour, as had Pavlov, but on the effects of the environment upon voluntary behaviour. His classic study of cats (Thorndike, 1911) resulted in the formulation of instrumental learning. Thorndike placed his hungry cats in a box from which they could escape by striking a release mechanism. The cats eventually succeeded in escaping and accessing food by initially hitting the release lever accidentally. After being repeatedly caged, the cats started to purposefully strike the appropriate lever, thereby opening the box and reaching the food. Thorndike labelled their unsuccessful and accidentally profitable escape attempts as trial-and-error learning. His law of effect proposed that behaviour which resulted in a positive consequence would be repeated in similar circumstances, as the cats had demonstrated by deliberately hitting the release mechanism with the positive consequence of food. As the action of hitting the correct lever was instrumental in the cats' escape, learning which focuses on behavioural consequences was termed instrumental learning, the forerunner of what is now known as operant learning theory.

Operant learning theory was developed by the famous American psychologist, Burrhus Fredrick Skinner during the 1930s and 1940s. Skinner, like his predecessors, insisted on a rigorous scientific approach to the study of behaviour; once again, the principles of this second example of associative learning originated from animal research. By analysing animal behaviour, Skinner sought to explain first the acquisition and maintenance of behaviour, and second, how behaviour could then be altered.

Operant learning theory is concerned with the relationship between voluntary (as opposed to reflex) behaviour and the environment. Operant behaviour refers to behaviours which are influenced by the consequences of the action. These operants are a substantial constituent of human behaviour. A spelling error while writing a letter is voluntarily corrected, a greeting is voluntarily acknowledged, such responses being operant behaviours in contrast to an eye blink or a knee-jerk action which are reflex behaviours. Operant behaviours are cued, as it were, by environmental stimuli. The green man on a traffic indicator sets the scene, so to speak, for the respondent behaviour of crossing the road with the likely positive outcome of reaching the other side safely. The cue of the red man can, of course, voluntarily be ignored and an attempt made to cross the street. The consequence of the behaviour on this occasion will probably be disastrous. Behaviours, therefore, which have a positive outcome will become stronger and likely to be repeated, whereas behaviours which result in negative consequences will be weakened and will be less likely to occur again. If, for example, the telling of a joke elicits a positive consequence – everyone falls about laughing – then that person is likely to tell the joke again at the next party. Conversely, if the joke only generates a blank stare, or a polite smile (a negative consequence), then the probability of the joke's being repeated will be decreased. Consequences then, of which there are four broad categories, are the key to operant behaviour. The laughter elicited from telling a joke is an example of a consequence described as a positive reinforcer. Punishment is the term applied to the aversive consequences of the joke's provoking only a blank stare. The same term can be used in a slightly different way to describe the removal of positive reinforcement. A teacher, for example, has the positive reinforcement of the class's attention. Her lecture, however, becomes increasingly disjointed if she loses the attention of her students. The fourth broad consequence category is that of negative reinforcement. Negative reinforcement encourages a behaviour by the removal of an aversive consequence which would occur if the behaviour was not carried out. A schoolboy knuckles down to his homework to escape from his mother's nagging – the aversive consequence is removed. If he then, the following evening, immediately after tea begins his school work, he will prevent his mother's tirade occurring; thus homework behaviour will be strengthened.

The technique use of the terms reinforcers and punishers are not exactly synonymous with the layman's rewards and punishments. Reinforcers are literally anything which increases the likelihood of a behaviour's being repeated; conversely, punishers are anything which reduces the occurrence of a behaviour. Both can be highly individualistic – what is pleasurable for one person can be unpleasant for another. An operatic performance for some is an exquisite experience, for others it would be positively painful.

The translation of Skinner's major developments in learning theory to human behaviour was not made for several years. Skinner himself did not publish a comprehensive conceptualization of operant conditioning to explain aspects of human learning until 1953 (Skinner, 1953). He had, however, perhaps uniquely illustrated his theoretical constructs within the fictional framework of *Walden Two*, a novel about a Utopian community, published in 1948 (Skinner, 1948).

The potential of operant principles was firmly established in 1959 with the publication of Ayllon and Michael's major study of the effectiveness of clinical methods derived from operant learning theory (Ayllon and Michael, 1959). Their study reported the therapeutic modification of behaviours such as hoarding, aggression and delusional speech, in a group of patients with a schizophrenic diagnosis (some, however, were classified as being mentally handicapped). The report is of further profound significance as it describes *nurses* implementing the treatment procedures. The conception of nurses as behavioural therapists has its origins in Ayllon and Michael's study.

Contemporary behaviour therapy draws, however, on learning theories other than classical and operant conditioning. As mentioned earlier, the late 1950s and 1960s saw the emergence of further advances in our understanding of the complexities of human behaviour. The limitations of the classical and operant models, in terms of their reliance on external, observable phenomena, focused attention on the role of internal behaviours, thinking, reasoning and imagining for example, and the way in which such covert processes influence the performance of behaviour. The resultant mediational theories of learning propose that environmental stimuli do not in themselves initiate overt behavioural responses; rather, the nature of the response is additionally influenced by cognitive or information processing elements.

An important feature of Bandura's social learning theory is the suggestion that learning can take place indirectly and not just through direct experience, as proposed by earlier theorists (Bandura, 1969). Indirect or vicarious learning can occur through the observations and experiences of others. The mimicry ability of children is well known and often a cause of adult embarrassment and amusement. Young girls learn how to apply make-up by observing and then imitating their mother; boys, through the same process, can replicate their father's shaving ritual. Moreover, as every parent knows, children do not just learn crude approximations, or the mere mechanics of behaviour. Their imitations will include subtle changes in facial expression or body posture. As with desirable behaviour patterns, maladaptive responses can be similarly acquired. A child who observes his mother's anxiety response to certain situations is likely to demonstrate equivalent behaviour when faced with analogous situations. Vicarious learning, however, involves more than simply watching. Bandura describes four cognitive processes, while acknowledging that there may be others, which mediate between the external event and the behavioural response, namely, attention, retention, reproduction and motivation. The child for, example, must be able to focus his attention on his father's behaviour; he must then retain what he sees, so that he can reproduce the action. Finally, but just as importantly, the child must be motivated to perform the behaviour. Bandura did not reject conditioning paradigms; rather, he added a further dimension to the established theories of normal and abnormal behaviour.

It would be simplistic to construe the rich complexities of human behaviour on the basis of one discrete model of learning. While each distinct learning theory is instrumental in illuminating facets of human behaviour, collectively they present a functional perspective from which the clinician can operate therapeutically.

The prominence given by Bandura to the internal or hidden processes generated prolific developments in clinical techniques explicitly directed at these covert behaviours. Mahoney (1974), for example, examined the relationship between perception and behaviour. He suggested that the interpretation of an event may not represent the reality of the situation. A train passenger who thinks an alteration in engine vibration means that the train is about to crash has not authentically interpreted what is happening. The concomitant effective and physiological responses are a consequence of his unrealistic perception of events. A few years later, Meichenbaum (1977) demonstrated how psychotic patients could learn to control disruptive cognitions.

Advances in the therapeutic manipulation of these mental processes not only enhanced contemporary knowledge of human behaviour, but also expanded the clinician's skills repertoire. The contemporary practice of behaviour therapy recognizes the contribution to individual problems of living of distorted or unhelpful cognitive functioning. Cognitive treatment approaches are increasingly combined with the more traditional behavioural methods of intervention to help people improve their quality of life.

Development of nurse behavioural therapists

Although much of the history of behaviour therapy originated from America, as did the first report of nurses functioning as behavioural engineers in Ayllon and Michael's previously mentioned study, the concept of behaviour therapy nursing is primarily a British one. Perhaps one reason for this apparent paradox lies in the different nursing traditions of the two countries. A significant characteristic of the British tradition has been its pragmatic and eclectic approach to nursing care. This is in contrast to the American tradition which reflects a greater centrality within a specific theoretical framework (Altschul, 1985). American nurses did, however, recognize much earlier than their British counterparts the therapeutic potential of their nursing interactions, or as Peplau termed 'the therapeutic use of self' (Peplau, 1952). The influence in the 1950s of psychodynamic theories on philosophies of nursing care, encouraged nurses to function with greater sophistication. The therapeutic manipulation of the patient's socio-environment, conceptualized for example in the milieu therapies (Jones, 1952), prompted American nurses especially, to adopt group therapist roles, although the value of such an approach, which continues to be widely promulgated, has yet to be systematically validated (Hauser, 1978).

In this respect, however, a certain vagueness pervaded the British scene where nurses continued (and still do to an extent) to opaquely describe their role in terms of caring for or looking after the patient. The therapeutic rationale of such fuzzy concepts can, not surprisingly, rarely be demonstrated.

Throughout their history, nurses have always been involved with changing behaviour, be it in the promotion of independence or alleviation of distress, under the broad umbrella of nursing care. Despite the potential for nurses to develop a behaviour therapist's role having long been present, it remained unfulfilled until quite recently. Many factors no doubt contribute to this latency in what would appear to be an obvious clinical progression. The interminable perception of nursing as a mere subsidiary of the medical profession, or of nurses as deliverers of medication, did not encourage nurses to view themselves as independent initiators of care. Behaviourism itself is perhaps at least partially responsible for this unrealized potential. To introduce a paper describing the therapeutic utilization of operant conditioning principles by the title 'Operant Conditioning of a Vegetative Human Organism' (Fuller, 1949) is unlikely to elicit a positive response from those involved in caring for others. A less emotive but equally relevant example is the use of the term behavioural engineer by Ayllon and Michael in 1959. While there is much truth in the old maxim 'don't judge a book by its cover', there have been occasions when the nature of the terminology used by behaviouralists, understandably, has raised the eyebrows of the uninitiated.

There was, however, a gradual realization of the significance of the findings being reported under such dehumanizing titles. That nurses could, without sacrificing their traditional caring role, successfully help disturbed and institutionalized patients by implementing behavioural concepts and practices, was clearly demonstrated by Ayllon and Michael. Their study carried out at the Saskatchewan Hospital in Canada, involved 19 patients of whom 14 were classified as schizophrenic. The remaining five were considered to be mentally handicapped. With the exception of one, all had been hospitalized for many years. Under the direction of these two psychologists, the nursing staff effected a therapeutic change in a number of behaviours which would not generally be considered as amenable to traditional psychotherapies. The nature of the problems described in the study are as familiar to present-day psychiatric nurses as they were to their colleagues of some 30 years ago: Helen's delusional speech, Dotty's aggression, Lucille's frequent visits to the nurses' office (she entered the office on average 16 times a day), Janet and Mary's refusal to eat unless fed by the nurses, and as a final example, Harry's hoarding of rubbish – to an extent which necessitated the nurses dejunking him several times a day.

The research of Ayllon and Michael, which illustrated the therapeutic benefits of modifying nurse–patient interactions, led others to examine the traditional caring orientation of nursing. For those who assumed that nursing care was intrinsically therapeutic or health promoting, Gelfand's graphic report in 1967 must have come as something of a shock (Gelfand, Gelfand and Dobson, 1967). In this highly critical study, Gelfand and her colleagues discovered that patients who demonstrated desirable or non-problematic behaviour were largely ignored by nursing staff. Conversely, a great deal of attention was given to those who were perceived as sick, or who exhibited disturbed behaviour. The rationale behind this selective concentration of nursing energies has its roots in the psychodynamic theories which continued to exert considerable influence. The nurse participants of Gelfand's study believed that withdrawn patients, for example, required support and sympathy to re-establish their self-esteem which had been eroded by negative self-evaluations. Such a view was by no means unique, as Gelfand observed from various nursing textbooks. The care of a mute patient for example was described in terms of sitting by him for long periods and doing little things like combing his hair or getting him a drink (Gelfand *et al.*, 1967). This interpretation of humanistic care, Gelfand suggests, results in the unintentional reinforcement of maladaptive behaviours and the promotion of the sick role. A few years earlier, similar anti-therapeutic effects of this caring approach were identified in studies carried out in mental handicap hospitals where, again, nursing practices were traditionally orientated. The prevalence of, for example, self-injurious, aggressive and destructive behaviours was shown to be greater among patients considered to be highly dependent upon nursing staff for the provision of basic care – dressing, feeding, personal hygiene (Klaber and Butterfield, 1965). Mental handicap nurses shared the view of their psychiatric colleagues that dysfunctional behaviour patterns were symptomatic of an underlying illness process. Within the nursing profession itself therefore, little consideration was given to the effects of environmental variables on behavioural performance.

Studies such as these illustrate the growing awareness that nurses are highly influential instruments of behavioural change. Their concept and delivery of care could, as demonstrated, promote either adaptive or maladaptive behaviours. The flood of research data following the Second World War unequivocally demonstrates the clinical effectiveness of behaviour therapy. Consequently the demand for this style of therapy to address a wide range of problems of living, rapidly exceeds the numbers of suitably trained therapists. The recognition that nurses were eminently positioned to contribute to this demand for behavioural services was realized in the early seventies by the establishment of training programmes for nurses to train as behaviour therapists. As such, nurse behaviour psychotherapists are a relatively new breed of clinical specialists. The first training programme for nurses to function not as psychologists' assistants but as independent practitioners of care, was established by Isaac Marks at the Maudsley Hospital in London and approved by the Joint Board of Clinical Nursing Studies for England and Wales in 1975. Recognition is deservedly given to this well known Professor of psychiatry by the subsequent research data which demonstrate the clinical effectiveness of nurses in this advanced clinical role (Marks, Hallam, Connelly and Philpott, 1977; Marks, 1985).

A concomitant development was generated in Scotland which likewise became an approved post-basic training course in behaviour therapy for nurses. It was not, however, a facsimile of the Maudsley programme. In contrast, the Scottish course originated under the auspices of the Tayside Clinical Psychology Department, who for over a decade sustained and nourished the philosophy of behaviourism taught in the training programme (McPherson, Barker, Hunter and Fraser, 1978). The quality of the commitment by Dundee psychologists to the role of nurse behaviour therapists enabled in recent years the creation of an independent behaviour therapy nursing service led by the well-known nurse consultant in behaviour therapy, Phil Barker, who has substantially contributed to the development and practice of behaviour therapy nursing (Barker, 1982; Barker, 1985; Barker and Fraser, 1985).

The full integration however of behaviour therapy into nursing practice despite the overwhelming evidence of its appropriateness and effectiveness, has yet to be realized. Resistance to and rejection of behavioural philosophy and even the concept of the nurse as therapist continues. Exactly why this should be so would be a valuable subject for research studies – although a variety of possible reasons have already been offered, for example, the clinical abuses of behaviour therapy and the erroneous belief that behaviourism and care are somehow mutually exclusive behaviours. Perhaps this negative response is primarily a consequence of the myths perpetuated about behaviour therapy which are perceptively discussed by Barker (1982) and by Barker and Fraser (1985).

Principal characteristics of behaviour therapy

According to the myth makers, the therapeutic style of behaviour therapy represents the antithesis of a holistic approach to mental health, which just goes to show that myths bear little resemblance to reality. Behaviour therapy is totally client-centred. It views the person as a unique individual with problems of living, rather than as a diagnostic category. This concern with the individual, not the diagnosis, is therefore opposed to the idea of treating a condition. Treatment interventions are designed, after extensive assessment, to meet the unique requirements of that particular person. Behaviour therapists do not control; they collaborate with the client and together problems are clarified, treatment goals identified, therapeutic strategies formulated and evaluated. The relationship more resembles that of coach and athlete, rather than therapist and patient. Genuineness, warmth, empathy and the therapeutic relationship are just as important to contemporary nurse behaviour therapists as they are to every other nurse, and full recognition is given to their significance as determinant variables of treatment efficacy. The therapeutic approach is based on a model which views human behaviour largely as a function of the individual's interaction with his environment. Furthermore, it suggests that maladaptive behaviours, reflected in problems of living, are primarily acquired through the process of learning, in the same way as adaptive behaviours are learned. It is the behaviour itself which is the focus of attention rather than any underlying psychopathology, with the emphasis on the here and now of the problem which detracts from the individual's quality of life. The principal characteristics of behaviour therapy can be summarized as follows:

1. Behaviour therapy is an empirical, scientific, client-centred approach to an individual's problems of living.
2. There is a rigorous systematic assessment process which precisely defines in operational terms the client's problem(s) and identifies environmental factors which influence the problem behaviour(s).
3. Explicit treatment goals are agreed upon and defined prior to treatment intervention. The degree to which these targets are met allows for accuracy in progress evaluation and treatment outcome.
4. The treatment techniques of behaviour therapy are not assumed to be effective because they are derived from this or that theory. They are, rather, developed from clinical and experimental research. Behav-

iouralists place great emphasis on scientific validation of their practices and on the individual appropriateness of the treatment methods selected.

5. During the assessment periods, observations are made of the problem behaviour which provide baseline measurements. These measurements are repeated at regular intervals during the treatment phase and again on completion of the intervention programme. This progress is rigorously monitored from start to finish. They are indicators for continuance or modification of the treatment package.

6. The collaborative nature of this style of therapy and the active participation of the client is strongly emphasized from the very beginning. Behaviour therapy as it is today, is all about helping people to change – the client does the changing, not the therapist.

7. Change, to have any real value to the individual, must be socially significant. Therapy cannot be said to be therapeutically effective if, on a practical everyday level, the client experiences no real improvement in his quality of life.

8. It is fairly common practice of behavioural interventions to involve the use of co-therapists who will assist in the delivery of the treatment programme. Co-therapists may be parents, nursing staff, spouses, friends or colleagues who, with the agreement of the client, make a structured contribution to the resolution of the problem.

Behaviour therapy has therefore a number of distinguishing characteristics. There is a clearly observable structure to this psychotherapeutic approach, which retains considerable flexibility and individuality. The assessment process and treatment strategies are tailor-made in accordance with individual circumstances and requirements.

Behaviour therapy and the nursing process

The similarities between behaviour therapy and the nursing process are striking. Indeed Altschul has referred to behaviour therapy nursing as an exemplary example of this approach (Altschul, 1982; 1984). The four principles of the nursing process, assessment of the patient's needs, planning appropriate nursing intervention, implementation of the nursing care plan and, finally, the evaluation of programme's efficiency, closely reflect the behavioural framework. Both approaches are firmly client-centred, rather than task-centred and are fundamentally concerned with assisting the patient to overcome his problems of living in order to maintain or improve his quality of life.

Although the nursing process has substantially enhanced the calibre of nursing assessment, there seems to be some vagueness about how to make the best use of assessment information. It is perhaps a deficit in technical psychiatric nursing skills which results in imprecise and shallow care plans, rather than a reflection of limitations on the nursing process itself.

The nature of behavioural assessment

Assessment is an intrinsic feature of everyday life. Each day begins with an assessment, an assessment for example about what to wear, consideration is given to the weather (which inevitably involves, at least in this country [Scotland], a fingers-crossed prediction), to the schedule of the day, to what's available in the wardrobe (the ironing might not be up-to-date) and accessory co-ordination. The way in which this dressing assessment is made varies enormously from the casual lucky-dip method, to the more studied, formal approach which precedes that special night out. A behavioural assessment reflects the latter.

One of the principal differences between traditional and behavioural assessment methods resides in the fundamental assumptions of the two approaches. In the behavioural approach, while acknowledgement is given to biophysical variables, behaviour is viewed primarily as a function of man's interaction with his environment. A contrasting assumption is interest in the traditional approach where psychopathology is regarded as the product of underlying intrapsychic conflict. Consequently, the emphasis is on interpretation of behaviour as indicators of those insidious variables. In traditional psychotherapy an enormous and diverse amount of information may be collected. Peterson (1968) suggested that three-quarters of assessment information acquired in traditional interviewing could probably be eliminated with no loss to the patient, which surely raises questions about efficiency and the ethical justification of enquiring into areas of the client's life when the information is irrelevant to treatment. What then needs to be known? According to Morganstern (1976), everything which directly relates to the development of an efficient, effective and durable treatment intervention and no more.

Behavioural assessment is viewed as a preparation for therapy. Broadly speaking, its objectives are: definition of the problem behaviour(s), selection of appropriate methods to measure the problem behaviour(s), identification of environmental variables influencing the target behaviour(s), construction of an individually appropriate treatment intervention which has a high probability of success, and finally, rigorous evaluation of treatment effectiveness. The approach is further characterized by recognition of the client's assets, as well as his deficits and the minimization of value or professional judgements and assumptions. Behaviours and emotional states are often attributed to patients with little or no verification. A patient who frowns or mutters to himself is likely to be described as annoyed or hallucinated and indeed he may be. Frequently however, such a judgement is based on the nurse's interpretation of what she sees or hears without collaborative evidence. In many instances, much time and energy are expended on making inferences; in comparison, little effort is made to collect objective data to support these conclusions. Paradoxically, this tendency to jump to conclusions is considerably less prevalent when the patient's physical state is the object of attention. Few nurses would assume that a patient who feels warm must automatically be pyrexial. The situation would be checked out, objective evidence would be obtained by taking the patient's temperature and then a conclusion would be reached. The procedure is not omitted just because on a previous occasion the patient's temperature had been raised. Yet, this formal, scientific approach is generally not adopted when the focus of concern is directed towards the mental condition of the patient. No psychological thermometer is used to verify the conclusion that a patient who talks to himself is hallucinating. While inferences are of course essential to the formulation of conclusions, if unsubstantiated by objective data, they can be unhelpful and misleading. The informality of this approach is somewhat inconsistent with the concept of professionalism.

The objectives of behaviour assessment can be briefly illustrated by the following example. The referral letter describes Mrs Smith's problem as disruptive, delusional behaviour. What is meant by disruptive and delusional must be defined. These terms can, after all, mean different things to different people. Mrs Smith's problem behaviour would therefore be translated into performance terms which allow for greater accuracy: thus, 'Mrs Smith attempts to engage the nursing staff in conversation about green men from outer space who are trying to abduct her. The frequency of the behaviour significantly inhibits the quality and the quantity of nursing interactions with other patients'. Not only is the behaviour clearly specified, but the nature of the definition allows the severity of the problem to be measured. Measurement may involve recording over a specified period of time how often the problem occurs or how much time is spent engaged in the behaviour. In addition to clarifying the size of the problem, measurement records also provide baseline material for the evaluation of treatment effectiveness. The conditions under which the problem occurs, and situations which increase or decrease behavioural performance will also be identified. Analysis of environmental variables might reveal a higher incidence of delusional verbalization when nursing staff are individually interacting with other patients, or when Mrs Smith is not involved in structured activity.

Behavioural assessment exemplifies a systematic, evaluative and functional analysis of an individual's problems of living in terms of his unique internal and external environment. Its person-centred orientation is repeatedly emphasized in its terminology, illustrated for example in the frequent use of the word appropriate.

Fundamental ethical issues are addressed in the avoidance of precipitous assumptions and inferences – problems are not presumed to be such until supporting evidence is obtained. Furthermore, the appropriateness of treatment intervention involves not only consideraton of the applicability of various clinical techniques, but also an evaluation of the likely costs and benefits to the patient of a successful outcome. Increased assertiveness in one partner, for example, may have a traumatic effect on the marital relationship. The effectiveness, however, of any credible process is finally determined by the skill and knowledge of its operator. It is of increasing concern that attempts are made to utilize the apparatus of behaviour therapy by those untrained in its application.

Behaviour therapy treatment methods

The acquisition of behaviour, be it adaptive or maladaptive, through a process of learning, is a basic tenet of behaviourism. In principle therefore, what has been learned, can be unlearned, but in practice, some problems are more amenable to intervention than others.

Problems of living can be classified as excesses or deficits of behaviour. The individual who experiences feelings of anxiety in non-threatening situations, or who is compelled to repeatedly check that all the lights in the house have been switched off before going to bed, is demonstrating behavioural excess. Conversely, difficulties in resisting unjust accusations, or distinguishing the appropriateness of various styles of dress, illustrate problems involving a deficit of behaviour. The consequences of behavioural excesses and deficits on the individual's interpersonal relationships, developmental potential and overall quality of life can be profound.

Behaviour therapy, as an exclusive or adjunct treatment measure, can be the medium by which an extensive range of problems, from single phobias to complex interpersonal or affective difficulties involving dysfunctional thinking patterns can, to varying degrees, be resolved. The extensive ambiance of behavioural intervention can be demonstrated by the following brief clinical reports.

Feared auditory hallucinations were reduced by satiation, a behavioural technique in which positive reinforcers, commonly related to the undesirable behaviour, are given to excess. Although the patient remained in hospital, his quality of life had been significantly enhanced by the removal of hallucinatory occurrences (Glaister, 1985). More recently, behavioural methods were again employed to obtain a significant decrease in verbally aggressive hallucinatory outbursts. In this instance the patient, who was considered to be chronically schizophrenic, resided in a nursing home (Belcher, 1988). A combination of two treatment measures was utilized to diminish incidents of verbal and physical aggression in a 69-year-old gentleman who had been hospitalized for 31 years. Differential reinforcement of other behaviours (DRO), which basically involves the contingent re-location of positive reinforcement from undesirable to desirable behaviours, was used in conjunction with an exclusionary time-out procedure in which reinforcement is withdrawn for a specified period of time. In this case, 10 minutes was determined as the time-out period (Vaccaro, 1988).

A multicomponent behavioural intervention, which included differential reinforcement, completely resolved bingeing and purging behaviour in a young woman with a nine-year history of bulimia (Posobiec and Renfrew, 1988). Encouraging results have been obtained by the use of behavioural strategies in patients suffering from irritable bowel syndrome (IBS), a gastrointestinal disorder. A behavioural treatment package commonly includes training in relaxation, cognitive coping strategies and education about IBS (Blanchard, Schwarz and Radnitz, 1987; Blanchard and Schwarz, 1988). While further research into the long-term effectiveness of behaviour therapy in this condition is required, the degree of clinical improvement which has been currently achieved is promising.

The wide applicability of a behavioural approach is finally demonstrated in a report which evaluates the long-term effectiveness of behavioural intervention in 15 male patients all of whom had been diagnosed as chronic schizophrenics. Target behaviours included, for example, verbal abuse, non-attendance at therapeutic activities and personal grooming skills. Treatment consisted of positive reinforcement and response–cost contingency techniques in which a positive reinforcer is permanently removed as a consequence of a target behaviour being exhibited. An everyday example of response–cost would be the imposition of a fine for parking on double yellow lines. The success of this intervention facilitated the discharge from hospital of all but one of the participants in the treatment programme (Peniston, 1988).

This compressed pot-pourri of clinical problems and discrete intervention methods attests to the scope of behaviour therapy. A number of the techniques mentioned, namely satiation, DRO, response–cost and time-out, could be classified as therapist controlled, as they tend to rely on the therapeutic manipulation of the patient's environment. Other methods, of which modelling is an example, reflect a more collaborative approach. The potency of modelling to effect behavioural change should not be underestimated. In crisis situations the behaviour of individuals to inspire others to heroic feats or generate pervasive panic is well recognized (Rachman, 1980). Modelling as a clinical technique can be used to form new behaviour patterns, increase existing skills or reduce avoidance behaviour. Invariably the target behaviour is broken down into a series of separate stages, graded in order of difficulty or distress. The first step of the hierarchy would therefore reflect the least difficult or least anxiety-provoking constituent of the behaviour. After observing the model perform the task in a controlled and safe environment, the client then imitates the model's behaviour. In participant modelling, the client and the model perform the behaviour together, prior to independent replication by the client. Bandura's description of fear reduction in snake phobics provides a classic illustration of the participant modelling technique (Bandura, Blanchard and Ritter, 1969). The appropriateness of the model is an important factor. Someone who not only demonstrates a coping rather than a mastery model (Meichenbaum, 1971), but is also perceived by the patient as credible, is likely to be more effective (Bandura, 1971).

A third category of behavioural techniques are those which can be described as covert methods of intervention. The three techniques which will be briefly summarized are examples of treatment strategies which actuate behavioural change through the use of cognition, imagery or fantasy. The treatment target may be an internal behaviour such as hallucinations and obsessional ruminations, or an external behaviour, for instance anxiety and habit disorders.

Systematic desensitization, developed by Wolpe (1958) to decrease avoidance behaviour, involves a hierarchy construction in which the anxiety-provoking stimuli are ranked in order of intensity, a training in relaxation and the imaginal pairing of the hierarchy items with the relaxed state. It is essential that the anxiety response is sequentially extinguished. A variant of systematic desensitization involves *in vivo*, rather than imaginal, exposure. As the literature documenting the success of this technique is so substantial, reference is restricted to two more unusual case illustrations, that of handwriting anxiety (Cornelio, Levine and Wolpe, 1980) and a mannequin phobia (Waranch, Iwata and Wohl, 1981).

Although Bain (1928) is credited with introducing the technique of thought-stopping, its history would appear to be at least a century old. An early precursor of contemporary thought-stopping in the case of a man obsessed by nude women and intercourse was used, according to Rosen and Orenstein (1976), in 1875. Wolpe (1958), however, popularized the present-day method of the technique. Thought-stopping (TS) has been widely used in the reduction of obsessional thought patterns (Horton and Johnson, 1977; Parenteau and Lamontagne, 1981). Less common applications include: hallucinations (Samaan, 1975; Lamontagne, Audet and Elie, 1983), phobias (Rimm, 1973), habit disorders such as smoking (Lamontagne *et al.*, 1978) and sexual deviation (Edwards, 1972). The mechanics of the technique are relatively straightforward:

1. First there is identification of the client's debilitating thoughts.
2. The client overtly verbalizes those thoughts as he imagines the problem scene.
3. The therapist interrupts the flow of thoughts by shouting STOP.
4. The client then interrupts his thoughts in a similar manner.
5. Finally, the client transfers the overt STOP into a covert utterance. This final stage enables the client to unobtrusively use the techniques as a self-control measure in everyday situations.

While the clinical effectiveness of TS, which is often used as an adjunct to other treatment techniques, has been widely reported in uncontrolled single-case studies, its effectiveness has not been confirmed by controlled, empirical research trials. This seeming contradiction in results may be partially due to the frequent amalgamation of TS with other procedures and the numerous variations in the technique. As the effectiveness of TS has not been conclusively demonstrated, despite its widespread use, further methodologically sound research studies are vital.

The final example in this third category of behavioural treatment techniques is covert sensitization, which was first described by Cautela (1971). This technique is often used in conjunction with other treatment methods; it involves the use of imagery that incorporates an aversive element and has been successfully applied to a variety of problem behaviours ranging from shoplifting (Glover, 1985) to self-injurious behaviour (Cautela and Barron, 1973). It has greater prominence, however, in problems of sexual deviation where contemporary behaviour therapy focuses on the development of alternative behaviour patterns (Hughes, 1977; Maletzky, 1980). In covert sensitization (CS), the therapist presents a scene for the client to imagine. The script will accurately reflect the problem behaviour and relevant environmental stimuli with a concomitant aversive element. The closing sequence of events described by the therapist always involves an aversion relief image in which the client turns away or desists from engaging in the undesirable behaviour. The imagined relief scene commonly involves a relaxation technique.

As any form of aversive therapy includes the deliberate introduction of an unpleasant element, it raises particular ethical considerations which must be addressed prior to such a treatment method being selected. Problem behaviours treated by aversion techniques are therefore often behaviours that have serious consequences for the individual and have not responded to other procedures.

The distinctive technology of behaviour therapy as an exclusive or adjunct treatment approach for a wide range of problem behaviours is continuously evolving as research probes and scrutinizes its validity and potentiality. Perhaps future advances will identify a prophylactic role for behaviour therapy in the prevention of problems of living.

Conclusion

The purpose of this chapter was to introduce the reader to a member of the therapy family. Even as an embryo, Behaviour was a cogent instrument in the remediation of problems of living. The overweight monarch of Kosala and the farmer who wanted the social competence to approach his king, both achieved their goals through the intervention of Behaviour. The 20th century announced the birth of Behaviour whose growth and development over the years gradually enabled him to function with greater sophistication, discretion and maturity. In the process, however, Behaviour did, on occasions, act imprudently and outrageously, but impropriety is not uncommon in the course of maturation. The character of Behaviour has been formed through the influence of discrete models of learning which, collectively, substantially contribute to our understanding of human behaviour and provide the means whereby distress and debility can be alleviated to varying degrees. Behaviour is never static, but is constantly evolving, always striving for greater competency and effectiveness in the promotion of an improved quality of life. Behaviour quite simply exists to help others and is available to those who contribute to patient care.

References

Altschul, A. (1982) Foreword, in *Behaviour Therapy Nursing* (ed. P. J. Barker), Croom Helm, London.

Altschul, A. (1984) A challenge to psychiatry. *Nurs. Times*, **18**, 49–51.

Altschul, A. (1985) Introduction, in *The Nurse as Therapist* (ed. P. J. Barker), Croom Helm, London.

Appel, K. C., Amper, J. M. and Schefler, G. G. (1961) Prognosis in psychiatry. *Arch. Neurol. Psych.*, **70**, 459–68.

Ayllon, T. and Michael, J. (1959) The psychiatric nurse as a behavioural engineer. *J. Exp. Anal. Behav.*, **2**, 323–34.

Bain, J. A. (1928) *Thought Control in Everyday Life*, Funk and Wagnall, New York.

Bandura, A. (1969) *Principles of Behaviour Modification*, Holt, Rinehart and Winston, New York.

Bandura, A. (1971) Psychotherapy based upon modelling principles, in *Handbook of Psychotherapy and Behaviour Change: An Empirical Analysis* (eds A. E. Bergin and S. L. Garfield), Wiley, New York.

Bandura, A. Blanchard, E. B. and Ritter, B. (1969) The relative efficacy of desensitisation and modelling approaches for inducing behavioural, affective and attitudinal change. *J. Pers. Soc. Psych.*, **13**, 173–99.

Barker, P. J. (1982) *Behaviour Therapy Nursing*, Croom Helm, London.

Barker, P. J. (1985) *Patient Assessment in Psychiatric Nursing*, Croom Helm, London.

Barker, P. J. and Fraser, D. (1985) *The Nurse as Therapist*, Croom Helm, London.

Beck, A. T. (1976) *Cognitive Therapy and the Emotional Disorders*, International University Press, New York.

Belcher, T. L. (1988) Behavioural reduction of overt hallucinatory behaviour in a chronic schizophrenic. *J. Behav. Ther. Exper. Psych.*, **19**, 69–71.

Blanchard, E. B. and Schwartz, S. P. (1988) Two year follow-up of behavioural treatment of irritable bowel syndrome. *Behav. Ther.*, **19**, 67–73.

Blanchard, E. B., Schwarz, S. P. and Radnitz, C. (1987) Psychological assessment and treatment of irritable bowel syndrome. *Behav. Mod.*, **11**, 348–72.

Cautela, J. R. (1971) Covert sensitisation for the treatment of sexual deviation. *Psych. Rec.*, **21**, 659–62.

Cautela, J. R. and Barron, M. G. (1973) Multi-faceted behaviour therapy of self-injurious behaviour. *J. Behav. Ther. Exper. Psych.*, **4**, 125–31.

Cornelio, R., Levine, A. B. and Wolpe, J. (1980) The treatment of handwriting anxiety in an in vivo desensitisation procedure. *J. Behav. Ther. Exper. Psych.*, **11**, 49–51.

Dhammapada Commentary Translation (1921) Buddhist Legends, translated by E. M. Burlingame, Pali Text Society, London.

Edwards, N. B. (1972) Case conference: assertive training in a case of homosexual paedophilia. *J. Behav. Ther. Exper. Psych.*, **3**, 55–63.

Ellis, A. (1962) *Reason and Emotion in Psychotherapy*, Lyle Stuart, New York.

Eysenck, H. J. (1952) The effects of psychotherapy: an evaluation. *J. Consult. Psych.*, **16**, 319–24.

Eysenck, H. J. (1960) *Behaviour Therapy and the Neuroses*, Pergamon, Oxford.

Fuller, P. R. (1949) Operant conditioning of a vegetative human organism. *Am. J. Psych.*, **62**, 587–90.

Franks, C. M. (1969) Introduction: behaviour therapy and its Pavlovian origins: review and perspectives, in *Behaviour Therapy: Appraisal and Status*. McGraw-Hill, New York.

Gelfand, D., Gelfand, S. and Dobson, W. R. (1967) Unprogrammed reinforcement of patients' behaviour in a mental hospital. *Behav. Res. Ther.*, **5**, 201–7.

Glaister, B. (1985) A case of auditory hallucination treated by satiation. *Behav. Res. Ther.*, **23**, 213–5.

Glover, J. H. (1985) A case of kleptomania treated by covert sensitisation. *Brit. J. Clin. Psychol.*, **24**, 213–4.

Gustavson, C. F. and Garcia, J. (1974) Pulling a gag on the wily coyote. *Psychol. Today*, August, 17–18.

Hall, M. C. (1984) Responsive parenting: a large scale training programme for school districts, hospitals and mental health centres, in *Parent Training* (eds R. F. Dangel and R. A. Polster), Guildford Press, New York.

Hauser, M. J. (1978) Nurses and behaviour modification. *J. Psych. Nurs.*, August, 17–18.

Horton, A. M. and Johnson, C. H. (1977) The treatment of homicidal obsessive ruminations by thought stopping and covert assertion. *J. Behaviour Ther. Exp. Psych.*, **8**, 339–40.

Hughes, R. C. (1977) Covert sensitisation treatment of exhibitionism. *J. Behav. Exper. Psych.*, **8**, 177–9.

Humphrey, C. (1967) *Buddhism*. Pelican Books, Harmondsworth.

Jones, H. M. (1924) The elimination of children's fears. *J. Exp. Psychol.*, **7**, 383–90.

Jones, M. (1952) *Social Psychiatry*, Tavistock Publications, London.

Jones, A. and Robson, C. (1983) Within-course effects of a training package for teachers of the severely mentally handicapped. *Spec. Ed. For. Trends*, **10** (Research Supplement), 17–20.

Kazdin, A. E. & Wilson, G. T. (1978) *Evaluation of Behaviour Therapy: Issues, Evidence and Research Strategies*, Ballinger, Cambridge, MA.

Klaber, M. M. and Butterfield, E. C. (1969) Stereotypic rocking: A measure of institutional effectiveness. *Am. J. Mental Deficiency*, **73**, 13–20.

Lamontagne, Y., Gagnon, M. A., Trudel, G. and Boisvert, J. M. (1978) Thought-stopping as a treatment for reducing cigarette smoking. *Int. J. Addict.*, **13**, 297–305.

Lamontagne, Y., Audet, N. and Elie, R. (1983) Thought-stopping for delusions and hallucinations: a pilot study. *Behav. Psychother.*, **11**, 177–84.

Levitt, E. E. (1963) Psychotherapy with children: a further evaluation. *Behav. Res. Ther.*, **1**, 45–51.

Liddell, H. S. (1938) The experimental neurosis and the problem of mental disorder. *Am. J. Psych.*, **94**, 1035–42.

Mahoney, M. (1974) *Cognition and Behaviour Modification*, Ballinger, Cambridge, MA.

Maletzky, B. M. (1980) Self-referred versus court-referred sexually deviant patients: success with assisted covert sensitisation. *Behav. Ther.*, **11**, 306–14.

Marks, I. (1985) *Psychiatric Nurse Therapists in Primary Care: The Expansion of Advanced Clinical Roles in Nursing*, Royal College of Nursing, London.

Marks, I., Hallam, R. S., Connelly, J. and Philpott, R. (1977) *Nursing in Behavioural Psychotherapy*, Royal College of Nursing, London.

Masserman, J. H. (1943) *Behaviour and Neurosis: An Experimental Psychoanalytic Approach to Psychobiologic Principles*, University of Chicago Press, Chicago.

Masters, J. C., Burish, T. G., Hollen, S. D. and Rimm, B. C. (1987) *Behaviour Therapy Techniques and Empirical Findings*, 3rd edn, Harcourt Brace Jovanovich, New York.

Matthews, A. M., Gelder, M. G. and Johnston, D. W. (1981) *Programmed Practice for Agoraphobia: Partners' Manual*, Tavistock Publications, London.

McPherson, F. M., Barker, P. J., Hunter, M. and Fraser, D. (1978) A course in behaviour modification. *Nurs. Times*, **74**, 1207–9.

Meichenbaum, D. (1971) Examination of model characteristics in reducing avoidance behaviour. *J. Pers. Soc. Psychol.*, **17**, 298–307.

Meichenbaum, D. (1977) *Cognitive Behaviour Modification*, Plenum Press, New York.

Mikulas, W. H. (1978) Four noble truths of Buddhism related to behaviour therapy. *Psychol. Rec.*, **28**, 59–67.

Morganstern, K. P. (1976) Behavioural interviewing: the initial stages of assessment, in *Behavioural Assessment: A Practical Handbook* (eds M. Herson and A. S. Bellack), Pergamon, New York.

Morton, A. M. and Johnson, C. M. (1977) The treatment of homicidal obsessional ruminations by thought-stopping and covert assertion. *J. Behav. Ther. Exper. Psych.*, **8**, 339–40.

Parenteau, P. and Lamontagne, Y. (1981) The thought-stopping technique: a treatment for different types of ruminations. *Can. J. Psych.*, **26**, 192–5.

Paul, G. L. (1967) Insight vs desensitisation in psychotherapy two years after termination. *J. Consult. Psychol.*, **31**, 333–48.

Pavlov, J. P. (1927) *Conditioned Reflexes*, Oxford University Press, Oxford.

Peniston, E. G. (1988) Evaluation of long-term therapeutic efficacy of behaviour modification programme with chronic male psychiatric inpatients. *J. Behav. Ther. Exper. Psych.*, **19**, 95–101.

Peplau, H. (1952) *Interpersonal Relations – Nursing*, Pitman, New York.

Peterson, D. R. (1968) *The Clinical Study of Social Behaviour*, Appleton-Century-Crofts, New York.

Pitts, C. E. (1976) *Behaviour Modification – 1787*. *J. App. Behav. Anal.*, **9**, 146.

Posobiec, K. and Renfrew, J. W. (1988) Successful self-management of severe bulimia. A case study. *J. Behav. Ther. Exper. Psych.*, **19**, 63–8.

Rachman, S. J. (1980) *Fear and Courage*, W. H. Freeman, San Francisco.

Reynolds, D. K. (1981) Morita psychotherapy, in *Handbook of Innovative Psychotherapies* (ed. R. Corsini), John Wiley, New York.

Rimm, D. C. (1973) Thought-stopping and covert assertion in the treatment of phobias. *J. Consult. Clin. Psychol.*, **41**, 466–7.

Rosen, G. M. and Orenstein, H. (1976) A historical note on thought-stopping. *J. Consult. Clin. Psychol.*, **44**, 1016–7.

Rosenthal, T. C. (1982) Social learning theory, in *Contemporary Behavior Therapy* (eds G. T. Wilson and C. M. Franks), Guildford Press, New York.

Samaan, M. (1975) Thought-stopping and flooding in a case of hallucinations, obsessions and homicidal–suicidal behaviour. *J. Behav. Ther. Exper. Psych.*, **6**, 65–7.

Shapiro, D. H. and Zifferblatt, S. W. (1976) Zen meditation and behavioural self-control: similarities, differences and clinical application. *Am. Psychol.*, **31**, 519–23.

Shapiro, D. H. (1978) *Precision Nirvana*, Prentice-Hall, Englewood Cliffs, NJ.

Sheldon, B. (1982) *Behaviour Modification*, Tavistock Publications, London.
Skinner, B. F. (1948) *Walden Two*, Macmillan, New York.
Skinner, B. F. (1953) *Science and Human Behaviour*, Macmillan, New York.
Smith, M. L. and Glass, G. V. (1977) Meta-analysis of psychotherapy outcome studies. *Am. Psychol.*, **32**, 752–60.
Stewart, M. A. (1961) Psychotherapy by reciprocal inhibition. *Am. J. Psych.*, **118**, 175–7.
Thorndike, E. L. (1911) *Animal Intelligence: Experimental Studies*, Macmillan, New York.
Twitmyer, E. B. (1902) A study of the knee jerk. Reported in *J. Exper. Psychol.*, (1974) **103**, 1047–66.
Vaccaro, F. J. (1988) Successful operant conditioning procedures with an institutionalised aggressive geriatric patient. *Int. J. Aging Hum. Dev.*, **26**, 71–9.
Waranch, M. R., Iwata, B. A. and Whol, M.K. (1981) Treatment of a retarded adult's mannequin phobia through in vivo desensitisation and shaping approach responses. *J. Behav. Ther. Exper. Psych.*, **12**, 359–62.
Watson, J. B. (1924) *Psychology from the Standpoint of a Behaviourist*, Lippincott, Philadelphia.
Watson, J. B. and Raynor, R. (1920) Conditioned emotional reactions. *J. Exper. Psych.*, **3**, 1–14.
Wolpe, J. (1958) *Psychotherapy by Reciprocal Inhibition*, Stanford University Press, Stanford, CA.

Chapter 5

Interpersonal relations model: theoretical constructs, principles and general applications

H. E. PEPLAU

In this chapter three key constructs – anxiety, self, and hallucinations – are explored within the theoretical framework of interpersonal relations (Peplau, 1987). Connections among these concepts are shown. Applications in clinical practice of nurses in psychiatric hospitals are described. These concepts pertain to phenomena commonly observed by nurses during their relationships with psychiatric patients. The nursing practices which psychiatric nurses provide are more likely to be remedial in intent and outcome when their work is guided by theory.

Definition of nursing

The definition of nursing which pinpoints the work of nurses and underlies this presentation is: '...the diagnosis and treatment of human responses to actual and potential health problems' (American Nurses' Association, 1980). Thus, the emphasis is on problematic, psycho-social, behavioural, human responses of patients rather than upon diagnostic categories of mental illness which are diagnosed and treated by psychiatrists. The theoretical concepts presented in this chapter refer to human responses of psychiatric patients that arise in day-to-day nurse–patient relationships, and which call for responsible, helpful nursing actions.

The nursing and medical professions

Psychiatric nursing is different from psychiatry. Both are branches of their respective professions. While both professions share the common mission of promoting health, and work collaboratively toward its achievement, each profession has a separate sphere of responsibility. The definition of nursing defines the focus of the nursing profession's work and the area of the expertise of nurses.

Psychiatric nurses have, as a primary responsibility, the nurturing and

aiding of psychiatric patients in their personal development through nursing services. The public expects psychiatric nurses to understand the
human responses of psychiatric patients and to use nursing practices
which will help to put patients in the direction of understanding and
resolving their human dilemmas. Nursing research, concerning the nature
of those human responses that are within the purview of nursing, provides theoretical constructs which nurses use to guide their observations,
inferences, and practices.

Psychiatric nurses also have secondary responsibilities which include
cooperative work with physicians who prescribe psychiatric treatments
for patients. Nurses voluntarily assist in the work of psychiatrists. For
example, nurses assist in carrying out various medical procedures; they
give medications, monitor reactions, record effects, and recommend adjustments in drug dosages; they discuss cases, share data and plan together
so that the patients' total programme makes sense and is as constructive
as possible. Nurses know that in addition to human responses, there are
physiological and biochemical reactions which occur, automatically, for
example, when a patient experiences pervasive, recurring anxiety or terror.
The medical treatment of these reactions by giving various pharma-
ceuticals or electroshock or other treatments prescribed by psychiatrists
are not included in the discussions that follow.

About theory for nursing practice

It is the contention in this chapter that each profession selects and defines
its theoretical constructs in ways most relevant for the profession's work,
using the best available scientific knowledge. That knowledge is obtained
from two sources: from nursing research, both empirical (clinical) and
controlled, and from the research findings published by all other basic
and applied sciences. Knowledge selected from these two sources comes
in the form of facts, principles, concepts, processes, models, general information, and the like. All of these forms assist nurses to know as much
as possible about the particular phenomena within the scope of their clinical work. For application of theory in direct clinical practice, however,
at least for novices in the profession, a particular format seems useful.

The three theoretical concepts in this chapter are described. They are
also shown in a serial order format which indicates two sequences: (1)
the consecutive order in which the essential characteristics of the phenomenon occur, and (2) the sequence of nursing actions addressed to the
various steps in the emergence of the phenomenon. Of necessity, these
are sometimes two different sequential orders. The three constructs and
suggested nursing practices were drawn from clinical data and scientific
literature and were tested, clinically, by many nurses for several decades.
Nevertheless, the reader is strongly advised to learn the concepts and
personally test them for effectiveness by reflection on personal experience
and in clinical nursing of psychiatric patients.

Interpersonal relations: The theoretical framework

Theory of interpersonal relations is of particular significance to nursing practice. Sullivan (1956) defined this framework as the study of what goes on between two or more people, all but one of whom may be completely illusory. Hallucinations, in this context, are to be viewed as interpersonal interactions between a real person and one or more illusory figures. Moreover, since nursing actions have consequences for patients, especially in terms of their impact on presenting psychopathology, nurses have a responsibility to study what goes on in their nurse–patient relationships. The results of such continuing study and the application of theory during practice afford choice rather than unwitting or routine nurse responses during interactions with patients.

Nurses lay claim to around-the-clock nursing care of in-patients. Their interactions with patients tend to occur with greater frequency, are of longer duration, and have more continuity than is true for the relationships patients have with all other health professionals. The potential is great for therapeutic benefits – as well as for illness-maintenance (Peplau, 1978). Interpersonal relations theories throw light on the quality of interactions (Peplau, 1988). Applications of interpersonal constructs enable nurses to become aware of, reflect on, and consider the possible consequences of the quality of their participation in nurse–patient relationships (Peplau, 1987). Thus, nurses gain a basis for choosing the behaviours they will use with patients in subsequent day-to-day interactions.

Uses of concepts and information in practice

Theoretical constructs are among the major tools which psychiatric nurses use during their work. At their best, such constructs describe and explain the origins and nature of the phenomenon or phenomena to which they pertain. Concepts also assist in making observations, by providing a general name under which certain raw data that have been noticed can, at least temporarily, be classified. For instance, on observing restless pacing in a patient, the application of the concept of anxiety would be considered. Concepts assist in making assessments, in that they supply – in their definition – clues to what to look for or to enquire about. The subsequent nurse observations or patient descriptions provide data which may confirm or disconfirm to the nurse the appropriateness of the particular concept chosen for use at that time. Nursing diagnoses of the human responses (needs, problems, dilemmas, etc.) of patients are also concepts. The current trend in this within-profession development is to identify, name, and describe indicators for each diagnostic category (Kim, McFarland and McLane, 1987). Theoretical concepts that are used to define a phenomenon also can be used to infer and design the nursing actions most likely to be corrective, remedial, or preventive of that phenomenon. Concepts are also used in planning nursing care, both the plan and the relevant constructs being further used in periodic and final evaluaton of outcomes of nursing care for particular patients.

In addition to theoretical concepts nurses need information. Effective nursing care is dependent upon nurses having maximum information about patients, which requires that nurses have full access to case history data contained in the hospital record, treating it with professional confidentiality. Additionally, a nursing history should be obtained. This instrument is constructed to obtain data directly pertinent to nursing's focus, as specified in the definition of nursing and amplified in a taxonomy of nursing diagnoses (Gordon, 1985; NANDA, 1987). This information provides background data – facts that may supply a context for enquiring about the life of the patient. These facts inform the nurse; however, if supplied by informants other than the patient they may not be wholly accurate.

Theoretical constructs, diagnostic terms, and life-history information are sometimes misused by professionals to the detriment of patients. The purposes of these data are to instruct and guide the private, professional, intellectual activity of nurses in determining the nature of dilemmas patients present to them and in choosing the therapeutic work that is necessary. Theoretical terms, diagnoses, and case history data are not labels or information to be used to intimidate, browbeat, stigmatize, label, or otherwise to be given to patients.

The tendency of all human beings is to seek explanations for their troubling experiences. Such explanations, however accurate or inaccurate they may be, provide a modicum of comfort – at last the dilemma has a name or a reason for it. Research suggests that people are more 'curious about causality when something unexpected or unusual happens' (Sears *et al.*, 1988, p. 121). Psychiatric patients are not exceptions in this matter. For them, explanations for their dilemmas which are given to them are often heard as epithets and they prematurely close off further work, which psychiatric patients must do in order to move toward and eventually achieve their understanding and their resolution of their difficulties.

The nurse–patient dialogue

Psychiatric nursing practices are primarily verbal. They consist mainly in talking with patients informally or in scheduled individual, group, or family interview sessions. Talking that occurs during these nurse–patient interactions serves such purposes as therapeutic work, teaching, planning or review of patient programmes or schedules, planning for discharge from hospital, and the like. All contacts which nurses have with patients are potential learning experiences for both parties: nurses enrich and refine their expertise, and patients expand and improve their competencies and their self-knowledge. In this sense, nursing care of psychiatric patients can be viewed as the provision of highly specialized learning events, in the verbal mode, that in a very personal way are educative for patients.

Psychiatric patients are embarked on a search for truth about themselves and their life experiences. This search is not for the literal, factual truths but rather for the inner truths about their perceptions and attributions of their experiences and the consequences in relationships with people. The term attributions refers to '. . . the process by which people arrive at causal explanations for events in the social world, particularly for actions they and other people perform' (Sears *et al.*, 1988, p. 117). Attributions about past events tend to influence expectations related to present and future events, and they also determine feelings, attitudes and behaviours.

Psychiatric patients are lacking in the intellectual and interpersonal competencies which are so necessary for the work involved in their search for self-understanding. It is the quality of the verbal participation of nurses in their interactions with patients – listening and posing investigative questions – that slowly but surely stimulates the development of these competencies in patients (Field, 1979). Competencies develop when latent capacities are used by patients; tapping into and thereby forcing patients to use these capacities is an aim of nurses when talking with patients.

Talking with patients in a professional mode is substantially different from customary social conversations, such as a nurse might have with family members or friends (Peplau, 1964). Nurse–patient discourse has as its purpose aiding a patient to gain the self-understanding and competencies required for living in the community outside hospital. Therefore, the focus is one-way, on the needs, concerns, and experiences of the patient; in friend-to-friend relationships the focus in reciprocal – on the needs of both parties. Considerable self-discipline is required of nurses in order for them to accomplish a shift from a customary social mode of talking to a professional stance.

Nurses are sometimes reluctant to seek maximum information from patients, for use within the nurse–patient dialogue. They consider this to be prying – which it would be in social situations with friends. Nurses have often been advised to be subtle and indirect in talking with psychiatric patients, who already have problems with ambiguity and lack of forthrightness of people in interpersonal situations. It is more useful when nurses are open, clear, simple, forthright, and direct with patients without being directive, autocratic and controlling.

Work of nurses with patients proceeds on the basis of information which is made available by the patient during nurse–patient relationships. In this regard, a general principle applies: anything that is going on, or that has occurred in the life of a patient, can be talked about openly and fully, reviewed, eventually understood, and then filed in the backlog among the patient's other past experiences. Conversely, anything that is not talked about but rather is merely acted out, is not likely to be understood by a patient. This principle suggests, for example, that when patients act out aggression the nursing interventions that are most constructive are: (1) stop the aggressive action, and (2) immediately sit down with the patient and require discussion of what went on by asking 'what was that all about?' With patients who are withdrawn and isolate themselves from others in the in-patient hospital unit, the principle suggests that periodically, every day, a nurse should be assigned to sit down next to the withdrawn patient. The nurse might initiate talking by saying: 'I have a half hour to talk with you,' and then wait for a response. Later on, the nurse might ask: 'what are you thinking about – say your thoughts out loud'. When the promised time period is up, the nurse would announce her departure and say when another half-hour of nursing time would be provided. Eventually, as the nurse's presence becomes familiar and expected, withdrawn patients will begin to talk but they very rarely initiate such effort. In other words, from the moment of admission to hospital the entire nursing staff ought to build-in the expectation that patients are there to resolve their problems which requires talking about their experiences, the nurse listening and being helpful as paients do their work.

Giving advice to patients is not what is being suggested here. To give advice is, in effect, to tell other persons how to live their own lives and is rarely welcomed or used. It can be assumed that psychiatric patients have already been given much advice and to no avail. Nurses who are over-eager in giving advice serve as reminders to patients of previously ineffectual advice-givers who most often were figures of authority.

Listening to patients attentively, all the while being intellectually active and considering privately which theoretical constructs help the nurse to grasp the import of what a patient is saying, and then posing a question that furthers the patient's effort is the nurse's work. However, words used in the nurse's questions do not magically produce constructive changes in psychiatric patients. Verbal interventions of nurses, intended to be corrective of the observed like-kind phenomena to which they are applied, must be repeated, sustained over time during recurring contacts with a given patient. In some instances considerable periods of time may be involved thereby testing a nurse's patience and resolve. Furthermore, repetition can become monotonous for nurses if not annoying for patients. Ingenuity, imagination, and flexibility in the use of words and their synonyms are indicated. The general principle is: vary the language but sustain the intended message. In this regard, a very useful exercise particularly for student nurses is to have them prepare a written list of all the different ways to ask a patient, 'Are you anxious?' which would illustrate the principle.

The questions that nurses pose to patients serve the purpose of investigation – aiding patients in their search for self-knowledge. Questions that begin with who, when, or what are to be preferred; why is an intimidating word in that it assumes that patients have reasons for their actions or experiences rather than being engaged in a search for them. The words 'can you' question a patient's ability to respond; 'will you' suggests the possibility of wilful stubbornness if the patient doesn't respond; the point being made here is that the language of the nurse conveys meaning and all too often patients are sensitively tuned to these nuances which they hear as references to them personally.

It is quite useful for nurses, particularly student nurses, to tape-record several sessions in which they talk with psychiatric in-patients. Review of these tapes afterwards provides an opportunity for nurses to hear and to become aware of their habits of speech, and to consider the short- and long-term impact of their words on the perceptions of patients. Exercises such as these provide a basis for nurses to begin to shift their mode of language usage from a social to a professional mode, and therefore to begin to audit and edit their verbalizations during nurse–patient dialogues.

The verbal nursing actions suggested below are primarily investigative. They are used to encourage the patient to do the problem-solving work in order to move toward resolution of his difficulties in living with people in the community, outside the hospital. The assumption is that the patient – and only the patient – has the data concerning his dilemmas. What the patient does not have is access to his data, nor methods for reviewing and making sense of it. Therefore, most psychiatric patients cannot extricate themselves from their difficulties without professional help. The professional nursing assistance to patients that is proposed in this chapter is that of helping patients to investigate their circumstances and to gain both a new perspective and the interpersonal competencies which result from that effort. Two major instruments which nurses use in this work are verbal facility and theoretical constructs which explain the phenomena that are problematic for the patient.

Anxiety

Introduction

The 20th century is often called the age of anxiety. The history of anxiety as a human experience is much longer. A recent publication devotes an entire chapter to anxiety as experienced by Calvin throughout his life in the 16th century (Bouwsma, 1988). Calvin recognized anxiety, his own and that of others, as a human condition. He discussed it often and the energy anxiety provided was a driving force in his life-long productivity as a religious reformer.

During the decade of the 1970s considerable research related to anxiety was conducted as reported in a conference report (Tuma and Maser, 1985). This publication raises important unresolved issues: what is the relation between fear and anxiety? Are there differences in the quantity and quality of general versus pathological anxiety? Does anxiety occur along a continuum or does a discontinuity paradigm pertain, panic being a unique episode rather than the extreme end of a continuum of anxiety? While the papers in this publication point to some areas of consensus, taken as a whole they suggest that theories explanatory of anxiety are as yet far from reliable and valid and that much more research into the nature of anxiety is urgently needed.

Laypersons and professionals often use the same terms but in different ways. Commonly, the laity use the word anxious when eager is what is intended; panic is a lay term to indicate being jittery or nervous. A characteristic of professionalism is precise definition of constructs which refer to phenomena within the purview of work of the profession and from which remedial interventions can be derived.

General characteristics   Anxiety is a universal phenomenon. Everyone experiences the discomfort of anxiety in some degree at some time during life. As a universal experience there are some general characteristics of anxiety that apply in all cases.

- Anxiety is a subjective, affective experience; it is felt as an unpleasant uneasiness, as apprehension, dread, or uncanny sensation.
- Anxiety is an energy and therefore it cannot be observed directly; what can be noticed are the effects of anxiety – the transformations of the energy into physiological reactions and behavioural responses which are the clues to the presence of anxiety.
- Anxiety is triggered cognitively by an input of real or imagined, internal or external, personal or situational information which is perceived as a threat to one's status or prestige or to attributions, beliefs, and expectations about oneself and one's world. Anxiety can also be triggered when a person feels the anxiety another person in the same situation is then experiencing; this transmission occurs by way of empathic observation, the ability to feel in oneself the emotions of another person during an interpersonal relationship.
- Anxiety triggers an immediate physiological reaction, automatically, as evidenced by increased heart rate, sweating, trembling, irritability, vertigo, etc. It may trigger a sense of foreboding, uncertainty about what might happen, anticipation of loss of control or an inability to cope or to survive.
- There is an awareness of apprehension, felt discomfort, and of physiological reactions but most often there is unawareness of and/or inability to formulate and verbalize the precise nature of the triggering cognitive input.
- Anxiety is adaptive in that it serves as a warning signal of impending threat to the organism's survival – particularly to the survival of the self-system; an immediate human response (other than physiological reaction which is automatic) is required to reinstate comfort and ensure survival. In this chapter these responses are called relief behaviours. The intention of relief behaviours is to reduce, relieve, and to prevent

escalation of anxiety. Psychiatric in-patients have many relief behaviours that are used automatically, without thought.

- Anxiety occurs in different degrees ranging from mild, to moderate, to severe, and to panic (terror, horror, awe, dread, uncanny sensation); escalation from lesser to greater degrees of anxiety can occur when the anxious person empathizes the anxiety of another or other persons in the same situation, and/or when the relief behaviours employed fail to work as intended.
- There may be a predisposition to anxiety within particular families.

The foregoing universal characteristics of anxiety include those common elements, regularities, which occur across cases, irrespective of ethnic and cultural factors. These latter factors, the particulars of a person's experience of anxiety, are inherent in the style, content, or behavioural acts illustrative of patterns of relief behaviour. The personal characteristics are also intrinsic to descriptions of the experience given by patients.

Definition of anxiety as a clinical construct The essence of anxiety abstracted from the foregoing general features, and confirmed in empirical–clinical psychiatric nursing research, has been formulated into a theoretical construct of this phenomenon (see Fig. 5.1). Nurses need to know the universal characteristics, as many facts and as much information as they

Figure 5.1 A concept of anxiety

Definition: sequence of steps in development of anxiety	*Information needed to understand a person's experience of anxiety*
1. *Expectations* are held, up front, in mind.	What expectations? Origins. How long held? How important? Can they be changed or given up? Was the expectation reasonable – capable of fulfillment?
2. *Expectations* held are *not met*.	What interfered? What happened instead? Who was to meet the expectation? When? How? What evidence?
3. *Discomfort* is felt.	Experienced in what part of the body? What degree? What was noticed by patient?
4. *Relief behaviours* are used.	What behavioural act or acts related to what pattern?
5. The relief behaviours are *justified* and rationalized.	

can obtain about anxiety as a human condition. However, for purposes of application during nurse–patient relationships, a succinct, practical-oriented, easy to recall, theoretical construct is required.

The concept definition in Fig. 5.1 asserts that anxiety is triggered when *expectations* that are operative, up front in mind, with or without the full awareness of the person, in a given situation, are *not met*. *Felt discomfort* is followed almost immediately by behavioural acts which provide *relief*, by reducing or preventing more anxiety, and which subsequently are justified or rationalized. The essentials in this concept, to be recalled and applied in clinical practice, albeit in a different order as shown in Fig. 5.2, are italicized.

The term expectations is a general classification which includes such similar but not identical cognitions as assumptions, preconceptions, attributions, wishes, wants, beliefs, values, hopes, desires, needs, goals, self-views and the like. The term expectations simplifies the nurse's conceptual task to recall of one overall rubric during clinical work. The following examples illustrate aspects of the essentials which define the concept:

A person assumes that the earth will remain firm; suddenly, unex-

Figure 5.2   Concept application in psychiatric nursing practice*

Nursing aim	*Nursing verbal interventions***
3. Get the operative expectations formulated and stated by patient.	3. After the patient is clearly aware of the relation between 1 and 2 below, ask: 'What were you thinking about *before* you felt upset?'
4. Get a formulation and recognition of the connection between expectations held and what happened instead.	4. When the patient has clearly formulated an expectation, then ask: 'What happened instead?'
5. Consider which factors in the sequence are amenable to control.	5. Then discuss what change in 3 or 4, above, might be possible.
1. Get patient to become aware of and name anxiety.	1. Ask the patient: 'Are you anxious?', 'Are you nervous?', 'Are you upset?', 'Are you tense now?'
2. Get the patient to become aware of, and state, the connection between the named anxiety and the behaviour used to relieve it.	2. When a yes answer has been obtained to (1), ask the patient: 'What are you doing now to relieve being nervous?'

*Note that the sequence of steps here is different from those in the definition in Fig. 5.1.
**Vary the language but not the message.

pectedly, an earthquake occurs; immediately the individual is awash with terror.

A patient feels a pressing need for a show of affection from her mother who, heretofore, has demonstrated a remarkable inability to express love to her daughter. The daughter telephones her mother thinking 'this time she will be nice to me'; on answering the phone the mother berates her daughter for this interruption in her day. The daughter cries, feels helpless, and berates herself for bothering her mother.

A psychiatric patient who has a very beautiful face claims loudly and frequently that she is ugly. Nursing personnel counter and rebut the patient's operative self-view and tell her, 'no, you are so beautiful', or 'I wish I had your lovely face'. The patient, using a razor blade, slashes her face (which both confirms the operative self-view in the effect of this action and relieves the anxiety evoked by the unmet expectation).

In therapy, a patient, with a rush of feelings of anger and rage, tells the therapist, 'my father hated me, my mother couldn't stand me, my sister was always disgusted with me, all my life nobody loved me.' The therapist then said: 'Well, I love you,' at which point panic ensued, the patient ran through the unit screaming, smashing furniture, and finally was restrained, taken to a closed unit and put into a seclusion room.

Not all unmet expectations lead to crippling anxiety. The energy of mild degrees of anxiety may rapidly be converted into disappointment, providing sufficient relief as well as a clear understanding of the expectations that were not realized. The use of annoyance and anger, in similar fashion, as energy transformations which afford relief is quite common. However, very minor incidents – often involving only marginal awareness of the operative expectations – do sometimes produce quite severe anxiety (see Fig. 5.3).

The expectations which a person holds, at any given time, may be unmet for many reasons. External circumstances may change suddenly, as in earthquakes, tornadoes, fires, car accidents, sudden death of a family member, and such. An individual may hold expectations that for their realization, involve competencies or capacities that he is lacking. Psychiatric patients particularly have sets of non-rational expectations of which they are largely unaware, but which nevertheless gain expression in their behaviour. Expectations are personal, situational, and socio-cultural or mixtures of these. While hospital personnel can make guesses as to what expectations are held by particular patients the accuracy of these estimates is debatable until a patient becomes aware of, formulates, and expresses his own expectations. Some of these patient-formulations may validate the guesses which staff have made.

The discomfort of anxiety is felt in some part of the body as are physiological effects. The extent of the discomfort is dependent upon the degree

Figure 5.3 Degrees of anxiety

Degree of anxiety	Effects on perceptual field and on ability to focus attention	Observable behaviour
+ Mild	Perceptual field widens slightly. Able to observe more than before and to see relations (make connection among data).	Aware, alerted, sees, hears and grasps more than before; usually able to recognize and name anxiety easily.
++ Moderate	Perceptual field narrows slightly. Selective inattention: does not notice what goes on peripheral to the immediate focus but can do so if attention is directed there by another observer.	See, hears, and grasps less than previously; can attend to more if directed to do so; able to sustain attention on a particular focus; selectively inattends to contents outside the focal area; usually able to state 'I am anxious now.'
+++ Severe	Perceptual field is greatly reduced. Tendency toward dissociation: to not notice what is going on outside the current reduced focus of attention; largely unable to do so when another observer suggests it.	Sees, hears, and grasps far less than previously; attention is focused on a small area of given event; inferences drawn may be distorted due to inadequacy of observed data; may be unaware of and unable to name anxiety; relief behaviours generally used.
++++ Panic (terror, horror, dread, uncanniness, awe)	Perceptual field is reduced to a detail, which is usually blown up, i.e., elaborated by distortion (exaggeration), or the focus is on scattered details; the speed of the scattering tends to increase. Massive dissociation, especially of contents of self-system, felt as enormous threat to survival.	Says 'I'm in a million pieces', 'I'm gone', 'What is happening to me?'; perplexity, self-absorption; feelings of unreality; flight of ideas or confusion; fear; repeats a detail; many relief behaviours used automatically (without thought); the enormous energy produced by panic must be used and may be mobilized as rage; may pace, run or fight violently; with dissociation of contents of self-system, there may be very rapid reorganization of the self usually along pathological lines i.e., a psychotic break is usually preceded by panic.

of anxiety. Where the discomfort is felt can only be determined by asking the patient. Some patients feel the discomfort in their gut, others in their genitals, some complain of feeling funny in the head or of blurred vision. Psychiatric patients tend not to connect these felt discomforts with being anxious. Similarly, the automatic physiological reactions, which are both felt and observable, are sometimes misnamed by the sufferer as a medical problem. For example, with severe anxiety or panic there is a sudden rush of adrenalin-related chemicals into the body which is accompanied immediately, automatically by various physiological reactions. Increased heart rate, felt constriction in the chest or throat, sudden dryness of the mouth, flushing and sweating, trembling of hands and legs, and dizziness are among the more common physical reactions. Panic can be felt as a blow on the head, severe anxiety may precipitate urinary urgency or activities involving the genitals, or an organic-like mental confusion can be experienced. These physiological effects are not specific for anxiety but may also be early warnings or symptoms of various diseases – such as heart disease, stoke, diabetes, etc. There are occasions when heart attacks and panic occur simultaneously. The general nursing background of psychiatric nurses informs their observations in this matter.

The definition of anxiety indicates that the energy of anxiety, signalled as discomfort, is more or less immediately transformed into behaviours that are intended to reduce, relieve, or prevent more anxiety. In most textbooks, these behaviours are called defence mechanisms or coping behaviours. In this chapter the term relief behaviours will be used. This designation pinpoints the functions served by the energy transformations. Psychiatric nurses who have witnessed sudden rage and violence of patients need to recognize that severe anxiety or panic are antecedent to these relief-giving outbursts. The rage and violence simultaneously relieve the antecedent anxiety while the staff response may evoke more terror.

Patterns of relief behaviour sort into at least three different major areas. (1) Psychiatric classification categories, such as neuroses, psychoses, and anti-social acting-out diagnoses. (2) Psychosomatic complaints, in which the body as a whole, a body part or an organ are used to transform the energy of anxiety into expression of symptoms of a physical illness – perhaps as a symbolic expression of a personal dilemma. Commonly, there are one or more complaints of physical dysfunction for which no hard evidence obtains after thorough medical investigation. (3) Generating learning products, by using the energy of anxiety in examining anxiety-evoking experiences in order to learn from them. This means being aware of and recognizing anxiety when it occurs, and being willing and able to manage the discomfort while transforming the energy into actions and use of resources, as required, for investigation of the personal and situational antecedents to anxiety (Burd and Marshall, 1963). Performing artists have long known that the energy of their pre-performance anxiety if sustained – and not

masked or blotted out by some immediate relief-giving action – can be used
to heighten their sensitivity and thereby enhance their artistic performance.

Adaptation and learning   The first two areas – psychiatric and psychosomatic – cover adaptive responses; the third area has to do with learning.
Adaptation and learning are two different human processes which persons employ when coping with the inevitable dilemmas of living. Synonyms for adaptation are to adjust, to fit, and to conform to environmental
conditions or to new stimuli. The physiological reactions to anxiety –
signals warning of a threat to survival – are immediate, automatic, and
adaptive. Learning is variously defined in the literature. For the purposes
of psychiatric nursing practice, the common meaning of this term is most
useful. The synonyms for learning generally include to find out about,
to ascertain, to study and to obtain knowledge or skill, and to gain understanding by investigation.

The descriptions of these terms define two processes which have significant differences. They differ in the extent of the cognitive effect employed,
in the patterning of energy transformation, and in the immediacy or delay
in gaining relief of anxiety. Anxiety influences both processes. It supplies
energy, the quantity being dependent upon the degree of anxiety that
occurs. That energy must be and is transformed either rapidly, into adaptive behaviours providing immediate relief, or more slowly, into cognitive,
problem-solving behaviours, the discomfort of anxiety being sustained
during a search for necessary information and until the learning products
obtain and eventually provide relief.

It is instructive to notice how quickly psychiatric in-patients adapt to
institutional requirements of them. The position taken in this chapter is
that psychiatric hospitals ought to be seen as special educational institutions which provide personalized programmes of educative events so
that patients learn about themselves and gain enduring competencies for
social living.

Relief behaviours of psychiatric patients   Anxiety is not in and of itself
pathological. Symptoms connected with pathology called mental illness
are evolved, initially, as coping behaviours. These often are actions at first
consciously taken in anxiety-laden situations, which are perceived as
threatening to the self-system. Persons who experience anxiety, particularly in severe degree, their own or the anxiety of others which they
empathize, tend toward avoidance. They move away from people and out
of situations that seem to evoke anxiety. This is an adaptive reaction. For
example, withdrawal, a common pattern of behaviour observable in psychiatric in-patients, is at first a conscious decision an individual makes
to remove himself physically from an anxiety-provoking situation. Such
behaviours are effective in terms of relief from anxiety. However, and

especially in persons who are psychologically vulnerable in ways other than recurring anxiety, they tend to become ineffective in terms of problem-solving and learning. If, for instance, withdrawal is used repeatedly as a coping behaviour, then the problem-solving that is attempted during withdrawal, becomes a highly private matter. It consists in autistic rumination about anxiety-laden experiences in which the individual not only has control over determining all dimensions of those experiences, but has such control under the condition of the limiting effects of anxiety, on his observation of what occurred during those events. The tendency is toward distortion of what was noticed, in the direction of self-interest and need. Moreover, the individual's perceptions and conclusions are unchecked, unverified, and unvalidated by discussion with another observer. The withdrawal, rumination, control, and distortion serve – unknowingly – to relieve the discomfort of anxiety which is the unwitting, immediate aim of the withdrawn individual. What goes on during withdrawal is more significant than is the pattern *per se*.

In this chapter withdrawal and other such behaviours are called relief behaviours, a term which designates their overriding purpose. The term is in keeping with the interpersonal theoretical framework. In an intra-personal framework, such as that of Freud and others, these phenomena are called mechanisms of defence.

The main utility of relief behaviours is to reduce, relieve, and to prevent more anxiety for the person using them. Relief behaviours have two main characteristics.

(1) Relief behaviours consist of overall patterns – such as withdrawal – each pattern having many separate acts which contain the same theme as in the pattern. There are many ways to withdraw; often there is a sequence of separate acts sometimes used in a particular serial order. When one action is challenged another will go into play. For example, a patient does not answer a question of a staff member who comments on that; the patient doesn't respond to the comment and looks away, then moves out of the situation; he then isolates himself from others as totally as possible. Psychiatric patients tend to have few rather than many patterns of behaviour as do healthy persons. In repetitive monotony most mentally ill patients tend to go round-and-round a circle of many acts related to few behavioural patterns. One patient, on recognizing it after considerable therapy, called this her trapadaptation, a very apt neologism.

Virtually any behavioural act can be used as relief giving. Consider the commonplace: 'I'm sorry'. At first the phrase was acquired consciously, usually in childhood with prompting from adults. Then it becomes an automatic, relief-giving verbalism used in many later situations in which anxiety is evoked when inadvertently, unexpectedly, giving offence, injury, or the like, to another person in a social situation. The phrase once uttered provides relief and closes off enquiry into the circumstances. At the other extreme, a delusion serves similar purposes. A delusion is an inadequate conclusion, inferred from insufficient data about an event observed and experienced under the conditions of panic, which at that time provided desperately needed explanation and relief from self-system disintegration consequent to panic. Patients resist investigation into their delusions because they urgently need them to prevent recurrence of panic of which they are unaware. The way back starts with recognition of anxiety (Fig. 5.2).

Psychiatric patients tend to have many anxiety-relieving behavioural acts as sets related to a few such patterns as: blame (self-blame or blame-avoidance), scapegoating (taunting, bullying, intimidating, etc), helplessness, dependency, concealment, shame–embarrassment, envy–jealousy, etc. For each pattern there is generally a characteristic repertoire of separate behavioural acts often used in a particular sequence – when one fails to work, another action automatically comes into play. For instance, an overall pattern of aggression can include, in an escalating order, annoyance, idling hostility, passive aggression, resentment, overt anger, rage, and impotent rage.

The language–thought process is quite frequently used by patients to evolve language–thought patterns which initially relieve anxiety. Anxiety disorganizes thought, a frequent occurrence in the pre-hospitalization experiences of psychiatric patients. Consequently, language–thought disorders are commonly observable – and in need of remedial assistance which nurses can provide (Field, 1979). For example, a pattern of overgeneralization can be noted in such separate language behaviours as global vagueness (everyone does that), erroneous classification, stereotypical clichés (time will tell), use of global, non-descriptive adjectives (e.g., good, bad, happy), and the like. Automatic knowing in which the patient assumes that another person knows something which the patient hasn't expressed, is the pattern of such phrases as 'you know', 'you see' etc. Anxiety also wipes out thought, as in blocking or blanking. All of these anxiety-related difficulties are relief behaviours which, by accretion form the syndrome called language–thought disorder so common in patients diagnosed as schizophrenics.

(2) A second characteristic of relief behaviours is their eventual involuntary nature following repeated use at the slightest felt discomfort related to anxiety. Such behaviours were at first consciously taken. By the time of hospitalization, psychiatric patients tend to be unaware of their original intent or use, their current utility, their self-limiting nature, or their original connection to anxiety – currently or in the past. Becoming aware of these points is part of the serious work which patients need to do, with the help of nurses.

(3) The third characteristic of relief behaviours is their tendency, at some time, to fail to work – at which point severe anxiety or panic is experi-

enced. Massive failure of sets of relief-behaviours to provide the assumed relief during panic precedes a psychotic episode.

Application of the construct Anxiety quite probably cannot be eliminated from human experience, yet it is a powerful energizer that demands transformation into behaviour – which can be in the direction of learning and personal growth or toward pathological adaptations as in symptoms of mental illness. Anxiety, however, can be amenable to personal control. The first step in that direction is to be aware of the presence of anxiety at the point of feeling the initial discomfort which it produces. Most psychiatric patients do not have this kind of control. Helping psychiatric patients to recognize and name anxiety as such, when it is occurring, is a learning experience which psychiatric nurses can provide (see Figs 5.2 and 5.4).

The learning experience may proceed somewhat in this sequence. The nurse will observe that a patient with whom she is talking is showing a physiological effect of anxiety such as flushing, hard breathing, or using a relief behaviour – such as restlessness, overtalkativeness, changing the subject of the conversation, etc. At that point, it is useful for the nurse to ask 'Are you nervous now?' (or some language variant of this message). If the patient says 'yes', the nurse can then ask 'What are you doing now to relieve it?' This question forces the patient to begin to notice the relief behaviour which the nurse has observed. If the patient says 'I'm breathing hard and I'm restless', then obviously the patient has made the connection between the felt discomfort of anxiety and the transformation of the energy of anxiety into the behaviours both the nurse and patient have observed. The nurse can offer validation, as in saying 'I noticed that too'.

What is more likely to happen, particularly with long-term psychiatric patients, when the nurse asks 'are you tense right now', is that the patient's response will be a vigorous 'no'. If the nurse persists and asks about anxiety in subsequent nurse–patient contacts, over as long a period of time as it takes, eventually the patient will give a 'yes' response. The usual sequence in getting to this affirmative response is: (1) unawareness – not noticing – the patient saying 'no' in various ways; (2) selective inattention (self-doubt), the patient responding variously with 'once I was', 'maybe I am', 'perhaps a little', and finally (3) awareness, i.e., the patient saying 'yes I am'.

No substantial therapeutic work can be accomplished until step 3 is reached. This is because the self-system (see later) is an anti-anxiety system which always operates to prevent anxiety, such as is involved in the therapeutically oriented self-disclosure work which patients must do in order to heal themselves. The very first step in such work is to have control over anxiety and its unwitting escalation by recognizing and naming anxiety when it is felt. But, initially, when a nurse asks 'Are you nervous now?' the patient's anxiety will increase. However, as the unfamiliar question

Figure 5.4   Nursing interventions related to degree of anxiety

Degree of anxiety	Nursing interventions
+ Mild	Learning is possible. Nurse assists patient to use the energy anxiety provides to encourage learning. See Fig. 5.2 – apply it in nurse–patient interaction.
++ Moderate	Nurse to check own anxiety so patient doesn't empathize with it. Encourage patient to talk: to focus on one experience, to describe it fully, then to formulate the patient's generalizations about that experience.
+++ Severe	Learning is less possible. Allow relief behaviours to be used but do not ask about them. See Fig. 5.2 – apply it in nurse–patient interaction. Encourage the patient to talk: ventilation of random ideas is likely to reduce anxiety to moderate level. When this is observed by the nurse, proceed as above.
++++ Panic	Learning is impossible. *Thereness*: nurse to stay with the patient. Allow pacing and walk with the patient. No content inputs to the patient's thinking should be made by the nurse. (They burden the patient who will distort them.) Use instrumental inputs only – the fewest possible and the least number of words: e.g., 'Drink this' (give liquids to replace lost fluids and to relieve dry mouth); 'Say what's happening to you', 'Talk about yourself', or 'Tell what you feel now' (to encourage ventilation and externalization of inner, frightening experience). Pick up on what the patient says, e.g., patient: 'I'm in a million pieces', nurse: 'Talk about that'; or, patient: 'What's happening to me – how did I get here', nurse: 'Say what you notice'. Short phrases by the nurse, direct, to the point of the patient's comment, and investigative, match the current attention span of the patient in panic and therefore are more likely to be heard, grasped, and acted upon with the patient's responses gradually reducing the anxiety in a helpful way. Do not touch the patient; patients experiencing panic are very concerned about survival, experiencing grave threat to the self, and usually distort the intentions of all invasions of their personal space. When the patient's anxiety is very obviously greatly reduced then apply Fig. 5.2.

and its requirement that the patient notice his anxiety become familiar, the patient will hear the question, take it in, and make an effort to act on it.

In working with psychiatric patients it is generally not useful to point out or to challenge their relief behaviours (or symptoms) especially in view of the unawareness of the patient and of his great need of these actions, as described above. Unawareness means that the patient is unable to notice these behaviours and that to do so would increase anxiety, which sometimes can escalate into panic. When a nurse asks (as in step 2 of Fig. 5.2) 'What are you doing to relieve your nervousness?' the patient's response will indicate the patient's ability to notice his behaviour. If the patient says 'nothing', then quite obviously he is not observing that he is pacing, trembling, or using some other relief behaviour which the nurse can observe. If the nurse asks 'What do you usually do to get comfortable?' or 'When upset in the past what did you do then?' again, the patient's response provides a clue to the patient's awareness. When the nurse persists with investigative type questions, as indicated above, in several contacts over time, eventually the patient will begin to notice his relief behaviour.

The nurse's questions, as phrased above, do not challenge or question the patient's ability as would phrasing such as 'can you tell me?' or 'will you tell me?', or still worse, 'why don't you tell me?', which is a question that is intimidating and a reminder of authoritarian persons known in the past; why questions are often heard as accusatory by psychiatric patients. The questions of a nurse to patients are, in effect, input appraisals, which must be heard, incorporated, and then acted upon by the patient (see section later on self-system).

Rationale for the nursing application   In Fig. 5.2, the sequence of nurse application of Fig. 5.1 is first to promote awareness and naming of anxiety by the patient. Naming – people, places, objects, events – is a very old competence, learned very early in life, as in naming 'mama', and rarely lost in psychiatric patients. Secondly, nurses ask patients to notice, name, and connect the relief behaviour being used in relation to the named anxiety. Identifying a relation between a current circumstance (relief behaviour) with its immediate antecedent (discomfort or anxiety) involves the competence of noticing a fairly simple, obvious before-and-after relation. It may not be an exactly simple task for the patient, given that psychiatric patients tend not to use relational thought for problem solving. The task, however, calls on a long-standing competence, known from childhood, as in observing and feeling a soiled diaper and having it changed.

The third step in nursing application of the construct of anxiety requires the patient to see and to state a more complex relation. The patient has to notice the connection between felt discomfort and relief behaviours, *and* between the antecedent unmet expectation and the consequent effects – a cause–effect relation. For psychiatric patients, this third step is complicated by their tendency to have fleeting thoughts rather than clearly formulated cognitions – such as of their expectations. Much effort usually is required on the part of the nurse in putting investigative questions such as 'What were you thinking of at the point you felt nervous?' (or 'felt anxious and then as you said, got restless'). Such questions serve as stimuli which, in time, encourage the patient to hang onto, notice, formulate, and state his fleeting thoughts. The sequence of nurse application shown in Fig. 5.2 is based upon the foregoing rationale.

Self

Introduction

Revision of the contents of the self-system is a crucial part of the self-development work which psychiatric patients must do. Problems related to self and to anxiety pervade the psychopathology of patients for which treatment programmes are to provide remedial assistance.

Currently, in the social sciences, there seems to be renewed interest in the self-concept. Gecas (1982) has recently provided a quite comprehensive review of conceptions of self, beginning with the work of Cooley (1902) and including contemporary research as well as an extensive bibliography. Wylie (1974) has also published a review of research on self.

The nursing literature on this phenomenon is not as extensive as this important aspect of nursing's work would suggest. The American Nurses' Association (ANA) has a publication on nursing diagnoses in preparation, in line with the definition of nursing cited earlier, which will include classifications of self-concept problems such as self-esteem, body-image, identity, and the like. In the work of various nurse theorists (King, 1981; Roy, 1984), and others, the self-concept is included.

General considerations   The self-systems of nurses and those of their patients are at interplay in all nurse–patient encounters. Moreover, psychiatric patients who are hospitalized invariably hold self views that are crippling, dysfunctional in social terms, and therefore are central among their many psycho-social problems. Nurse–patient interactions provide nurses with many opportunities to be instruments for constructive changes. Nurses have the function of helping psychiatric patients to revise their self-views more in accord with their inborn capacities and in the direction of views that enable living comfortably and productively with other people in the community. This nursing responsibility is likely to be accomplished when nurses have and use a viable theoretical construct concerning the self-system, as Sullivan called it (Sullivan, 1956). Nurses need theoretical understanding about what the self is, how one gets a self-system in the first place, how it functions and what purposes it serves, what the observable phenomena of self are as involved in mental illness, and, finally, how such theory informs and guides the nursing interventions during nurse–patient relationships.

In order to be helpful to patients, nurses need to obtain a general idea of the nature, dimensions, and general orientations of the contents of the self of each patient. However, it would be a serious error to believe that complete knowledge can ever be secured about the total contents of any person's self system. At best, only an approximation can be obtained. This caveat applies in work with psychiatric patients especially, for they tend toward private thought and concealment rather than toward public expression and self-disclosure. According to Sears *et al.* (1988, pp. 269–73), self-disclosure serves uses such as expression, self-clarification, self-validation, social control, and relationship development. Psychiatric patients need therapeutic help in order to attain these purposes.

Psychiatric patients do make comments about themselves and others from which the general tendencies in their self-system contents can be inferred by nurses. Nursing's work cannot proceed effectively without some general hypotheses about the self-views of patients. Such a working hypothesis can be obtained by nurses from data patients present to them, in nurse–patient talks, on admission to hospital and within the first few days thereafter. It is useful to nurses to notice and write down verbatim statements which patients make with reference to themselves. These concrete items can then be classified into I, maybe me, and not me self-views along lines of Fig. 5.5. These data can also be sorted further into those pertaining to family, friends, strangers; one's intelligence or competence; or into major patterns which the language used suggests: derogation, accusation, belittling, blaming, concealment, and so forth.

Developing a working hypothesis of the contents of self of each patient can be a staff effort which generates a shared understanding as a basis for the joint, remedial verbal nursing approaches to be used. It is difficult to see how patients whose self-views are primarily derogatory can be helped without the nursing staff having an understanding that such is the case, and of knowing the what and why of remedial nursing interventions. Nurses, of course, do not change the self-views patients hold – only patients can do that; nurses, however, through their verbal approaches in nurse–patient dialogues, do provide instrumental inputs intended to stimulate patients to do the necessary work of self change.

What is the self?　The self is an abstraction; it is a convenient way of describing a function of the total person. It is not a thing, nor a body part, nor a place in the mind. The self is a function of the mind – which is a more comprehensive function of the entire human organism. The self is something like a theoretical framework in that it serves as an organizing structure through which experiences, events and people are perceived and known, accepted or rejected. The self is a conceptualization of one of the most important human functions.

In the literature the self is alternatively referred to as ego, personality, identity and such. These conceptions are not precisely synonymous with self-system as defined in this chapter. The construct provided below is presented in a format considered to be most useful for purposes of both observation and intervention in psychiatric nursing practice.

The self is viewed as a system because of the interlocking nature of its many functions and the tendency toward maintenance of equilibrium or stability. As with all systems, a change in one self-system function, constructive or otherwise, impacts upon all other functions. It is for this reason that helping patients to revise handicapping self-views which they hold and to aid them to embrace constructive ones, in accord with their capacities, is a most difficult, time-consuming, piecemeal task.

Parsons (1961, p. 38) in another context identified four 'essential functional imperatives of any social system: pattern-maintenance, integration, goal attainment, and adaptation'. These formulations apply as well to the self-system. The self expands, contracts, changes, and is otherwise revised as it functions, particularly in maintaining security. Security obtains through intellectual activity and interpersonal security operations (or relief behaviours) which simultaneously sustain system integration and prevent anxiety.

When a psychiatric patient, who is experiencing panic and/or terror, says 'Where am I, I'm all over the place – in a million pieces', he is at that point saying that integration of the self-system has been gravely threatened or is being lost. Security of the self-system which is assumed, and is felt when the interlocking functions are maintained, is, during panic and terror, replaced by enormous, felt, insecurity, disintegration and dysfunctioning of the self. The security operations (relief behaviours) that previously had worked successfully to maintain system stability are now failing to do so. Terror arises during this shift from expected integration to perceived disintegration of the self. Panic and terror cannot be sustained for very long, for in effect the individual is for that duration without an integrated self-system. Therefore, the self reorganizes swiftly, and if the person is unaware at least of the anxiety experienced at that time, or if the interventions others provide in the situation are not cognizant of the nature of terror and act accordingly, the reorganization will be along lines of psychopathology. Panic precedes a psychotic break (see Fig. 5.5).

Sullivan (1956) defined the self as an anti-anxiety system. In this regard, beginning in infancy and continuing throughout life, the self – in accord with whatever stage of intellectual and interpersonal development of the person – polices its owner's behaviour in interpersonal situations. This vigilance occurs in the interest of maintaining security and the previously mentioned functions, and in order to reduce, relieve, and prevent more anxiety. For example, the self audits and edits out errors of speech – slips of the tongue – so as to prevent anxiety, subsequent humiliation, or embarrassment, and therefore loss of prestige (see Fig. 5.6).

The self-system is a product of socialization, a function which humans evolve and revise, along constructive or destructive lines, during interper-

Table 5.5   Dimensions of the self

In awareness: I	*Selectively inattended: maybe me*	*Dissociated: not me*
Up front in mind	On or near the margin of attention and awareness	Excluded from awareness
Easily recalled, noticed, talked about	Can recall if attention is directed to do so	Unable to notice or accept these self-views without experiencing severe anxiety or panic
Fully accepted self-view	Only partially accepted self-views; doubt	Unacceptable self-views
Views are owned and presented in using pronouns such as I, me, my and mine.	Views are partly owned. Views are presented with qualifiers such as maybe me, sometimes I, once I was.	Views are disowned. Prefixes to convey exclusion include negatives such as not me, at no time, never did, no way, etc.
Anxiety: none	Anxiety: mild to moderate	Anxiety: severe to panic
These views are reflected appraisals deriving from input appraisals from people and experiences that were the most *frequently recurring* designations, definitions of self and *perceived* as me – i.e., approved.	These views are reflected appraisals derived from input appraisals from people and experiences that were infrequently occurring designations, definitions of self and *perceived* as disapproved.	These view are reflected appraisals derived from input appraisals from people and experiences that occurred rarely, were connected with great pain, punishment or panic, and *perceived* as aspects of self to be ignored or be indifferent to.
In psychiatric patients these views tend to be mainly derogatory, destructive to self-development.		In psychiatric patients these views tend to be ones in accord with capacities for self-affirmation and for constructive self-development.
Sets up situations to confirm and get affirmation of others of these self-views.		Sets up situations to maintain exclusion of these views from awareness.

Figure 5.6 Major components of self-systems

Interrelated functions	*Contents*
Sustain integration of self-system	Self-views
Maintain equilibrium and stability	Self-images

Prevent anxiety
  Police attention; and audit and edit
  errors and slips of tongue
	Self-worth
	Self-respect
	Self-esteem

Monitor relation between focal attention and security operations (patterns of relief behaviour)	Stature Status
Manage incongruence, i.e., conflict among self-system contents	Prestige
Maintain boundaries between self-in- awareness, selectively, inattended contents, and dissociated contents of self	Supervisory personifications (if not edited out)
Allow acceptable incremental revisions and avoid massive change in self- system	
Monitor self in interpersonal interactions to gain confirmation of self- system contents and to maintain exclusion of dissociated self-views	

sonal relationships throughout life. Mead (1934) suggested that '. . . selves exist only in relation to other selves', that individuals have within-person concepts, the 'generalized other', by which they imagine the views and reactions of others in relation to their own behaviour. This conception is in accord with Sullivan's (1956) later definition of interpersonal relations. The lonely isolate who hallucinates invented figures does so, in part, so that his self-system relation to other selves can be maintained, and he draws his characterizations of the figures from the incorporated generalized other.

Origins of the self-system Infants are not born with a self-system, which is an anti-anxiety system evolved as a product of socialization. Infants do bring their own resources – inborn capacities and tendencies – into the interactions they have with socializing agents, the first of which are their primary care-takers. These resources include genetic endowment, gender, temperament, body characteristics and body build, bodily rhythm, a level of capacity for intelligence, various capacities such as for speech, hearing, vision, and bodily movement. In a self-system that functions constructively there is, at least in adulthood, awareness and acceptance of the nature of one's resources and a match between them and operative self-views that are held in awareness. At birth, however, these resources are merely potentials, capacities that are transformed (or fail to be) into interpersonal, intellectual, and other social competencies as are required for social living within a community.

At birth, the most important ability which an infant has is the ability to cry. This pre-speech instrumental ability is the only one which the infant has to call the attention of others to his needs for food, warmth, and other forms of comfort. The responses to the infant's cry, of the mothering one, parenting ones, primary caretakers and/or significant others begin the process by which the infant evolves a self-system.

The structure of the self-system process, its phases and steps, are of particular interest to psychiatric nurses. When nurses assist psychiatric patients to become aware of and to revise the contents of their self-systems, the same structure and the same sequence of its phases as these evolved in infancy are utilized. The process evolves in the following manner (see Fig. 5.7).

Sullivan (1956) claims that the self is an anti-anxiety phenomenon having its earliest roots in mother–infant interaction in the feeding situation early in life. The interactive sequences during the first few weeks of life go like this: the infant cries, signalling an operative need; the mothering one responds, accurately inferring and then meeting the infant's need; mutual satisfaction is felt by both infant and mother, both of whom have had their different but complementary needs met. However, at some time during this same time period a change occurs. The sequence now goes like this: the infant cries, signalling an operative need; the mothering one responds as before except that this time the mothering one is anxious; using an inborn capacity for empathic observation, the infant feels the anxiety as extreme visceral discomfort and stops feeding and instead cries more; the mother's anxiety increases; the infant now evolves new, unique, adaptive behaviours: he cries until exhausted and sleep occurs, or he cries, eats, cries, and then vomits. In this sequence, both infant and mother are left with their needs unsatisfied.

It is assumed that the infant discriminates between the differences in the two sequences just described, at the level of feelings, sorting them in some way into felt satisfaction and felt discomfort. Thus, the infant, perceiving a felt relation, sees the mothering one in two ways: as good mother and as bad mother, and himself as good me and bad me. The main question, in terms of the developing self-system, is: which sequence becomes the prevailing, recurring, expected experience? It can be taken for granted that all mothers will experience anxiety at some point during the feeding experience; other questions are: how frequently and to what degree?

Infants go through a period of pre-speech vocalizations and then the

Figure 5.7 Components of evolving self-systems: process and nursing applications

Process components	*Nursing applications*
1. Felt relations: Infant feels satisfaction and shares mutual satisfaction with mother in feeding situation	1. Nurse evokes trust in patient, as a felt relation, as the patient perceives that the nurse does what she promises the patient that she will do.
2. Empathic observation: Infant feels mother's anxiety in the feeding situation.	2. Nurse controls her own anxiety and assists patient toward control of this anxiety (Fig. 5.2).
3. Input appraisals of defining others Child hears appraisals, repeats appraisals verbatim, incorporates appraisals of others as his own views – which are now reflected appraisals.	3. The form and language of the nurse's questions and comments are investigative, thereby not colliding with or confirming self-views of patient. Nurse inputs are unfamiliar to patient who experiences anxiety; nurse applies Fig. 5.2 and then repeats investigative input. Patient hears nurse input. Patient incorporates nurse input as his own stimulus to enquire and think about his circumstances; nurse inputs are reflected back by patient.
4. Actions to go with reflected appraisals (self-views) are acquired.	4. Patient gradually acts on incorporated investigative nurse inputs.
5. Sets up situations to maintain contents of the self-system.	
6. Supervisory personifications are incorporated.	

capacity for language development ripens. Most parents are eager for their children to talk, they encourage verbalization, and eventually children say 'mama' or 'dada'. At this point, perhaps more so with first-born children, most parents respond verbally and with attention, pride, pleasure, and approval. On the basis of a felt relation (a connection experienced at a feeling level rather than as a thought) the child recognizes that something important has occurred. In order to call out similar parental responses the child tries harder and more often to hear, form, and say the words which adults in the situation use.

As the child becomes mobile, the adults make more defining statements about the child which are designations of the child and estimates or appraisals of the child's ability or worth. The toddler pays attention to these input appraisals of significant others for otherwise he has no views of himself. These become the initial contents for his self-system. The mode of imitative learning is used along with ability to focus attention as the toddler hears and repeats verbatim what others say that seemingly refer to him. For example, the parent says 'Johnny is a bad boy'. Gradually, the toddler incorporates the input appraisals. This occurs through revision of the language used, with adult help, in three observable steps: the child will reflect back (1) 'Johnny is. . .,' (2) 'me is. . .,' then (3) 'I am. . .'. When the personal pronoun I is used, the defining input appraisals of others have been incorporated, have become beginning contents of the self-system, and have been accepted as baseline self-views.

The child now begins to watch in order to notice those behaviours which he uses that evoke specific defining appraisals from adults; by watching and by trial-and-error he gets the actions that go with the appraisals of adults which now are self-views incorporated into the self-system. The tendency thereafter is to set up interactive situations with adults which are more rather than less likely to confirm and maintain the reflected self-appraisals.

Self-system maintenance involves the prevention of anxiety by accepting appraisals into the existing system that are congruent with already incorporated views. Revision is possible but anxiety is experienced with it. Important as this early period is in laying down a baseline of self-views, every subsequent major new experience – entering school, various church activities, getting into a peer group, having a chum, being hospitalized, getting into college, various achievements or failures, marriage, etc. – has the potential for forcing changes, constructive or not, in the self-system.

Child rearing and childhood education involve the use of three major patterns in the behaviour of adults toward children, namely approval (praise, compliment, reward), disapproval (blame, punish, rebuke, castigate), and indifference (ignore, banish, dismiss, reject, ostracize, expel, abandon). Very young children do those things of which they are capable, the pleasure being in the discovery and use of their capability. In these matters they are often unaware of risks and dangers that may be involved. Parents and teachers, on the other hand, know the possible untoward consequences of some child actions and so they interfere and begin to shape the child's behaviour, using one of the three patterns. For children, in general, it is more comfortable for them to be liked, rather than disliked or not noticed. They tend to work for approval, that is, to please parents and to be what parental defining inputs suggest.

Parents and teachers use disapproval to force the child to give up disapproved behaviour and behave in ways that adults want, expect, and can approve. Hochschild (1986, p. 57) has written a poignant biography in which he describes the awesome, lingering effects of parental disapproval experienced in the absence of directly expressed affection and approval. However, when disapproval becomes the recurring, predominant pattern of the adults, some children lose hope or interest in gaining approval and instead tend to work for disapproval. This tendency is commonly seen in psychiatric patients. Similarly, the child who commands almost no attention, being treated with indifference by adults, is also very likely to work for disapproval. To be ignored imputes the self-view 'I am nobody' on the child, an anxiety-evoking experience; at the least, being punished implies being noticed for something. Very withdrawn psychiatric patients however tend to accept indifference and to make it a mutual pattern integration – they ignore others who ignore them.

Thus approval, disapproval, and indifference by adults – upon whom the child is in some way dependent – impact on the child's evolving self-system. They are in effect input appraisals and they become self-system contents in the same way: they are heard (noticed), incorporated, reflected back as self-appraisals, and actions to confirm these self-views are acquired. (As a folk-saying puts it: 'You get the name and then get the game'.)

The point needs to be emphasized that what gets up front in awareness as accepted, owned, self-views, consists in the most frequently recurring appraisals (see Fig. 5.5). Toddlers and young children think 'that's me' in terms of what adults say they are, and in terms of their own experiences. It is in this sense, to the child, that adult verbal appraisals such as you are stupid, you can't do that, bad, etc., and teacher as well as self-appraisals derived from personal failure in efforts toward achievement – as in physical activities and school work – are perceived as approved views. The disapproval or indifference of others, adults and peers, becomes approved self-views (as in psychiatric patients), when the evolving individual accepts these appraisals as 'that's me – I'm stupid, I'm a failure, I can't do anything.' It is important to note the distinction between what others, external to the psychiatric patient approved, disapproved, or ignored, and what the patient, earlier in life, perceived, internalized, classified, and incorporated into his self-system.

The destructive effects of input appraisals of adults that have been primarily derogatory in content, incongruent with inborn capacities, and of a preponderant use of disapproval or indifference, as patterns used by parents and teachers, especially early in the child's life, can most clearly be seen in psychiatric patients, juvenile offenders, and prisoners.

The significant persons in the life of a growing child are also incorporated into the self-system as supervisory personifications; a Sullivanian term. Parents particularly, but also other adults significant to the growing child, supervise their children by telling, warning, ordering, forbidding, punishing, and by conveying principles or other guidelines for living. Later on, in the absence of these significant others, most children recall both the parental figure (or teacher, or clergy, etc) and the guidelines, and utilize these incorporated inputs in making judgements and decisions, particularly in stressful situations. This is useful in that children, some more so than others, up to reaching adulthood, become more aware of the risk element in situations they get into. This identification with parents should be transitory, so that when full adulthood is reached the supervisory personifications are edited out. Actions are then based upon self-discipline and responsibility, and not on 'my mother told me to...'.

Psychiatric patients invariably sustain autistically controlled interpersonal relationships between themselves and their incorporated supervisory personifications. This remnant of earlier self-system development is employed in the production of hallucinations. It is also an anxiety-maintaining phenomenon, especially when the parent (now an illusory supervisory figure) peppered the guidelines given to the patient as a child, with shoulds, oughts, musts, cannots, don'ts and the like, and without practical instructions to go with these injunctions. These words generally accompany expectations that were and still are unlikely to be met by the individual.

Stability within the self-system also requires a sorting out of incongruent views into separate categories, the figurative boundaries between them being a function of attention and its relation to the overall anti-anxiety performances of the self (see Fig. 5.5.). Those self-views which have been accepted into awareness, i.e., focal attention, are easily noticed, openly claimed, and comfortably expressed – usually with the use of personal pronouns such as I, me, mine. Originally, these were input appraisals, defining statements, which defining 'others' made to the person, which subsequently were accepted and incorporated into the person's self-system. These were the recurring, frequently repeated, defining statements which adults made of the infant and then of the growing child. In this sense they were perceived as approved – what others said the child was. They may have been primarily affirmative *or* destructive inputs to the child's evolving self-system. This distinction is worth noting; most so-called social rejects – prisoners, juvenile offenders, psychiatric patients – experienced an overload of destructive input appraisals early in life; these then tend to be the contents of their self-system that is up front, in awareness.

While early infancy and childhood are crucial in self-system development, all later experiences also influence the self. The growing child gains self-esteem and many competencies when acceptance by his peers is forthcoming. Age mates, especially during the first six years of school, are all seeking to establish their position – status – among peers and to gain acceptance into the peer group of their own choice. They are usually brutally frank with each other – name-calling is common. For some children, these peer definitions become self-views. Others gain strategies to avoid incorporating peer designations; the phrase sticks and stones will break my bones but names will never hurt me is one such tactic. Children often ignore or are totally indifferent to those children who act helpless and who are unable to compete, compromise, and cooperate in relation to the needs of the evolving peer group. These latter rejects may have growth-enhancing make-up experiences later on although some become isolates and vulnerable, at risk of psychiatric problems. In describing his experiences through seventh grade a scientist says 'I was *really* left out' (Wright, 1988, p. 35).

Self-worth is further influenced by success in a chum relationship (best friend) and by achievements in school, sports, and community affairs. However, the contents of self which a child brings into these opportunities, for enlargement and revision, weigh heavily in determining how situations will be set up – in the direction of success or failure, peer acceptance or rejection, or to be a winner or a loser.

Self-views are also sorted into categories called selectively inattended and dissociated. In order to prevent anxiety individuals inattend to aspects of what's going on including not noticing some of the self-system contents. These are generally self-views perceived as disapproved. The characteristic of selective inattention is that the degree of anxiety involved is minimal, so it is possible for the individual to notice whether attention is directed to it by others. Dissociation, the tendency not to notice and to be unable to do so without experiencing severe anxiety or panic, is a more difficult attention problem. The security of the self-system is maintained by not noticing these aspects of self (see Fig. 5.5).

The contents of the self-system are conveyed, wittingly and unwittingly, in relationships between people, by language usage, actions, body gestures, appearance, and the like. For instance, psychiatric patients most often will say freely, directly, 'I am no good, stupid, worthless', etc. Some prisoners say without a trace of anxiety 'I am a killer'. These statements, to which the personal pronoun I is attached, are the operative self-views of the persons involved. For most people the mere thought 'I am a killer', is so abhorrent that it raises a touch of uncanny sensation (sometimes experienced as shivering or goose bumps). Since it collides with and is inadmissible to self-views in awareness it is a dissociated, not-me self-view.

Contents of self-system   The major contents of the self-system include the following:

Self-views are definitions, conceptions, of oneself, which consist in the base-line reflected appraisals, inputs originally from caretakers early in life, and incremental additions, elaborations, and revisions resulting from the person's subsequent life experiences. Aims, attitudes, opinions, goals, etc are also among these contents (see Fig. 5.6).

Self-images are imagined pictures of oneself, drawn from memory or fantasy, which are projected onto or otherwise conveyed to the outside world. Images are generally representations of how one wishes to be seen by others and, therefore, may not always be congruent with self-views and other self-system contents.

Self-worth is originally a by-product of an interpersonally intimate, two-person, same-sex, best friend, chum relationship, usually experienced around ages 9 to 12, in which validation of personal worth outside the family, by a peer, occurs (Sullivan, 1956). Self-worth includes the extent of personal liking or valuation of oneself, one's characteristics, talents, abilities, etc. The ability to evoke meritorious valuations from others, with regard to personal attributes, performance levels, moral or principled actions, or usefulness to others, are also aspects of self-worth. Self-worth judgements are acceptable when they are in accord with the prevailing self views. Self-respect is an ingredient of self-worth.

Self-esteem, which is an internal sense of self-regard, includes confidence in one's abilities and judgements, and serves as a measure of self-praise or the favourableness which the person attributes to himself. Estimates of self-esteem tend to be higher when the person has self-reliance, awareness of and confidence in his own powers and resources, and when there is self-determination: inner control, self-regulation and self-discipline. Self-control over one's actions and feelings requires an awareness of them in current situations, reflection on their consequences for self and others, and self-discipline in subsequent situations. No one, of course, is totally self-sufficient. Interdependence among persons is a condition of social life. But, recognizing one's separateness (and) independence, is an important aspect of self identity.

The major source of self-esteem is achievement, socially acceptable accomplishments, recognized by oneself and others, which result from using one's capabilities. *Stature*, within a field of endeavour – an occupation, profession, or social group – derives from estimates of achievements attributed by others and the importance assigned as to their merit or usefulness. Intrinsic and assigned merit are not always identical. *Status* refers to the official and informal position or rank of an individual, in relation to others, in a group such as the family, workplace, social group, and the like. Official and informal status may not be similar or identical. *Prestige* means having the personal and/or social power to command admiration or esteem of others and thereby to maintain status. Prestige includes one's reputation and ability to influence others, particularly in terms of successful achievements of interest to them.

Nursing applications   Nurses have the difficult work of aiding psychiatric patients to change their socially dysfunctional self-systems which inherently resist change. The construct presents the structure which is employed in establishing a self-system and which suggests the nursing applications (Fig. 5.7) that can be drawn from it. The work of both nurse and patient goes on during verbal interactions in nurse–patient relationships.

In this work nurses are, in effect, definers of patients. Such definitions are inherent in statements made to, about, or in response to patients. What is being suggested in this chapter is that these input appraisals of nurses be oriented primarily to the patient's capability rather than being of defining content. When a nurse says 'describe what happened' or 'illustrate that', the verbalization rests on the assumption but does not say directly that the patient has the necessary capability which the patient's response requires. If the patient doesn't respond as asked, the nurse then assumes on the basis of Figs 5.5, 5.6 and 5.7 that the input has not yet been heard – because it is unfamiliar. Later on, as the same messages are posed, the patient will hear, eventually incorporate, and make the necessary effort to describe or to illustrate. Timely repetition of such instrumental nurse inputs eventually serve the patient as internalized stimuli for self-change. It is in this sense that nurses are definers who are significantly different from the defining others who, during pre-hospitalization, applied content appraisals to the patient. The theoretical constructs regarding the phenomena to which the nurse's verbal actions are being addressed suggest the design of the nursing intervention most likely to move the patient in a remedial direction.

Verbal statements made to patients can collide with, confirm, or stimulate change in a patient's self-views. Collisions occur when what the nurse says disputes, refutes, or otherwise disconfirms a self-view which is inherent in what a patient says to a nurse. Such collision will evoke anxiety in some degree in the patient. Confirmation of a patient's self view means that the nurse's response conveyed agreement with what a patient has just said with reference to himself. This is problematic on two counts. Patients become dependent upon the nurse's agreement or praise or approval, rather than developing ability for self-evaluation. Moreover, if the patient's self-reference is derogatory, the nurse has confirmed a dysfunctional self-view. In both cases, collisions and confirmation, constructive change has not been aided in the patient.

The self-system is resistant to change; it functions to maintain the existing system. Therefore, nurse statements in relation to self-views expressed by patients should bypass the operative system. Instrumental inputs by nurses are more likely to serve this purpose. Instrumental statements serve as the means by which nurses address the components of the process rather than the contents of a patient's self-system (see Fig. 5.7). They are designed as verbal contrivances most likely to evoke interest, effort, and eventually use of latent capability for self-change by patients.

Instrumental inputs are investigative questions which are put at the point when a problematic, self-view is being presented by a patient to the nurse. Such enquiries include, but are not limited to queries such as 'When did you get that idea?', 'What's the source of that notion about you?', 'When did you first think of yourself in that way?', 'Who called you that?' (when, where, circumstances) 'Who referred to you that way?', 'What's the evidence for that self-reference?', 'Illustrate that', 'Describe one time that view applied to you.', 'What do you get out of thinking that about yourself?', 'What's the point of classifying yourself that way?', etc. Such questions require the patient to do his work – to recall, to think, to formulate, to express, and to reflect upon what he has said.

Investigative questions seek the origins of, evidence for, and purposes of patients' presenting self-views. It is quite likely that the language, form, and intent of these instrumental inputs will at first be quite unfamiliar to psychiatric patients. The prevailing tendency in social situations is to ignore or to agree, or disagree with the self-views which people present to others, rather than to investigate them. Thus, anxiety is likely to occur as the patients do not expect questions of this type. The patients' awareness and ability to name anxiety (Fig. 5.2) therefore are important antecedent factors to be accomplished. As the nurse's questions become familiar, expected words, the patient will begin to hear, incorporate, and then act in terms of these inputs. At first, this remedial effort, which proceeds quite slowly, will be primarily attempts on the part of the nurse to put the patient in a direction: toward having within himself the incorporated instruments necessary for self-change. In time, as these instruments are internalized the patient will initiate his own use of them as more generalized problem-solving tools.

Hallucinations

Introduction

Everyone has the human capacities that are employed in the development of hallucinations (see Fig. 5.9). Only those persons who have need of interpersonal relationships with illusory figures invent and sustain them. In psychiatric nursing practice hallucinations are most commonly observed in patients diagnosed as having schizophrenia although they also occur with other diagnoses such as alcoholism. There are several types of hallucinatory experience all of which involve the senses: visual (seeing invented images), auditory (hearing invented voices), gustatory (taste), olfactory (smelling invented odours), and tactile (inventing crawling things such as bugs, felt on the skin along with uncanny sensations). It is not uncommon for auditory and visual hallucinations to occur simultaneously. Auditory hallucinations are discussed in this chapter.

There are various definitions of hallucinations in the literature. Some authors refer to these phenomena as 'inner speech' (Johnson, 1978). Arieti (1959) defines hallucinations as 'an inner experience expressed as though it were an external event'. Gould's research demonstrated that halluci- nations were 'automatic speech' which employed the 'vocal musculature' (Gould, 1948, 1949, 1950). Two social workers designed and tested a tech- nique by which several patients were taught to control their voices at the point of hearing them by employing their vocal cords in activities such as talking or gargling water (Erickson and Gustafson, 1968). The nursing literature generally defines hallucinations as need-based perceptions hav- ing no basis in reality (Beck *et al.*, 1988). Nursing texts usually suggest reality testing, decoding the verbalized hallucinatory content, and express- ing doubt when patients indicate hearing voices.

Definition For purposes of this chapter, hallucinations are defined as follows: visual and auditory hallucinations consist of illusory figures, perceived as if they were real persons. Interactions between the individual and his autistically invented images or voices serve to maintain his self- system, the precarious stability of which is increasingly threatened by the effects of social isolation. The figures are invented, initially, for purposes of avoiding anxiety-evoking social situations and to mitigate loneliness. The individual attributes human characteristics to his figures drawn from data derived from past experience. These characteristics change, over time (from helping, to derogatory, to terrorizing, and then to pleasant but ever-present), their nature being determined by the person's changing circumstances – particularly, competencies which the individual loses through disuse, distortion of data due to lack of social checks and vali- dation, and the evident display of this pathology to external observers who intervene. In the absence of professional psychotherapeutic assist- ance this psychopathological process evolves toward its endpoint in chronicity (see Fig. 5.8).

Human capacities employed in hallucinations The development of hallucinated figures makes use of capacities developed early in life (see Fig. 5.9). For instance, it can be observed that children, particularly before the age of six, are able to move freely between autistically invented play and interactions with real people. For them, there is no figurative line of demarcation between fantasy and reality, interactions that involve private or public thought. Small children invent playmates, endow them with names, roles, and personal characteristics, share experiences and have conversations with them. In effect, the children thus have total con- trol of both sides of these self-and-other interactions in which one is real, the others are illusory. Moreover, there is no observable anxiety-related discomfort as the children move from the imagined to the real world, when

Figure 5.8 The hallucinatory process and nursing interventions

Phases and steps in the process	*Nursing interventions*
Phase I. Problem-solving reveries	None
1. An individual who is alone, lonely, undergoes great stress or severe anxiety, and/or feels some large and burdening responsibility.	Be aware of this as a personal experience.
2. Being unable to command attention of a real person in the situation, the individual recalls a helping person, known in the past, and thinks about the help this person would give.	
3. The memory assists the individual in enduring the stress and in at least partially resolving the stress-producing problem.	*General considerations*
4. The foregoing steps lead to a definite experience of felt relief. All steps in this phase are within the awareness of the individual.	1. Identify the phase of hallucinations. 2. Identify and name anxiety (Fig. 5.2). 3. Provide opportunities with real people to mitigate loneliness.
Phase II. Courting similar relief	
1. In a subsequent experience of stress, whether it be in greater or lesser degree than in the previous phase, the individual recalls that relief followed an autistic reverie about a particular helping person.	
2. In stressful and non-stressful periods the individual now sets up the situation to spend more time in private thought of like kind.	Observe tendency toward withdrawal.
3. The increased time spent in isolation from people – particularly in persons who are lacking in social skills – affords additional, though temporary, relief from even minor anxiety. The relief occurs because the interpersonal strains with real people are reduced. As an aspect of courting this considerable relief, however, a listening state	Provide opportunities for development of social skills. Encourage interactions with family and friends. Observe listening state (patient alerted; face averted slightly – to hear). Provide opportunity to talk with a professional.

Figure 5.8 (cont.)

Phases and steps in the process	*Nursing interventions*
develops. Anticipatory anxiety arises of the kind: 'Will I or won't I be able to think of him today?' The answer hinges on intrusions of daily social life which must be reduced to a minimum. In search of relief from the now added anxiety more time is set aside for autistic reveries. As a result there is a consequent adaptive beginning loss of ability to control focal attention and the contents of thought, for such abilities are sharpened by use in verbal interactions with real people, rather than by private thought unchecked by others.	Observe and intervene to avoid increased moving away from real people. Intervene to reduce withdrawal time and solitary activities.

Phase III. Marked loss of ability to discipline focal awareness

1. The need for the relief afforded by the autistically invented interactions with illusory figures becomes more compelling as the time spent with real people decreases markedly. In one contact with a real person, often a family member, there is a sudden breakthrough of the autistic reverie. The individual will hear the illusory figure say something to which the person responds verbally; the family member will notice and question this behaviour, the breakthrough signals the individual's loss of control over focal attention and over the person's discrimination of the difference between private and public fields of interactive discourse.	Observe inappropriate laughter, which is appropriate to the content of the interaction of patient and illusory figure. Ask a neutral question: 'What's going on now?' Respond to such breakthroughs in the least threatening manner; provide non-threatening discussion with a professional. Schedule activities and interactions with real people to provide compelling pulls toward control over focal attention.
2. The individual feels embarrassment and shame for revealing private behaviour to another person who has called attention to it (most often in derogatory terms such as 'Are you crazy or something?').	Avoid evoking these emotions. If evoked, aid person to recognize and name them, and to connect them to their antecedents. Work on getting anxiety and loneliness named.

3. The individual now becomes more guarded and secretive, using previously acquired techniques of concealment, which every human being has developed to some extent. Concealment is used to prevent the terror of being noticed publicly again and to sustain the hope of relief through continuing use of the autistically invented relationship with illusory figures.

Use of 'thereness' instead of prying

4. More time is spent in isolation from real people. Plausible excuses such as 'I'm tired', 'I have a virus', 'I feel sick' are used to ensure maximum time for autistic activity to go on uninterrupted. As a consequence there is an even greater loss of ability to control thought, that is, to choose what to think about, to audit (notice) and edit (change) the contents of thought, now that the voices become much more definite and pop into the mind. In the sense that the individual can no longer control his thoughts (the voices) at will, the so-called voices control him (i.e., splitting within the self-system, has also occurred).

Medical assessment of illness-complaints is in order.

5. There is some dim awareness by the individual and perplexity concerning the loss of ability to discipline thought (control the voices); this increases anxiety which is now almost constantly of severe degree. Terror is also felt from noticing the concern shown by others as the excessive withdrawal hallucinating behaviours become more self evident. (If the techniques of concealment work, the process in this phase may go on for years; if they do not the individual may seek therapy and if not treated as sub-human will respond quickly.)

If the individual mentions voices, ask for description of 'these so-called voices you say you hear' (i.e., separate the nurse from the patient's experience linguistically).

Figure 5.8   (cont.)

Phases and steps in the process	*Nursing interventions*

Phase IV. Failure of concealment techniques

1. Generally, when the efforts at
   concealment fail, a family member
   will hospitalize the patient. This
   procedure adds new stress and
   may give rise to panic (see Figs 5.3
   and 5.4). Hospital admission
   disrupts the individual's control of
   his situation and his inept efforts
   to obtain relief particularly from
   loneliness; it also again evokes
   embarrassment and shame and
   imposes care by strangers in a
   totally unfamiliar environment.
   Heroic measures are now needed
   to obtain relief and for the
   self-system to survive.

2. The individual has heretofore
   narrowed his adaptive powers
   down to one pattern: austistic
   reveries in isolation from real
   people. As a next adaptation,
   under the new circumstances of
   hospitalization and in the same
   direction as the previous one,
   the patient taps aspects of the
   self-system and experience having
   to do with failure (rather than
   helping); the voices now become
   derogatory, accusatory, and/or
   persecutory. This shift in content,
   and the patient's inability to edit it
   out of his thoughts, and the further
   failure to experience relief, is felt
   as terror – generally projected (the
   patient will say 'The voices
   terrorize me').

3. If the process goes on without
   corrective professional intervention
   the terror will persist – disturbing
   eating and sleeping patterns – until
   the derogatory content attributed

to voices becomes familiar and
accepted by the patient as his view
of self. Chronic patients (before the
days of psychotropic drugs) in
seclusion rooms could be heard,
at this point in the process,
pleading, negotiating, bargaining
while screaming with terror at their
voices. Finally, a compromise
would be reached: 'I won't talk to
staff if you don't leave me', etc.

---

adults address them and thus distract their attention from the invented to the actual situation. Children often re-enact parent–child scenes, taking the role of parent, for example in beating a child (doll), in order to experience what it feels like to be the beater rather than the beaten one.

Once children begin school their teachers require them, in the classroom, to give full attention to their school work. This work, which is the same subject matter for all of the pupils, may be said to be in the public mode. Private mode – autistic thought – such as imaginary play, is more or less discouraged during classroom hours. Some teachers are more lenient, others are more severe and punitive, in their efforts to get children to discipline their attention and to focus their thoughts on the common subject matter under consideration at a given time.

Teachers use various disciplinary strategies: calling on a child unexpectedly to read something; using a facial gesture of forbiddance while saying 'pay attention', or using some form of disapproval. Most children somehow adapt; they voluntarily give up private mode thought while in the classroom and focus on teacher-directed lessons. There may be lapses but if caught by the teacher the child may be subjected to humiliation and experience shame and embarrassment in front of age-mates who have become important to him. Slowly, a figurative boundary separates fantasy and reality as these powerful emotions spur the child toward more actively policing his attention. Or, they may increase feelings of inferiority, distance from peers, and new ways to act as if attending while daydreaming.

Failure to gain acceptance into a peer group of age-mates, or to successfully have a chum relationship (a best friend), as noted earlier in this chapter, or to achieve something of interest in an enduring way, makes private thought much more enticing than discussions with others of one's generation. Some of these individuals by the time of adolescence are loners. Some isolates may eventually have make-up experiences with people, find satisfaction in solitary pursuits, or otherwise be successful in some way. Still others become experts in private thought. They ex-

Table 5.9 Comparison of selected competencies and purposes of children, adults, and hallucinating patients

Pre-school children	Normal adults	Hallucinating patients
Move freely between autistically invented play and interactions with real people; no anxiety.	Maintain an imaginary boundary between fantasy and reality and are aware of fantasying when it occurs – anxiety if caught.	Loss of the figurative line between the autistic and public mode; no anxiety until voices threaten to leave.
Invent figures, endow them with human characteristics; converse with figures; take role-of-other to test roles in imagination; no anxiety; total control over all components of interaction.	Relationships with real people; some control of interaction and potential for anxiety.	Invent illusory figures using data from past experience, figures are given human character-istics, have interactions with figures; no anxiety – unless figures threaten since have total control over all components of the interaction.
Purpose: to use evolving capacities, developing ability to focus attention, testing in imagination, learning the dimensions of observed adult roles, exercising developing verbal and social abilities in safe, self-controlled situation.	Purpose: to use competencies to meet personal needs and to establish and maintain social relationships. Some social control.	Purpose: to avoid people as relief-behaviour; to attenuate loneliness by having invented interactions; to mitigate powerlessness socially by control over autistic invention.
Beginning in school years shifts interests to interactions with real people – peers, chums, adults.	Interactions with real people, in home, work, and social situations.	Isolate: invents relation-ships based upon need: (1) for help – invents helping figure; (2) derogation as failure, shame, embarrassment, occur – invents derogatory figures.

perience anxiety and loneliness (Peplau, 1964; Peplau and Perlman, 1982). They are labelled isolates, rejects or loners.

As described previously, individuals who experience high anxiety in recurring situations tend toward avoidance of such anxiety-evoking situations. Loneliness, an intense, unpleasant, affective, emotional experience, tends to drive the lonely person toward people – at any price, as observable in public places such as bars, brothels, clubs, gangs, etc. Persons who experience both of these powerful affects and have a history of spending much time in private thought, are at risk of hallucinatory experience. They are, in effect, pulled away from and toward people simultaneously, a circumstance which is initially attenuated by withdrawal and by hallucinating helping figures – a safe way initially to relieve both anxiety and loneliness.

Clinical examples of phases of hallucinations Hallucination is an interpersonal process having four phases. Each phase has its own characteristics. Each succeeding phase in the evolving process is heralded by new interpersonal circumstances which intrude and change the hallucinating person's patterns of trying to meet his needs. Those needs include avoiding anxiety, relieving loneliness, and maintaining a precariously integrated self-system. The intrusions are experienced as failure of previously effective, relief-giving concealment and autistic resolution of personal need. As with all psychopathological processes the patient cannot extricate himself from the hallucinatory experience without effective psychotherapeutic help. Therefore, in each subsequent phase in the process, the hallucinating person employs more drastic measures to obtain more desperately needed relief, but to no avail. Without psychotherapeutic intervention the process moves inexorably toward its inevitable end in chronicity.

Phase I of the process of hallucinating is illustrated in the following vignette in which an operative need for help was relieved and met by an autistic reverie. The wife of a farmer became critically ill in the middle of the night. Her husband and their three children drove her to the hospital, quite a distance from their farm. At the hospital, the husband attended to arrangements for his wife's care, with staff, the physicians and nurses. He left his nine-year-old daughter in charge of her siblings, ages 4 years and 1 year, in the waiting room alone. The two younger children were very irritable and crying, and the nine-year-old felt her great burden of responsibility and was very worried about what might happen to the children and her mother. Then, she remembered a girl she knew at church – they used to talk amiably together when she went to Sunday school. She invented a conversation with her remembered friend, consulted her on what to do to comfort her small siblings, and sought her approval for actions taken. All went well. At daylight the father returned and was pleased that the children were alright.

An eleven-year-old schoolgirl's experience illustrates phase II in the hallucinatory process, her need evolving out of her failures in earlier developmental events and a very deprived socio-economic home situation. On arrival in the office of the school nurse, Mary asked: 'May I talk with you about something that's bothering me?' Mary then told the school nurse: 'There is this other girl who goes everywhere with me. She sleeps in my bed, she reads my school books, she walks to school with me, she's a real friend. But now she's telling me what to do and says if I don't do it she'll go away and never come back'.

Intervention at the phase II point in the hallucinatory process is most likely to be effective. In the case cited, the school nurse arranged ten talking sessions with Mary, during which she discussed her need for real friends, her difficulties in making them, and the way in which she recalled and courted an illusory, make-believe friend. The school nurse also talked with the schoolteachers and the child's mother, and without revealing to them the confidential data obtained in her talks with Mary, she made suggestions to them about including Mary in school group activities, and for talks between Mary and her mother during shared activities at home.

Phase III of the hallucinatory process evolves when interventions into phase II have not been carried out, or have not been effective, or when the occurrence of phase II behaviour has not been recognized as such by persons who could be helpful. It is at this point that withdrawal behaviour becomes most prominent. It is not the withdrawal behaviour *per se* that is problematic, but rather what goes on during such retreats from the social scene. Since the individual has felt helpless in regard to having some felt power and control in social situations with real people, interactions with autistically invented figures become more attractive. The person exercises much ingenuity in finding time, places, and excuses that seem plausible to others, in order to be alone. In other words, he/she sets up situations to court and to have extensive interpersonal interactions with one or more illusory figures. In so doing, what is missing that would ordinarily be provided by real people is checking, challenging, validating or invalidating the highly private thought which the person is using exclusively, thereby having total power and control over self and invented others. This experience relieves the previously felt helplessness and powerlessness.

The problem that arises, however, as a consequence of disuse, is the loss of control over the contents of awareness. This is manifested when so-called voices arrive uninvited by the person, 'pop into mind', and conversations with them are held so as to be heard; often this occurs in the presence of other people. As one patient put it, 'I was outblued' (the nurse, at first mentally spelled this verbalization as 'outblewed', and decoded it as a blowout, but then she asked the patient to spell the word, at which point the patient also told her that the 'voice came in out of the blue').

Whereas previously the person was able to conceal interactions with figures when real people entered his situation, with a beginning loss of control over focal attention his efforts at such concealment fail to work. Anxiety, shame, and embarrassment rather than relief are felt when a real person observes the individual's hallucinatory behaviour. These powerful emotions call out an even greater need for relief from such overwhelming discomfort, which is achieved by almost complete withdrawal from real life situations.

Phase III is a very good time for interpersonal intervention, particularly by a professional who is thoroughly knowledgeable about the free constructs presented in this chapter and one who uses an investigative psychotherapeutic technique (Field, 1979). Great increases in shame and embarrassment, the escalation of anxiety into panic, and enormous fear generally occur when hospitalization occurs at this point, making the relief-giving symptoms even more important to the survival of the person as he/she perceives it. The careful use of psychotropic drugs to take the edge off anxiety is helpful. Long-term help, however, requires psychotherapeutic work and social interaction by persons sensitive to what is going on in the thought processes of a very troubled person.

Without effective intervention psychopathological processes continue to evolve toward an end point of chronicity. Phase IV, in which the person's loss of control over focal awareness is almost complete, means that inappropriate behaviour – such as talking to so-called voices – becomes quite obvious to all observers. With increasing anxiety, more felt shame and embarrassment, and a dimly perceived sense of failure of patterns of relief behaviour that had previously worked, derogatory elements of the self-system come into play. The so-called voices, previously helpful and friendly, now become angry, threatening, and derogatory. The voices threaten to go away, make demands, and terrorize the individual who now becomes quite confused. Survival looms as the major goal. Hospitalization generally occurs at this point. The people who observe such irrational behaviour usually become very anxious and fearful; their expectation to maintain the figurative boundary between public and private mode thought and behaviour is being threatened. The hallucinatory individual empathizes the anxiety of others which tends to increase his own and quite frequently panic ensues. All too often the hallucinating individual at this point converts his escalating anxiety into enormous rage, acted out as violence, and requiring physical restraints applied by others.

The end point of phase IV generally is reached during hospitalization. Ineffective available treatments, insufficient knowledge, insufficient or unqualified staff, staff unable to use current knowledge fully, and unwitting symptom-reinforcement (illness-maintenance) by persons in the patient's environment all are aspects in the production of the patient's chronicity. For the patient, the need for relief from terror is very great. This is achieved by the patient's reaching compromises with his so-called voices. These compromises – negotiations – are along the lines of 'I won't...if you won't'. Most frequently, the patient promises not to talk with or obey the hospital staff if the so-called voices don't derogate, threaten to leave, or make demands. Since the patient is in charge of his part and that of his autistically invented figures in this interpersonal transaction, it could be said that the patient achieves peace with himself – but forever remains mentally ill.

Nursing interventions   There are some general guidelines for working interpersonally with patients who hallucinate (see Fig. 5.8). For the patient, the experience of hearing voices (or, less frequently also seeing illusory figures) seems real; however, the nurse knows from the theoretical construct that they are illusory figures autistically invented for the twin purposes of avoiding anxiety and mitigating loneliness. This distinction between the patient's and nurse's perception should be clearly emphasized in what the nurse says to the patient. For example, when a nurse says 'tell me about the voices' she has, in effect, linguistically accepted the voices as real. It is possible to maintain the distinction when the nurse says 'tell me about these so-called voices of yours', or 'talk about the voices you say you hear', or 'when did you first notice these so-called voices of yours?' These verbalizations are cumbersome. Their merit is threefold: it lies (1) in shedding doubt on the reality of the hallucinatory figures; (2) in attributing them solely to the patient – the nurse neither confirming nor denying them, and therefore not agreeing to their reality; and (3) in keeping the perceptions of nurse and patient completely separate. If the nurse uses verbal inputs such as suggested, sustaining the message but varying the language, eventually the patient will hear, incorporate, and act on – that is, begin to question or doubt – the reality of his/her so-called voices.

Sometimes, particularly with patients in phase IV, the so-called voices interfere and tell the patient not to talk to the nurse; patients tend to convey that message. A useful nurse response is some variant of: 'You tell your so-called voices they have 23 hours of your time while I have only this hour with you, so the least your so-called voices could do would be to go away while you and I talk.'

Eventually, patients must dismiss their voices – which they can and will do only after they have generated awareness of their anxiety and loneliness, and of their behaviour responses to these powerful energizers. Usually many hours of therapeutic work precede dismissal of voices in phases III and IV. In the meantime, along with and not as a substitute for therapy, engaging patients in physical activities with staff and with other patients – such as throwing a ball – is remedial, for this engages their attention in watching for the ball in play. Talking about anything helps as it is almost impossible to hallucinate while talking with another person.

The way out of their trapadaptation is long, and the work is difficult and can be accomplished only when knowledgeable, sustained professional assistance is provided for hallucinating patients.

Summary

Three complex interpersonal constructs have been presented. Pragmatic definitions and nursing applications have been supplied, along with partial descriptive information regarding each term.

References

American Nurses' Association. (1980) *Nursing: A Social Policy Statement*, ANA, Kansas City, MO.

Arieti, S. (1959) Schizophrenia: the manifest symptomology, the psychodynamic and formal mechanism, in *American Handbook of Psychiatry*, Vol. 1, (ed. S. Arieti), Basic Books, New York, pp. 455–84.

Beck, C. K., Rawlings, R. P. and Williams, S. R. (1988) *Mental Health – Psychiatric Nursing*, Mosby, St Louis.

Bouwsma, W. J. (1988) *John Calvin: A Sixteenth Century Portrait*, Oxford University Press, New York, pp. 32–47.

Burd, S. and Marshall, M. (1963) *Some Clinical Approaches to Psychiatric Nursing*, Macmillan, New York.

Cooley, C. H. (1902) *Human Nature and the Social Order*, Charles Scribners' Sons, New York (reprinted in 1964 by Schocken Books).

Erickson, G. D. and Gustafson, G. J. (1968) Controlling auditory hallucinations. *Hosp. Comm. Psych.*, **19**, 327–9.

Field, W. E., Jr. (1979) *The Psychotherapy of Hildegard E. Peplau*, PSF Productions, New Braunfels, TX.

Gecas, V. (1982) The self-concept. *Annu. Rev. Socio.*, **8**, 1–33.

Gordon, M. (1985) *Manual of Nursing Diagnosis*, McGraw-Hill, New York.

Gould, L. N. (1948) Verbal hallucinations and activity of vocal musculature. *Am. J. Psych.*, **105**, 367–72.

Gould, L. N. (1949) Auditory hallucinations and subvocal speech: objective study in a case of schizophrenia. *J. Nerv. Mental Dis.*, **109**, 418–27.

Gould, L. N. (1950) Verbal hallucinations as automatic speech: the reactivation of dormant speech habit. *Am. J. Psych.*, **107**, 110–19.

Hochschild, A. (1986) *Half the Way Home*, Viking–Penguin, New York.

Johnson, F. H. (1978) *The Anatomy of Hallucinations*, Nelson-Hall, Chicago, pp. 1–40.

Kim, M. J., McFarland, G. K. and McLane, A. M. (eds) (1987) *Pocket Guide to Nursing Diagnosis*, 2nd edn, Mosby, St Louis.

King, I. M. (1981) *A Theory of Nursing*, John Wiley, New York.

Mead, G. H. (1934) *Mind, Self, and Society*, University of Chicago Press, Chicago.

NANDA (North American Nursing Diagnosis Association) (1987) *Classification of Nursing Diagnosis: Proceedings of the Seventh National Conference*, Mosby, St Louis.

Parsons, T. (1961) *Theories of Society*, Vol. 1, Macmillan, New York.

Peplau, H. E. (1955) Loneliness. *Am. J. Nurs.*, **55**, 244–8.

Peplau, H. E. (1963) Interpersonal relations and the process of adaptation. *Nurs. Sci.*, **1**, 272–9.

Peplau, H. E. (1964) Professional and social behavior: some difference worth the notice of professional nurses. *Quarterly* (published by the Columbia University Presbyterian Hospital School of Nursing Alumni Association, NYC), **50**, 23–33.

Peplau, H. E. (1978) Psychiatric nursing: role of nurses and psychiatric nurses. *Int. Nurs. Rev.*, **25**, 41–7.

Peplau, H. E. (1987) Interpersonal constructs for nursing practice. *Nurs. Ed. Today*, **7**, 201–8.

Peplau, H. E. (1988) *Interpersonal Relations in Nursing*, Macmillan, London, (re-issue of 1952 book).

Peplau, L. A. and Perlman, D. (1982) *Loneliness: A Sourcebook of Current Theory, Research, and Therapy*, John Wiley, New York.

Roy, C. (1984) *Introduction to Nursing: An Adaptation Model*, 2nd edn, Prentice Hall, Englewood Cliffs, NJ.

Sears, D. O., Peplau, L. A., Freedman, J. L. and Taylor, S. E. (1988) *Social Psychology*, 6th edn, Prentice Hall, Englewood Cliffs, NJ.

Sullivan, H. S. (1956) The interpersonal theory of mental disorder in *Clinical Studies in Psychiatry*, (eds H. S. Perry, M. L. Gawel and M. Gibbon), W. W. Norton, New York, pp. 3–11.

Tuma, H. and Maser, J. D. (eds) (1985) *Anxiety and the Anxiety Disorders*, Lawrence Erlbaum Associates, Hillsdale, NJ.

Wright, R. (1988) Did the universe just happen? *Atlantic Monthly*, **261**, 29–44.

Wylie, R. (1974) *The Self Concept*, revised edn, Vol. 1, University of Nebraska Press, Lincoln, NB.

Chapter 6

General systems model: principles and general applications

S. A. SMOYAK

Overview

How one views the world is a complex outcome of both primary and secondary socialization processes. Psychiatric nurses need to know not only how their clients, patients or families view the world, but how they, themselves, see things. It is very useful for nurses, who choose to work with the complicated, multidimensional natures of human personalities, to also know about themselves. In this chapter, the aim is not to provide material about how primary socialization shapes and forms the human personality, but rather to focus on the secondary socialization process – how our education, as professionals, leads us to think in particular ways about how the world works, and how the human personalities within it think, feel and act.

Basic nursing curricula include views of human behaviour and psychosocial functioning selected from the fields of psychology, social psychology, psychiatry, anthropology and sociology. Theories in these fields are relatively new, having emerged only in this century, and they are quite diverse in terms of scope and explanatory foci. Before explicating the manner in which general system theory (von Bertalanffy, 1956; 1968) can serve as a useful theoretical base for psychiatric nurses, a very short history of the available theories in the earlier part of this century will be presented. Then systems concepts will be described and discussed. Specific applications will follow, derived from clinical cases.

Earlier theories to explain human behaviour

Background

Before the development of scientific theories to explain human behaviour, there were many directions, admonitions, principles and rules suggested by classic writings. For example, in Genesis, in the Bible, the story about Noah's sons, and what they did when they found him lying naked and drunk outside his tent, gives direction for how fathers and sons are supposed to relate to each other. The two sons, who laughed at his drunkenness, and did not choose to help or to be respectful, are portrayed as deviant and certainly not humane. The son who provided consideration and care is the one we are told to emulate. The focus of the story is filial respect, and how this assures the continuity of care in families; the moral of the tale is not that drunkenness is to be condoned, as some might be tempted to conclude.

Also in the Bible, in Leviticus, there is a tale about how conflicts in marriages ought to be handled. Here, the story is ostensibly about keeping a fire in a hearth burning brightly, and how this can be assured by cleaning out the ashes daily and making sure that there is an adequate foundation for the fire. Couples who prefer to keep all the ashes in place, never shovelling them out, can predict difficulty (less warmth and light) in the marriage.

Themes of how family issues and couples' relationships ought to be handled, and what happens when agreed-upon or tradition-driven norms and values are violated, appear in the works of great writers such as Dostoyevsky and Shakespeare. In fact, some graduate courses in family therapy begin with an examination of these early roots of family dynamics in literature.

Intrapsychic, or psychoanalytic theories

The first scientific theories to explain human behaviour appeared in the literature at the turn of this century. The earlier textbooks for psychiatric nurses gave a synopsis of the work of Freud and his followers, which actually provided very little practical help in the day-to-day management and care of acutely and chronically ill psychiatric patients. Freud's theories were rooted in very early developmental moments of infants and children, and were deterministic in their design. The operative ideas suggested that specific early trauma produced specific later, troubled outcomes. Further, the nature of the concepts was abstract and not directly observable, thus requiring interpretation, inference and judgement on the part of the clinician choosing to use these in practice with patients. Freud's theories were read and quoted widely in the Western world, and were almost the only available source of understanding and influence in psychiatry for the first two decades of this century.

Libido, superego, ego and id, while not visible directly, were presumed to be necessary for clinicians to use as operative explanatory constructs. Nurses were supposed to know what these concepts meant, but were taught that only more knowledgeable professionals, such as psychiatrists and psychoanalytically-trained psychologists, could apply them in practice situations with patients. Unfortunately, severely ill psychiatric patients could not be treated by analytic methods. In mental hospitals and asylums, as they were called then, nurses relied on basic skills learned in fundamentals classes, and concerned themselves with keeping the environment safe, and providing a physical and social milieu where natural healing could occur.

When psychoanalytic theories were the only explanatory ideas available, no one scrutinized the behaviour of nurses or other professionals in terms of the potential impact of their behaviour on the course of the client's illness. The illness was presumed to have occurred in the far past of the patient's life; psychoanalytic techniques and strategies merely made these early traumas available to recall and rethinking. No one, for the first half of this century, thought that nurses or others could actually create or maintain an illness in a psychiatric patient, or make matters worse for the patient by what the care provider said.

Psychiatric treatments which were provided in in-patient settings had very little to do with the psychoanalytic concepts. Strategies to contain bizarre behaviours were used pragmatically; these included physical restraints of various kinds, isolation and seclusion, and calming devices such as hydrotherapy or wet packs. Electro-convulsive and insulin shock treatments were also used, and criticized even then by professionals who worried about the fact that healthy tissue was being damaged, that the treatments were frightening, and that patients really disliked them greatly, but felt helpless to object.

Interpersonal theories

World War II was the impetus for some very practical changes in the way psychiatrists treated military men who became psychiatrically disabled. Rather than taking intrapsychic approaches, strategies closer to the present time were used, basing the analysis and treatment in the here and now. Grinker and Spiegel, in *War Neuroses*, described their discovery that commanding officers were precipitants of psychiatric casualties, and that group processes could be helpful in ferreting out the present connection to past faulty learning. The search for causes of psychic distress or mental illness shifted from the very far past, intrapsychic area (the mind, abstract constructs) to the present, where interactive phenomena could be directly observed, classified and organized into hypotheses about specific dysfunctions.

In the United States, the National Institute for Mental Health, a federal government agency, was created in 1946. Through this agency, scientists were funded to pursue study of the causes of schizophrenia and other severe mental illnesses. Bateson, Jackson, Weakland, Fry, Watzlawick, Haley and Satir are recognized names in the arena of scientists developing interpersonal theories to explain dysfunctional human behaviour.

The double-bind hypothesis, connected with schizophrenic pathology, emerged in the 1950s as a very popular idea and was used widely by clinicians for the next two decades. The work of Harry Stack Sullivan was also widely quoted and used as a framework to teach psychiatric professionals to work with the mentally ill.

When interpersonal theories were applied in clinical settings, and served as the basis for treatment strategies for patients, the professionals' behaviour was also examined. The new thinking was that the professionals, engaged in therapeutic encounters with patients, were significant others and equally influential in labelling and defining behaviour as the patients' earlier significant others, such as mother, father, relatives and other authority figures.

Psychiatric nurses used interpersonal theories in in-patient and community settings, and published reports of their work in journals and books. The most often quoted and most highly regarded work of this period was published in a book edited by Smoyak and Rouslin (1982): *A Collection of Classics in Psychiatric Nursing Literature*. Hildegard E. Peplau is recognized as a key figure in the development of the clinical practice of psychiatric nurses; her analysis of the historical developments in psychiatric nursing appears in the collection.

The emergence of systems thinking

When the only scientific theories about human behaviour available to nurses and others who work directly with patients were framed and focused as inside the mind or between persons, the view was necessarily very limited. Systems thinking allows a broader, more encompassing view of why people do as they do within families and also in other contexts. The earlier dyadic conceptualizations limit the analysis to one person and an interacting other; systems thinking captures entire units, or holons, as the field for analysis.

Ludwig von Bertalanffy, born in Austria in 1901, was a leading contemporary biologist, with wide-ranging scientific and cultural interests. His first works appeared in the twenties and were devoted to problems of growth and form, the theory of organic gestalt, and general philosophical problems in biology. In the first issue of a journal, *General Systems*, which began being published in 1956, von Bertalanffy states: 'General systems theory is a new discipline whose subject matter is the formulation and derivation of those principles which are valid for systems in general.' He defines a system as sets of elements standing in interaction. The theory is a logical–mathematical field which deals with scientific doctrines of wholeness, dynamic interaction, and organization.

General systems theory was not formulated by von Bertalanffy all at once, but rather emerged from a long and interesting evolution of views, including two major concepts, organismic biology, about which he wrote in 1928, and the theory of open systems, appearing in 1932. The concept of general systems theory (referred to by him as general system theory) was not published until 1945. It received almost instant receptivity among scientists in many fields, since a new climate had emerged wherein model building and abstract generalizations had become acceptable. His work was seen as providing a bridging framework, so that specialists in diverse fields could communicate with one another. Some referred to his work as a language rather than a theory. Others called it a Meta-theory, since it provided a way to think about theories.

Overview of systems theory

Another way to view the theories categorized above as intrapsychic and interpersonal is to recognize that they are causal, if–then, or linear theories. When one thinks causally, only two or more variables can be handled at one time; when more than two are considered, they need to be grouped in chains of reasoning, or summed together, always with a sequencing structure in mind. When, as is the case with the complexity of human personalities, a large number of interacting or even unknown variables is in the field, then these causal models actually do not allow an accurate or fruitful analysis of the situation. One cannot isolate a few variables, and predict the outcome for a human being, unless there is a trivial event or overly simple formulation. To understand the interactions of biological, social, ethnic, religious, racial, and psychological factors, systems thinking is needed.

Since von Bertalanffy's efforts to provide this type of systemic approach, applications and extensions of his work have burgeoned. Probably the best known application of general systems theory to psychiatry has been the collected work of Gray, Duhl and Rizzo (1969) where contributors, including Menninger, Arieti, Miller, Ruesch, Scheflen, Marmor, Paul and Laqueur, described their particular uses and elaborations of the original work.

In this chapter, the social interaction theories of Harry C. Bredemeier are used in an integrative fashion in order to demonstrate the application of the modified theory to the understanding of normal and troubled families. In the next section, basic systems principles will be described, followed by the paradigms adapted from Bredemeier.

Systems principles

1. The whole is greater than the sum of its parts Probably no systems principle has been repeated more often than this one, or is so poorly understood by lay people and professionals alike. What it means is that there is an entity, a quality, an abstract essence in a system which cannot be understood as simply an additive, mechanistic operation. Some attempts at explicating this idea take the approach: two plus two sometimes equal five. That is a step in the right direction, but still conveys a summing or linear, as opposed to a systems, idea.

The key to understanding this principle is to see the 'greater than' as symbolizing 'organization'. Parts of anything, without organization, remain just parts. They become an identifiable system only when they are organized.

Consider an old-fashioned watch or timepiece, the kind with gears and wheels and springs, instead of chips. If a watch-maker were to take the watch apart, and place all the parts on a table, it would no longer be a watch. Even if the watch-maker arranged the parts artfully and aesthetically, or glued them down, or put them in a container, it would not be a watch. It becomes a watch only when organized in a particular way; the organization makes it recognizable as a system, a watch.

To use another non-living system example, musical notes written on a page are not a musical piece or tune; they become one only when organized in a fashion agreed upon by other musicians. Ballerinas standing about in costume on a stage become an identifiable system when organized by music and a choreographer's instructions.

Since this chapter is about living systems, all other examples will be from that domain. However, bear in mind that systems principles can be applied to any system, living or non-living, and at any degree of size and complexity. Physicists today use systems language when they talk about quarks, and astronomers use systems theories in considering planet and star problems.

2. Rules of organization Systems theorists and clinicians working with troubled human systems have found it useful to describe the concept discussed above as a set of rules by which the parts of the system, or players, or actors, or family members arrange themselves. Rules of organization are not directly visible, yet they can be relatively easily inferred or discerned by asking. A family's rules of organization are determined by their culture, embodying ethnic, religious, and social factors. Tradition is a ritualized, remembered, and practised set of rules of organization which serve to place people in their proper roles, by age, gender, and generational place in the family or community. Everyone in a particular social group or family system understands these rules, and also understands how violations of them will be perceived, tolerated, dismissed or punished.

Rules of organization are what aid identification of a particular system, making it recognizable over time, even when there are numerous entries and exits of members from the original system. A hospital department, as a system, is recognizable as a very particular entity; it has its own rules of organization and a sense of continuity over time. Staff members and patients know what to expect, in terms of services offered and the general ambience of the setting. Similarly, families continue as recognizable entities through the years; one knows what to expect from the Smiths, or the Joneses, or the Reynolds. Other systems, such as football and soccer teams, university departments or national political parties are also continuous and recognizable because of these ongoing rules of organization, even though members may come and go. Through generations of births and deaths, a family's rules of organization provide a continuity of expectations, organizing them and providing meaning for their environing others.

3. Janus effect and hierarchical order   A system is a set of interacting parts, organized by rules. The boundaries or parameters of these systems vary in size and complexity; they may be as little as two small parts of something (a cell nucleus and its environment, within a cell) or may have thousands of parts, scattered geographically, as in a nation. Holon is the term used for a system under analysis; it means the interacting parts, and their boundary. The analyser, or theoretician, or clinician determines what constitutes the holon; there are no exterior methods for determining how to think of this arrangement.

A system, or holon, has sub-system parts; further, the holons, at another level of analysis, may be sub-systems of a still larger system. These system arrangements have a hierarchical order – sub-system, system and supra-system.

The concept, Janus effect, reminds the systems theorist to keep in mind that any given holon has sub-system parts, but, on the other hand, is a part, also, of a larger system, or supra-system. For instance, John may be considered as a holon; his sub-systems then might be his superego, ego and id; or, his thoughts, feelings and actions; or his respiratory, circulatory, digestive, reproductive and neurological units. John, as a holon, might be a part of a supra-system of a marriage, a nuclear family, or a family of origin. Another way of organizing the analysis would be to view John's work unit as the system or holon; then John would be a sub-system worker in that holon. The decision to view one or another level as the primary unit of analysis depends entirely on the purposes to which the analysis is to be put.

Sub-systems, systems and supra-systems are arranged in a hierarchical order. For family systems, it is tempting to think of a generation as being a hierarchy, but this is not necessarily so. An entire, two- or three-generational system may be a holon, or one hierarchical level. On the other hand, a large sibling system may have an internal hierarchical arrangement. The idea of hierarchies will become more clear when exchanges are discussed further on.

4. Depth and breadth of hierarchies The arrangements of systems, in terms of the breadth and depth of their hierarchies, yields a clue to complexity. For instance, there may be only one unit at a particular level, and hundreds at another, when the system being analysed is the governance structure of a city or nation. Most hospital systems are seven levels deep, with most work units arranged laterally with fewer than 20 sub-systems.

For the first time in history, families today may be five generations deep, if the analysis warrants viewing a generation as a level. At the turn of the century, most families had only three generations alive, and these were very likely to be organized as two-levelled decision systems. Grandparents tended to live apart from the nuclear family, and attempts were made to see them as outside the given nuclear units.

The concept of breadth and depth of the hierarchies is generally used more in organizational, agency, and institutional analyses than in family work or other dimensions of psycho-social treatment. However, when the analysis includes families interacting with school systems, or governments, or legal systems, then these ideas may be salient.

5. Adaptation In common usage, adaptation means that an object, or an act, or a process is measured or brought to bear against an external standard of some sort. For example, a two-pronged electrical plug may need an adaptor to fit a wall receptacle that has three prongs, one being an earth. Or a nursing action may be evaluated or measured against an agreed-upon Standard for Nursing Practice, or Manual of Procedures. With this sense of adaptation, the act or the object is viewed as having to be tailored to the external thing – which is presumed, in a sense, more correct or right. The idea of standard has an uprightness about it.

The idea of adaptation, however, in systems usage, has an entirely different meaning. The context is two units or sub-systems interacting with each other, by exchanging matter, energy or information. Sub-system A and sub-system B, to be adapted to each other, need to perform a series of exchanges. A diagram (see Fig. 6.1) will be helpful as a reference for the exchanges which will be described. It was first developed by Harry C. Bredemeier in the context of his theory-building in the area of understanding social interaction of systems of various size, relatedness and complexity, in the early 1960s, and has been adapted for use as a family therapy tool, to aid in the assessment of maladaptation of family units.

Sub-system A and sub-system B might be a husband and wife, or siblings, or any two members of a system engaged in a social interaction. The matter, energy and information is the what of the exchange; the amount of what exchanged also is important to consider, as is the timing. A needs to obtain matter, energy or information from B, in order to survive, or carry on, or do his or her work; A also needs to contain out from his or her sub-system those things that B would like to give over to A, but which

Figure 6.1 Social exchange paradigm

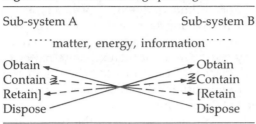

Sub-system A   Sub-system B

········matter, energy, information········

Obtain
Contain
Retain]
Dispose

Obtain
Contain
[Retain
Dispose

A does not want or need; *A* needs to retain within his or her system those things which *B* might like, but which *A* does not wish to give up to *B* (or cannot afford to), and *A* needs to dispose of to *B* those products *A* wishes to give, or energy or information. Likewise, *B* needs to obtain matter, energy or information from *A*, in order to survive, carry on, or do his or her work; *B* also needs to contain out from his or her sub-system those things that *A* would like to give to *B*, but which *B* does not want or need; *B* needs to retain within his or her system those things which *A* might like, but which *B* does not wish to give up to *B* (or cannot afford to), and *B* needs to dispose of to *A* those products *B* wishes to give, or energy or information. When the matter, energy or information that *A* and *B* each need, or need to contain out or retain in, is exchanged at the appropriate level and in the mutually desired time frame, then the two sub-systems are understood to be adapted to each other. Maladaptation occurs when any one or several of the exchanges does not occur, or is blocked, or a transaction is attempted which is not wanted by either sub-system. Neither *A* nor *B*, as sub-systems, is thought to be wrong; the error or the problem is conceived of as a faulty exchange. When clinicians employ this kind of thinking, they are able to manage a no-fault or non-blaming analysis of a difficult situation. The conflict is reframed as a systemic issue, which can be analysed and changed by the two sub-systems. *A* and *B* are less likely to continue conflictual or adversarial stances when invited to rethink the issue in exchange terms. Therapists are less likely to hold a view of intrapsychic pathology, ill-will or malevolence when using an approach which requires analysis of exchanges.

A and *B* might be a husband and wife, in a traditional marriage, who at first engage in the following exchanges. *A*, as husband, obtains from *B*, his wife, expressions of love and loyalty, and energy directed at childbearing and child-rearing activities (these are what *B* disposes of to *A*); *A* contains out of his sub-system news of the bad behaviour of the children, or trouble with tradesmen, since *B* is willing to retain in such data, classifying it as entirely her territory; *A* retains within his system fears of losing his job because of mergers at his company, and also information about his on-going interest in his secretary, while *B* is willing to contain out this knowledge, by not asking; *A* disposes to *B* a weekly pay cheque, expressions of admiration, and public acknowledgement of her household management going well, which *A* is willing to receive or obtain. Thus these two sub-systems are adapted to each other. Maladaptation may occur when either *A* or *B* changes any one or more of the exchange patterns. For instance, *B* might decide that she wants to return to school and earn a professional degree, thus requiring a different type of output or energy allocation from *A*. *A* might decide to take the information he has so far retained, that about his fears of losing his job and add this to the information he disposes of to *B*, thus interfering with what has been previously contained out of her system. The system is now maladapted and needs to be re-equilibrated.

The Social Exchange Paradigm provides a framework for analysing the substance of exchanges between sub-systems. An associated paradigm, which has as its focus the modes or the ways in which the exchanges might be handled was also developed by Bredemeier. Interacting sub-systems each try to persuade the other to comply with wishes, needs, requests and so on. In order to gain compliance, each engages in a series of tactics or strategies to convince the other that non-compliance with its needs will reduce the other's gain or profit from the continued relationship, and that compliance will improve the relationship and guarantee future fruitful interchanges. Each needs to know what the other values and respects in order for these persuasive moves to go well. These tactics or strategies are categorized into five broad groups, called modes of transaction.

The *bargaining* mode of transaction is frequently used in market-place exchanges, with markets thought of as an applicable idea for workplaces and home environments, as well as the usual commercial notion. If *A* says to *B*: 'I want you to do *X*', *B*'s question would be: 'Why should I?' A bargaining persuasive response could be: 'Because it will be well worth your while in the long run. It's a bargain you can't let go by; do this for me and you'll really be gaining a lot.'

The *legal–bureaucratic* mode of transaction is formalistic and relies on the two interacting sub-systems valuing the notion of rules, duties and job descriptions, associated with a formal status or office as in the Weberian sense of bureaucracy. If *A* says to *B*: 'I want you to do *X*', *B*'s question: 'Why should I?' would be answered in legal–bureaucratic terms, suggesting that a duty is to be performed. For example, *A* might say: 'Because it's your job – your duty. You agreed to do this as part of your work.'

The *gemeinschaft* mode of transaction is a familistic stance, wherein warmth, affection and interpersonal bonding are relied upon. If *A* says to *B*: 'I want you to do *X*', *B*'s question: 'Why should I?' would be answered by a response reminding *B* of the family bonds. For instance, *A* might say: 'Because you love me and I love you', or 'Because we're sisters.'

The *team-cooperative* mode of transaction suggests that the interacting members are part of a group or team effort to accomplish a task, which won't be completed unless the members pull together to get the work done. If *A* says to *B*: 'I want you to do X', *B*'s question: 'Why should I?' would be answered in terms of a common goal being at stake. For instance, *A* might say: 'Without you, we'll never win this', or 'I need you to help because I can't get there [goal] without you.'

The fifth mode of transaction, *coercion*, operates when the two subsystems do not belong to a larger system which has an available and operative set of rules for interacting short of force, fraud, deception or violence. It is a default category, called into play when the other four cannot be used. If *A* says to *B*: 'I want you to do X', *B*'s question, 'Why should I?' would be responded to with some type of force. *A* might say: 'Do it or I'll hurt you', or even, 'Do it or I'll kill you.'

Families tend to prefer one of the modes more than the others, but rarely use one of them exclusively. Rather, depending on the nature of the interaction and where it is taking place, one or another of the modes would be used. For example, within the family's home, parents of teenagers might be willing to bargain as a mode of transaction, but in public would rely on the gemeinschaft or the team-cooperative mode. In some cultures, married couples rely on gemeinschaft interactions, while in others legal–bureaucratic tactics might be more commonly found.

For use in systems analysis, the modes of transaction are placed on a grid, with *A*'s five choices across the horizontal and *B*'s expectations about what mode *A* ought to be using on the vertical (as shown in Fig. 6.2). If *A* and *B* agree on the mode to be used, then they are adapted to each other. When *A* is using an inappropriate mode, in *B*'s view, then the system becomes maladapted. On the diagram, it appears that there are only five chances out of 25 that the two interacting sub-systems will be adapted to each other. However, bear in mind that these interactors have probably been socialized to the same set of values and norms, including the appropriateness of the rules for conducting their interchanges. Conflicts do occur, but they are still the exception rather than the rule.

The two paradigms, together, are very useful tools for clinicians in both the assessment and treatment phases of the work with clients in the context of systems, whether those be family, school or work systems. While the clinician would not necessarily use the language of modes or exchanges *per se*, the system framework is invaluable.

In an introductory text of this type it is impossible to describe all the variants in given systems, how they operate and what the nature of the dysfunction is. What can be made clear, however, is that using systems theory as a framework for understanding what, why and how people do what they do provides a rich, non-judgement approach. Symptoms used as diagnostic signs in psychiatric diagnoses no longer can be viewed as being owned by an individual, but rather become statements about system maladaptation or signals of distress for the system.

Figure 6.2 Modes of transaction

	Sub-system A				
Sub-system B	Bargaining	Legal–bureaucratic	Gemeinschaft	Team-cooperative	Coercion
Bargaining	×				
Legal–bureaucratic		×			
Gemeinschaft			×		
Team-cooperative				×	
Coercion					×

These concepts are broad enough to be applicable to systems of any size, in any context. Their use is determined by the purposes to be served by the systems analyser, whether that person is a student, an advanced professional, or simply someone trying to understand the complexities of human beings interacting with each other in daily life.

These ideas of system maladaptation are less pejorative and blame-laying than the diagnostic systems such as ICD-9 or the DSM III-R, which are popular assessment devices in psychiatric practice. The more familiar diagnostic systems see the dysfunction as within an individual; systems analysis focuses on violations of rules and failed expectations instead.

6. Decision-making   The rules of organization, described above, may be thought of as a kind of regulator of a system's functioning. However, when the system is maladapted, or confronted with a new or different situation of some kind, decision-making functions are called into play.

In human systems, decision-making is closely related to power issues. The work of Caplow is useful as an organizing framework, allowing an analysis of power dynamics in the context of triangles.

Comparison of intrapsychic, interpersonal and systems views

An illustrative case. Mrs Jones is a 50-year-old woman, married, and the mother of two adult children, neither of whom lives at home. Her daughter has decided to drop out of college and see the world; she occasionally sends a short note from her travels. The son is divorced, is in graduate study, and is trying to manage weekend care for his five-year-old son. Mr Jones is a minister aged 62, and is considering a missionary second career in Africa, post-retirement. During the past year, Mrs Jones has gained 20 pounds, experienced sleep disorders, cries frequently, and has thoughts of ending her life.

If intrapsychic perspectives were used to explain Mrs Jones problem, she might be diagnosed as depressed, and analytic formulations used to guide her psychotherapy. The psychodynamic theories regarding the dynamic structure of depressions have their roots in Freud's early paper 'Mourning and melancholia' (1917). Freud differentiated between normal grief and depression, identifying complex mechanisms such as oral dependency, identification with a lost object, anger turned inward, and inhibition. Mrs Jones' treatment would be individual analysis and her prognosis would be guarded.

If interpersonal perspectives were used to explain Mrs Jones' problem, she might still be diagnosed as depressed, but the therapist would bring her husband into the assessment and treatment. A focus might be on how her response to his changes is a pattern learned in other relationships. Their interactive strategies with each other would be viewed as causal of her present mood state, and also as a focus for potential change.

If a systems perspective were used to explain Mrs Jones' problem, her entire family would be considered as part of the assessment strategy. The therapist doing the intake or evaluation interview would construct a genogram and use it as the basis for discovering rules of organization and patterns of maladaptation. The symptoms would be reframed as signals of distress in the family system, not as owned by Mrs Jones. The treatment would be centred around identifying and changing the system's rules of organization.

The above comparisons highlight the differences in focus and thinking among the three approaches. Further, the thinking about affective illness has been changed because of other developments since the turn of the century, beyond the psychological or socio-cultural theories. These changes include the discoveries related to genetic transmission of certain affective disorders, the discovery of psychopharmacological agents which dramatically alter depressed mood states and the experience with treating severely depressed patients outside of the hospital. The dominant principles for classifying non-organic or functional mental illnesses had been the psychotic versus neurotic distinction. This distinction is rarely used any longer, regardless of which theoretical formulation is being used by the clinician.

The three broad approaches to understanding human behaviour – intrapsychic, interpersonal and systems – can be compared by raising the question: 'Why do people do what they do?' The answer, in intrapsychic terms, is: 'Because mind determines this. In interpersonal terms, it is: 'Because people learned to interact that way'. In systems terms, it is: 'Because of the structure of the situation in which people find themselves, and the rules of organization that operate in that structure'. Here, structure is understood as the family system, with all its members and their relationships to each other considered, for all generations, even those where there may now be no living members. This family structure is best depicted using a genogram.

Use of genograms for assessment of family systems

Families are very complex systems which change structurally through time, but which are held together by unwritten, but understood, rules of organization. These rules are the collection of values, norms, traditions, rituals, religious ceremonies and rites, and day-to-day expectations regarding how things are to be done, and who may do what to whom under specified conditions or situations. The structure can best be seen by making it visible through the use of a genogram. The genogram captures all of the structural information about a family, including, for each member, age (birth date/death date), sex, ethnic/religious origin, education, and occupation. The relationships of members to each other are portrayed by using a system of hierarchically organized lines and symbols.

Genograms are used by family therapists in many treatment settings today, such as in-patient units, mental health centres and clinics; other practitioners, such as family physicians, public health nurses and social workers use the tool to aid their understanding of their clients, and to help to systematically plan treatment goals. Family sociologists use them in their basic curricular planning in universities and anthropologists use them for research purposes.

The directions for constructing genograms, as described in this chapter, were developed by Smoyak at Rutgers, The State University of New Jersey, in the course of teaching psychiatric nursing graduate students to be family therapists. The work began in the early 1960s, when students worked with the early wave of de-institutionalized mental patients and their families in a public health setting. Early versions of purple ditto or mimeographed instructions for the genogram were used widely by agency personnel. A published version appeared in *Proceedings: Brooks Air Force Base* in 1978, and an expanded version was printed in Clements and Buchanan's *Family Therapy in Perspective* in 1982.

The value of genograms over voluminous paragraphs of written histories in patient records becomes clear very quickly. It is usually possible to capture, on one 8.5 × 11 inch page, the needed data about most three-generation family systems. When there are many children, or four or more generations alive (or still very relevant to the present system), or complexities such as many divorces, remarriages and so on, then a legal-size paper or additional sheets, as extensions, can easily be used.

The following set of directions gives a synopsis of what is needed to construct the diagram. Pencil and eraser, instead of ink, will reduce the frustration of first efforts to arrange the data for the best possible representation.

General directions for constructing a genogram

1. Use a plain, white sheet of paper, turned sideways. Imagine it divided into a top, middle and bottom third, as general areas for the grandparent, parent and child generations.
2. Men are placed in squares; women are placed in circles.
3. The family name is printed above the top generation; the first name of each member is written within the square or circle.
4. Men are on the left, and women are on the right in marriages. A marriage is depicted by a horizontal, solid line. The marriage date is written on the horizontal line, preceded by an *m*. A living-together or serious dating relationship is depicted by a horizontal, broken line. A child line is a vertical, solid line from the marriage or living-together line; when more than one child is in the family, a horizontal line appears under the child line, to accommodate the others.
5. Birth dates are written, preceded by a *b*, under the square or circle.
6. Death dates are written, preceded by a *d*, under the birth date. In the square or circle, when a death occurs, a slanted line is drawn through.

7. The date on which the genogram is first constructed is written in the lower left corner, with the constructor's initials. The present age of family members in active therapy might be written under the birth date, and changed as birth dates occur.
8. A pregnancy in progress is depicted by a triangle; an aborted fetus is a triangle, with a line drawn through it.
9. Adoption is depicted by a vertical, broken line drawn from the marriage line down to the circle or square for the child. The adoption date is added, with an *a* preceding it.
10. The years of education, or final degree, are shown to the right of the square or circle.
11. The present occupation is noted to the left of the square or circle. Abbreviations can be used.
12. Twins are depicted by adding a rocker or curved line between the member symbols.
13. When a separation or divorce occurs, the date is noted above the marriage date, and two short lines are drawn on either side of the child: vertical lines if there are children, and in the middle of the marriage line if there are no children.

Depending on the uses to which the genogram will be put, the constructor can vary the information, or the way it is abbreviated, or add other notations. It is generally a good idea to first display the basic data, as described above, and then add any variations on a photocopied version, leaving the original pencil version intact. The photocopy versions can be colour-coded (for instance, all suicide attempts can be circled in red; all depressives can be coloured blue, etc).

The Jones family genogram is provided to illustrate the directions above. It represents a three-generation family system, wherein John, the second child and only son of John and Phyllis Jones, marries Jane, the second daughter of John and Mary Smith. There were twin girls born to John and Mary Smith on New Year's Day, 1945; they both died within hours of their birth. John and Jane Jones have four children, three sons and an adopted daughter. Only the daughter lives at home. Also shown on the genogram are everyone's age, educational level and occupation.

What is not shown, but could be added on a photocopy, are the people diagnosed or showing symptoms of depression. The older Mary Smith is described by her daughter, Jane, as having a life of depression. She goes on to say: 'My mother never got out of bed after the twins died; she just vegetated. My father, who was very busy with being a judge, just got various ladies from the church to come in and care for her and for us. I never saw my mother dressed up. I don't think she owns a dress!!' Her husband adds: 'When I first went to my in-laws' house, it was to discuss our wedding. Jane had told me that her mother was strange – but I

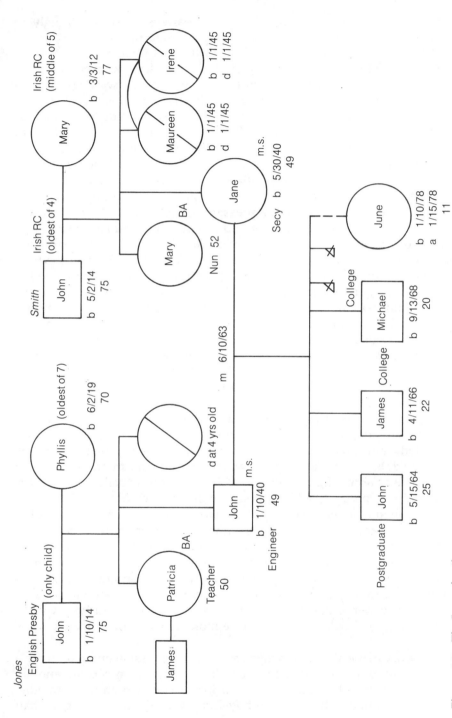

Figure 6.3 The Jones family

wasn't prepared for *that* strange!' John's parents objected strongly to his marrying Jane, but finally reluctantly gave their blessing.

John and Jane had three sons. Their births and their childhoods were uneventful. John had promotions at work, and Jane worked part-time as a secretary. When Michael was five, Jane had a miscarriage. Within a year, she had a second miscarriage. Directly after this, she began to experience night terrors and various forms of somatic distress, such as hyperventilation and tachycardia. She felt unable to work, and spent longer periods in bed. Her husband at first was sympathetic, but then demanded that she get help. When she refused, he stayed longer hours at work, sometimes not returning until everyone in the house was asleep.

Jane sought help, after about a year, from the family physician, who suggested that she take an antidepressant. After several months, on several drugs, with no lightening of mood or affect, Jane refused to take any more medication, and returned to bed. At Christmas, 1976, Mary, her older sister, a nun, visited for a two-week period. She, John and the boys badgered, cajoled, pleaded and argued with Jane about seeking another kind of help. Jane's belief was that she was destined to be just like her mother, and that nothing would help. Her husband's parents were advising him to leave, with the boys, and start a new life. Sr Mary, through her order, investigated a range of psychiatric referrals. Jane, insisting that she was not mental – but just living out God's will, refused them all. After the holidays, John and the two younger boys left to live with his parents. A tense, angry 'status quo' arrangement lasted for most of 1977. At the end of the summer, John III, the son staying at home, told his mother that one of his friends had made a girl pregnant, and that her parents were looking for a private adoption to solve the problem. Jane saw this as a message from God, and hired a lawyer to arrange the necessary legal work. The girl's due date was January 1, 1978, which, for Jane, meant more than ever that God was arranging this for her. Baby Jane was actually born January 10th, and was brought to Jane's house within the week.

Rather than that being the end of the story, another phase began. John, her husband and the boys returned, and things were fairly normal. The two older boys left for college in distant cities. The autumn that Michael was to leave for school, John announced that they were in serious financial trouble because his company was being merged with another, and he was being forced to take a salary cut in order not to lose his job entirely. He began to experience gastric symptoms, sleep disorders and very volatile mood swings and outbursts. Jane, once more, felt she could not get out of bed.

The new variable this time, when stress and depression entered into this unit, was little Jane's school system. The younger Jane became another signaller of distress by wetting her pants in third grade, fighting with other children, announcing that she was boy and not a girl, and twirling her hair until she made a bald spot. The school insisted that the family seek help, and they were referred to a community mental health centre. After many cancellations of appointments and tearful, troubled sessions, a systems therapist persuaded them to become scientists and examine their own system, using the exchange ideas and modes of persuasion viewpoint in the paradigms described above. One session was conducted with Grandfather Smith present; he made the two-hour trip from his home to 'help end this nonsense, once and for all'. The outcome of that session was that a referral was made for someone to work with the elder John and Mary, in their own town. Jane agreed to try a new antidepressant drug; she also started to work as a teacher's aide in her daughter's school. After six months, the younger Jane was symptom-free, and the older Jane adjusted to the new requirements of her. New family rules included that the boys had to contribute financially to the household, even though they were living away, and that the younger John and Mary would accept financial help from the elder John Jones to clear some debts from the education bills.

For this family, the new views were in the area of how symptoms were to be understood and dealt with, and what expectations of each other (using the Bredemeier paradigms) could be altered. Drug therapy alone had not helped Jane, nor had the situational solution of adding a child to the system. Only when the ways in which the family members dealt with each other were analysed, and their belief systems regarding what was and what was not possible and acceptable scrutinized and evaluated, were they able to shift their thinking and their actions. The tendency toward depressive states may be inherited genetically, but people need not succumb to total immobilization and demoralization.

Application of general systems theory

Many agencies are reluctant, and some are adamantly opposed, to using a systems orientation as a framework for the service they provide. The older intrapsychic and interpersonal models are still more familiar and comfortable, and an easier match for reimbursement methods. Nonetheless, there is a rapidly growing literature about systems theory and family therapy, and an interest among clinicians in understanding its application in various clinical settings. There are handbooks, monographs and journals devoted exclusively to the field, and major conferences to share research findings and new clinical directions. Further, psychiatric nurses in the United States are concerned with defining the appropriate educational bases for different levels of their clinical practice, and discuss the preparation and the clinical skills of baccalaureate as opposed to master's-prepared psychiatric nurses. There is a certification process both levels, beyond the initial licence to practise as a professional nurse. Psychologists, for the most part, are doctorally-prepared, and many used modifications of systems theory in their work. Psychiatrists are trying to regain their position as physicians, first, and tend to medicate almost all their patients, yet some find systems approaches useful. Social workers, who work in community settings, apply systems principles with organizations and agencies, as well as families.

Some major sources of reference are listed in the bibliography. The student should appreciate the fact, however, that clinical skills can never be learned from a text such as this. This chapter should serve only to whet the reader's appetite and to serve as a stimulus to seek more knowledge from a live supervisor/teacher in the field.

References

Bredemeier, H. C. (1968) *Social Systems Integration and Adaptation*, doctoral seminar and lecture, Rutgers, The State University of New Jersey, New Brunswick, NJ.

Buckley, W. (ed.) (1968) *Modern Systems Research for the Behavioural Scientist*, Aldine Publishing, Chicago.

Burgess, A. W. (1985) *Psychiatric Nursing in the Hospital and the Community*, Prentice Hall, Englewood Cliffs, NJ.

Carter, B. and McGoldrick, M. (eds) (1988) *The Changing Family Life Cycle: A Framework for Family Therapy*, 2nd edn, Gardner Press, New York.

Clarkin, J., Haas, G. and Glick, I. (eds) (1988) *Affective Disorders and the Family*, The Guilford Press, New York.

Freud, S. (1917) Mourning and Melancholia, **14**, Hogarth, London.

Freud, S. (1955) *Complete Psychological Works of Sigmund Freud*, Hogarth, London.

Gray, W., Duhl, F. and Rizzo, N. (eds) (1969) *General Systems Theory and Psychiatry*, Little, Brown & Co., Boston.

Koestler, A. (1967) *The Ghost in the Machine*, Macmillan, New York.

Laszlo, E. (1972) *A Systems View of the World*, George Braziller, New York.

Like, R. C., Rogers, J. and McGoldrick, M. (1988) Reading and interpreting genograms: a systematic approach. *J. Fam. Pract.*, **26**, 408.

Miller, W., Hedrick, K. and Orlofsky, D. (1981) The Helpful Response Questionnaire. Unpublished paper, Univ. New Mexico, Albuquerque.

Smoyak, S. (1969) Toward understanding nursing situations: a transaction paradigm. *Nurs. Res.*, **18**, 405–11.

Smoyak, S. (ed.) (1975) *The Psychiatric Nurse as a Family Therapist*, John Wiley, New York.

Smoyak, S. (1982) Family systems: use of genograms as an assessment tool, in *Family Therapy in Perspective* (eds I. Clements and D. Buchanan), John Wiley, New York.

Smoyak, S. and Rouslin, S. (eds) (1982) *A Collection of Classics in Psychiatric Nursing Literature*, Slack, Thorofare, NJ.

von Bertalanffy, L. (1956) *General System Theory: General Systems*, Vol. 1, No. 1.

von Bertalanffy, L. (1968) *General System Theory*, George Braziller, New York.

Chapter 7

Rogers' client-centred model: principles and general applications

W. REYNOLDS

The Rogerian model is essentially an approach to counselling. Implicit in the theoretical constructs contained within this model is the notion that the helper (therapist) should allocate time for one-to-one verbal talks and group discussion with the client. This approach to counselling, that was at first called non-directive (see Rogers, 1951), but is now called client-centred, is still best represented by the writing of its originator, Carl Rogers (1957, 1961, 1975).

The stimulation of teaching and research at Ohio State University and the University of Chicago, and Rogers' continuing experience in practising psychotherapy resulted in the development of Rogers' approach in theoretical formulation of the nature of therapy, and in a tentative theory of personality. In later years, Rogers became involved in the group movement and extended his theory to encounter groups and other treatment modalities such as play therapy. He also became interested in the application of his theory to education, and extended it to interpersonal relations in general (see Rogers, 1960 and 1977).

General principles

One concept of people is that they are by nature irrational, unsocialized and destructive of themselves and others. Conversely, the client-centred point of view sees human beings, on the contrary, as basically rational, socialized, forward moving and realistic. Furthermore, people are said to be basically co-operative, constructive and trustworthy, when they are free of defensiveness. As individuals, we possess the capacity to experience, and to be aware of, the reality of our psychological maladjustment, and have the capacity and the tendency to move from a state of maladjustment toward a state of psychological adjustment. These capacities and this tendency will be released in a relationship that has the characteristics of a helping (non-threatening) relationship. This type of relationship may also be described as a therapeutic relationship.

Characteristics of the therapeutic relationship

From time to time we all claim that we have good relationships with our clients, but what do we mean by good, and how is the quality of that relationship assessed? Closer examination of those relationships might reveal that, in some cases, they actually damage the mental health of those they purport to help.

One definition of the therapeutic relationship, which may be used to identify and measure the successful ingredients of a helping relationship, was provided by Kalkman (1967, p. 226):

> Relationship therapy refers to a prolonged relationship between a nurse therapist and a patient, during which the patient can feel accepted as a person of worth, feels free to express himself without fear of rejection or censure, and enables him to learn more satisfactory and productive patterns of behaviour.

Kalkman's description of the helping relationship emphasizes that this form of treatment, which is often referred to as a form of psychotherapeutic activity, involves the provision of relationships within which the conditions exist (for example, mutual trust) to promote growth and behavioural change. Because the primary goal of psychiatric nurses is to provide services that assist in moving clients to their optimal health levels, helping relationships form the cornerstone of all interventions with the client. The provision of a caring atmosphere, or helpful interpersonal experiences can, and should, occur in various forms, one-to-one verbal talks (counselling), psychodrama, or during various types of group activities.

The core conditions of the helping relationship

If Kalkman's description of the helping relationship is carefully examined, it is clear that it describes a *non-threatening* experience for the client, in which problem solving is possible. That is another way of saying that the conditions to promote growth and behavioural change should exist within the relationship. Kalkman's description is very compatible with Rogers' view that human beings are basically co-operative and constructive when they are free of defensiveness. The questions that we need to ask ourselves are: how does non-defensiveness occur, or, what are the key nursing behaviours which create a non-threatening relationship that enables the client to study the effectiveness of his coping strategies?

Numerous contributors to the literature have suggested that certain core helper strategies are necessary and sufficient for client growth. Rogers (1957), the strongest advocate of that view, proposed that the techniques of psychotherapy are less important than what he has described as the facilitative conditions for therapeutic change. The necessary and sufficient conditions which have received the greatest amount of attention all relate to the therapist's attitude and behaviour. Rogers argues that the client learns to change when the helper is warm, empathic and genuine. Rogers' theory states that when the client experiences those conditions in abundance, he is enabled to feel non-defensive and to be able to consider, and experiment with, alternative coping strategies. Those conditions are, therefore, facilitative conditions, in other words, conditions which build the type of relationship described by Kalkman (1967).

The relationship of empathy to warmth and genuineness

Rogers' statement would appear to imply that the core facilitative conditions of the therapeutic relationship are separate and independent. However, many theorists, including Rogers, suggest that they are interrelated. For example, Rogers and Truax (1967) state that the three conditions have an interlocking nature, and Muldary (1983) argues that they interact in such a way as to increase and complement each other. For instance, the communication of empathy (the ability to see things from another person's point of view) can be hollow or threatening if the empathizing individual is not without facade and is not genuine.

While impressive evidence exists within the literature to support the view that empathy may be the most important facilitator of a therapeutic relationship (see Gurman, 1978; Reynolds, 1987; Reynolds and Presly, 1988), warmth and genuineness may be of equal importance to therapeutic outcome. Reynolds and Cormack (1987) suggested that warmth (spontaneous commitment to the therapy interaction) and genuineness (being your real self) contributed towards empathy and, were therefore, part of empathy. The close association between the three facilitative conditions was demonstrated by Reynolds and Cormack (1987, p. 131) when they described key helper behaviours and the operational conditions which build the type of helping relationship described by Kalkman (1967). Reynolds and Cormack's (1987) discussion suggests that it is somewhat artificial to separate the three conditions, and suggests that empathy cannot exist in the absence of the other two conditions (see Fig. 7.1). For example, it was difficult to see how the nurse would be able to understand the feelings behind the client's words (empathy), if external stressors such as dissatisfaction or anger, prevented her seeking clarification when the client's message was unclear, or focusing on the here and now message as it was being communicated to her.

Possibly, as a consequence of the voluminous amount of research findings supporting empathy as being the most critical ingredient of the helping relationships (see Carkhuff, 1970; Kalish, 1971; La Monica *et al.*, 1976) numerous instruments purporting to measure empathy have been

Figure 7.1   The interpersonal strategies associated with relationship building

Empathy (understanding)	Warmth (respect)	Genuineness (trust, openness)
Accurate perception of current fellings/concerns, and communication of this understanding to the patient	Commitment by the therapist in his effort to understand. Involves spontaneous participation	Therapist is without facade or pretence. Involves being real self and non-defensive
Key behaviours: Conveying empathy	Conveying warmth	Conveying genuineness
1. Listen for the feeling behind words	1. Focus on the here and now (immediacy)	1. Apply 1–3 under 'Warmth'
2. Attend to non-verbal communication	2. Use open rather than closed questions	2. Avoid frequent inter-ruption of silence, but sometimes use it as a focus
3. Avoid taking on the patient's feelings as if they were your own	3. Remain neutral and accept the patient's reality	3. Respond to direct questions, then re-focus on the patient
4. Reflect the patient's own feeling tone and language	4. Allow the patient to make the decisions, avoiding advice or manipulation of their thoughts	4. Be consistent and predictable
5. Convey impressions in a manner which allows the patient to refute your observation if you are wrong	5. Focus on the patient rather than yourself	5. Don't allow external stressors to alter your behaviour
	6. Seek clarification when message is unclear	

developed. However, close examination of some of the available instruments suggests that they may measure all of the facilitative conditions associated with therapeutic change. Of particular interest to nursing is an instrument developed by La Monica (1981) called the empathy construct rating scale (ECRS). La Monica developed the instrument for use among nursing and other health professionals who are in a position of giving help, and who are in positions of authority relative to the recipients of care. The scale is concerned with initiating supportive interpersonal communication, and the focus of empathy is the other person who is in need of affective support. Thus the scale appears to measure what Cormack (1985) refers to as the unique use of interpersonal skills in nursing, in that the use of interpersonal skills is built into the normal day-to-day contact between nurses and clients. This contact may occur during the delivery of physical care and the administration of medication, as well as one-to-one talks (counselling), or group, verbal interactions. The ECRS also offers great flexibility in view of its potential use as a self-report, client or associate/observer measure of empathy.

The empathy construct rating scale (ECRS)   La Monica's (1981) definition of empathy, which is operationally described by the items (questions) on the empathy construct rating scale (ECRS), tends to support Reynolds and Cormack's (1987) view that warmth and genuineness are part of empathy. La Monica considered empathy to be a sequence of perceptual and interactional events (state empathy) which involved both verbal and non-verbal behaviour on the part of the helper. She operationally defined empathy as: 'Empathy signifies a central focus and feeling with and in the client's world. It involves accurate perception of the client's world by the helper, communication of this understanding to the client, and the client's perception of the helper's understanding.' (La Monica, 1981, p. 398).

Examination of the scale items (questions) on the ECRS suggests that the empathy scale measures all of the facilitative conditions identified by Rogers (1957). Examples of scale items include:

Empathy   Accurate perception of current feelings/concerns, and communication of this understanding to the client.
Item 1   Places herself in another person's shoes.
Item 2   Is able to feel with another person.
Item 5   Seems to understand even when people do not talk.
Warmth   Commitment by the helper (therapist) in her effort to understand. Involves spontaneous commitment.
Item 11   Does not wait for a person to ask for help, but anticipates needs and offers assistance.
Item 20   Helps a person to realise that options are available.
Item 51   Makes time in a busy ward schedule to talk to someone who is upset.
Genuine-   Helper (therapist) is without facade or pretence; involves being
ness   real self and non-defensive.
Item 19   Allows people to cry and offers support.
Item 30   Counsels others without imposing personal feelings or values.
Item 39   Respects the values of others.

It can be seen from the items selected from the 84 questions on the ECRS that the scale measures all of the facilitative conditions of relationship building, and that warmth and genuineness cannot be separated from empathy. Furthermore, factor analysis of the combined responses of 900 nurse subjects to the ECRS found that empathy is comprised of five identified elements, namely honest, non-verbal behaviour, sensitivity to another, responding and respect. This provides further support for the view that all of the facilitative conditions are strongly interrelated.

The centrality of empathy to helping

Irrespective of the interrelationship between the facilitative conditions, empathy represents the final therapeutic intervention that makes therapeutic change possible. It has earlier been suggested that impressive research evidence exists to support the hypothesized relationship between empathy and therapeutic outcome. In order to examine the available research evidence, it is useful to return to Kalkman's definition of the helping relationship. Examination of that definition and the research literature reveals that there is considerable evidence to support the view that high levels of empathy may well be the most critical variable in determining the outcomes postulated by Kalkman (1967, p. 226). For example, Kalkman states that: 'Relationship therapy refers to a prolonged relationship between a nurse therapist and a patient, during which, the patient can feel accepted as a person of worth and feels free to express himself without fear of rejection or censure.'

Reynolds (1986) found that as clients' ratings of student nurses empathy increased between repeated measures on the empathy construct rating scale, their anecdotal descriptions of students behaviour during a series of counselling interviews suggested that they felt more able to be open with their students. Typical examples included: 'It's hard for her to understand me, but she is trying very hard.' (second counselling interview), 'I can talk freely to her, there is no barrier.' (fifth counselling interview).

Lyons-Halaris (1979), commenting on non-verbal behaviour, reported that low-empathy nurses mainly exhibited listening via non-verbal communication – for example, avoidance of eye contacts, eyebrows down, wrinkled forehead, and the crossing and uncrossing of legs. Those non-verbal behaviours tend to convey a lack of respect, interest and support, according to client reports.

Zoske and Pietrocarlo (1983) reported that all nurse subjects in a dialysis unit who were provided with intensive empathy training, reported that they had gained greater awareness of the client's experience, an essential prerequisite of promoting feelings of self-worth. The explanation for that outcome may be related to the studies conducted by Rotheman (1978) and Boremand (1979). Those researchers demonstrated a significant positive correlation between empathy and the ability of subjects to rate themselves and others on several psychological traits. Self-awareness is another pre-requisite of the helping relationship.

Another essential feature of building a trust relationship is the ability to anticipate the needs of others. Hogan and Henley (1970) found that those who are highly empathic anticipate the information requirements of their listeners more effectively than low empathizers, and guide their remarks accordingly. That outcome may explain why Hogan and Manikan (1970) found a significant high correlation between likeability and empathy. This tends to support Hogan's view that empathy facilitates an attractive inter-personal style.

Finally, Stotland *et al.* (1978) studied the behaviour of nursing students, relative to empathy and helping. During clinical experience, they observed students who had been tested regarding their ability to empathize. By the end of a semester, the hypothesis that high-empathy students would spend more time with clients than would low-empathizers was supported. That finding is important in view of Kalkman's assertion that a prolonged relationship is necessary in order to create a climate in which problem solving is possible.

Kalkman's description of the helping relationship also suggests that it is a purposeful activity which has, as its final objective, client growth. She states that: 'Relationship therapy enables the client to learn more satis-factory and productive patterns of behaviour.' (Kalkman, 1967, p. 266).

Numerous studies have established a correlation between empathy, the helping relationship, and measures of therapeutic outcome (see Feitel, 1968). Examples include a study by Gerrard (1978) who showed a positive relationship between the core interpersonal strategies and client responses. Such responses included relief from pain and distress, improved pulse and respiratory rates and client reports of reduced worry and anxiety.

Truax and Carkhuff (1967), in a study known as the Wisconsin Project, investigated the relationship between therapists' interpersonal behaviour and the outcome of long-term counselling with chronic schizophrenic patients. High empathy produced the most reduction in schizophrenic pathology. Furthermore, Truax (1970) reported that clients who had been treated by high-empathy therapists had the most time out of hospital in the following nine years.

These results are congruent with many other studies. For example, Siegel (1972) found improvement among children with learning disabilities in both verbal and behavioural spheres, related to time in play therapy, and therapists levels of empathy, warmth and genuineness. Additionally, Kendall and Wilcox (1980) demonstrated a significant relationship between empathy and therapist effectiveness during their treatment of hyperactive and uncontrolled children.

Evidence that empathy may be a more important facilitator of a helpful (therapeutic) relationship than the helper's ideological orientation came from a study by Miller *et al.* (1980). That study found that behaviour therapists who scored high in empathy, were more potent reinforces of adaptive behaviour than therapists who were low empathizers.

Finally, with respect to confrontation of unpleasant or maladaptive behaviour, Mitchell and Berenson (1970) found that during the first counselling session, highly empathic therapists, significantly more than low-empathy therapists, used confrontations which provided important information about the therapist, focused on the here-and-now relationship between therapist and client, and emphasized the client's resources. On the other hand, low empathizers were more likely to confront clients with pathology rather than their resources.

Application of empathy, warmth and genuineness

The initial phase of the relationship

During this phase, which is often referred to as the orientation phase (see Rogers, 1951; Peplau, 1960 and 1962), the nurse and the client are strangers to each other. At this point the nurse is confronted with several interferences or barriers, which hinder the formulation of accurate empathic responses to the client, and the subsequent development of a problem-solving relationship. Overcoming interferences is an integral part of eliciting the client's story. At this point the nurse's objectives are to become known to the client and to establish a climate for trust, where at some future point, when the client feels comfortable, it is possible to work with the client on the issues that concern him.

Interferences to trust and empathy lie partly in the nurse's and partly in the client's world. The major barrier to empathy during the initial phase of relationship results from the helper's lack of personal knowledge of the client's world. Additional problems are that the client is often unaware of the purpose of the relationship, and he has not yet learned whether his nurse helper is genuinely interested in him, is consistent, and can be trusted. These barriers can be overcome once trust has been established. Trust is the foundation of the helping (therapeutic) relationship and consistency (a key component of genuineness), and commitment to the client (a key component of warmth) are the building blocks. Empathy, the final and most potent phase of the therapeutic intervention, becomes possible when the client perceives the helper to be genuine and warm. In other words, warmth and genuineness allow the nurse to learn experientially about another person, they are part of the empathic process and a prerequisite to accurate understanding of what it is like to be that person. When this final phase is complete, the nurse has passed beyond the orientation (stranger) phase. To quote Rogers (1975):

The way of being with another person which is termed empathic has several facets. It means entering the private perceptual world of the other and becoming thoroughly at home in it. It involves being sensitive, moment to moment, to the changing felt meanings which flow in this other person, to the fear or rage or tenderness or confusion *or* whatever that he/she is experiencing. It means temporarily living in his/her life, moving about in it delicately without making judgements, sensing meanings of which he/she is scarcely aware, but not trying to uncover feelings of which the person is totally unaware, since this would be too threatening. It includes communicating your sensings of his/her world as you look with fresh and unfrightened eyes at the elements of which the individual is fearful. It means frequently checking with him/her as to the accuracy of your sensings and being guided by the responses you receive. (Rogers, 1975, p. 4).

When this is possible, the nurse is moving towards a problem-solving phase of the relationship. However, before this can be achieved, it is necessary to utilize interventions that build the climate for trust, openness and deeper understanding.

Orientating yourself to the client: creating a climate for trust

In the beginning, the nurse helper must take the initiative, for many clients will avoid contact with their nurse, or be confused about the purpose of the nurse–client relationship. While all contacts with clients may be utilized for the purpose of building a relationship, it is often essential to provide time for one-to-one verbal talks (counselling). Unfortunately, the research and non-scientific literature has indicated that clients view some nurses as being insufficiently available, and perceive such nurses as being insensitive, hostile, manipulative and untrustworthy. For example, Denny and Denny (1980, p. 1806) observed: '...there was a lack on the nurse's part of a psychodynamic exploration of the patient's behaviour. The usual response to unacceptable behaviour was admonishment to cease. When this was unsuccessful punitive measures were suggested'. Subsequently, this problem was confirmed by Cormack's (1983) study of psychiatric nursing. To quote from Cormack's data: 'There was a time when I was depressed and inwardly crying out for someone to talk to. The staff nurse was not prepared to give up even one minute of her time to discuss my feelings. I know they all do a marvellous job, but there are times when you need to talk.' (Cormack, 1983, p. 72).

While these examples relate to psychiatric nursing in Scotland, the author has observed similar nursing behaviour in an American state mental hospital, and a New Zealand psychiatric hospital. The essential point is that time must be allocated for verbal interaction, in order to allow your client to learn that you can be trusted and to enable you to gain understanding of his world.

Verbal strategies during the initial phase of the relationship

At this point, the client needs to be provided with an explanation for one-to-one verbal talks (counselling interviews) with his nurse helper. Because nursing is unlike the role of other helpers (who may provide only formal, time-limited and private counselling interviews) and because nurses often engage clients in social chit chat during the working day, the client may often be unclear about *why* the nurse is talking to him. As the eventual outcome of the nurse–client relationship is unknown at this point, it is sufficient to provide a simple explanation that does not produce unrealistic expectations. For example the nurse helper might say: 'I would like to talk about yourself as a person. This will help me to understand your nursing needs as you see them'. It is important that your client talks as freely about himself as possible and, for this reason, it is best to initiate counselling interviews with open-ended questions which invite expanded responses. For example: 'Tell me a bit about yourself.', or 'Describe how you feel.' This strategy of asking open questions also provides the client with the opportunity to choose the response which is most comfortable for *him* at that time. Typical responses are for the client to ask the nurse direct questions about herself, which indicate an attempt to test her (i.e., to find out whether she means what she says), or to say 'I'm not very interesting nurse.' That may indicate low self-esteem on the part of the client. Alternatively, the client might say: 'What do you want me to talk about nurse?' This suggests that he is unclear about the purpose of the relationship.

At that point, because very little is known about the client, the nurse is limited to such straightforward, uncomplicated statements, which seek to focus on the here-and-now (a component of warmth). Examples include: 'You seem uncomfortable?', and 'Talking is not comfortable?' Such statements which stem from the nurse's observations of the client's current behaviour, when delivered non-judgementally in a tone which also expresses puzzled interest, are usually sufficient to generate a dialogue or remove the barriers to open communication. Frequent direct questions, which invite a limited response, and create an interrogative atmosphere, should be avoided. Examples of questions to be avoided are: '*Why* do you feel depressed?', and '*Why* can't you sleep?' These questions are often too difficult for the client to answer. At this point, patience is required, particularly when progress *seems* to be slow. However, it is best to remember that objectives associated with a more advanced phase of the relationship may be unrealistic and unattainable at this point. The nurse helper, by consistently displaying her willingness to make herself available to the client (for the purposes of talking), by her tendency to be neutral and to focus on the here-and-now, is demonstrating that the client is important to her.

In conclusion, in respect of the verbal strategies during the initial phase of the relationship, the intervention should begin with clearly stated observations which allow the client the opportunity to refute the nurse's observation, or to clarify what he really means. Rogers (1975, p. 4) put it this way:

> To be with another in this way [empathy] means that for the time being you lay aside the views and values you hold for yourself in order to enter another's world without prejudice. In some sense it means that you lay aside yourself and this can only be done by a person who is secure enough in himself [genuine] that he knows he will not get lost in what may turn out to be the strange or bizarre world of the other, and can comfortably return to his own world when he wishes.

Elaborate interventions are the end result of a complex understanding of the client, they are based on accurate (insightful) empathy, and are appropriate only in the later phases of the relationship. Presenting clients with complex interpretation, or explanation, infantilizes them at this point (orientation phase) and may be based on incorrect assumptions. Particularly in the initial phase of a relationship, interventions need to be tempered by the ever present awareness that the client perceives the nurse to be both a confidant and an intruder. For that reason he needs to be provided with the time to talk and to experientially learn that his helper is consistent.

The problem-solving phase of the relationship

Once a climate has been established for open communication it is possible to move toward a more insightful, problem-solving phase of the relationship. In this phase the nurse confirms the client's reality and passes beyond it to a deeper understanding. Remember, that as your personal knowledge of the client's world increases, the more complex and accurate one's empathic understanding becomes, and it is possible to present more detailed and comprehensive evidence of your comprehension of the client's world. While this transition from stranger to working phase is sequential, these phases of the relationship often overlap, and vary in respect of time span and the degree of difficulty that exists within each individual relationship. Interferences or barriers to progress tend to be fewer during the problem-solving phase, but they can re-emerge from time to time.

Key therapist behaviours Broadly speaking, the nurse helper's aims within the problem-solving phase of the counselling relationship may be summarized under six categories of intervention. They are:

1. observing and listening;
2. exploring feelings;
3. responding to feelings;
4. exploring personal meaning;
5. responding to feeling and meaning;
6. providing your client with direction.

These interventions require the nurse to utilize all of the key therapist be-haviours that have been identified by Reynolds and Cormack (1987) (see Fig. 7.1).

Observing and listening to your client These behaviours are placed first because the nurse's responses to the client should be determined by the client's perception of the world, *not* the nurse's view of how the world is, or should be. The nurse observes and listens not only to the words, but also to the nuances (feelings behind the words) and to the client's expression and posture. In this way the nurse is impressed by her recogni-tion that much of what she knows about her client is a function of what she had observed in his behaviour and heard in his expression. There is a dif-ference between the client who is slumped forward, looking at the ground, and the client who sits rigidly erect. There is a difference too, between the listless 'What do you mean?', and the spontaneous, 'I know, I know'.

Often non-verbal aspects of behaviour negate verbalizations. As the nurse listens to, and observes her client, she appreciates that the feelings being expressed through all channels of communication influence her behaviour. When verbal messages are not synchronized with non-verbal behaviour, or voice tone, listeners may become confused. If the speaker does not clearly express the emotional content, the listener is not likely to respond in the manner intended by the speaker. When your client states 'I'm not angry', and emphasizes this by crashing his fist down onto a table, what do you respond to? Is it his verbal statement, or the gestural message? Often when this occurs, helpers choose to talk about themselves as a person rather than focus on the client.

Exploring feelings This means that the nurse encourages her client to describe or evaluate his feelings. Roger's (1961) proposed that the major barrier to empathy is our very natural tendency to approve or to disapprove. Rogers suggests that this tendency to judge another's statements becomes even stronger when feelings and emotions are involved. When our feelings (disinterest, confusion, anger or disgust) influence us to evaluate another's statements, we shift from listening to a person to a preoccupation with our own judgements, which precludes understanding of the other person's point of view. When this happens, and we become defensive, it is often transmitted to the client through unwanted advice, failure to respond to direct questions from the client, or curt unfriendly voice tone. At that point, the client is experiencing rejection and the nurse helper has switched from being his helper to being his adversary. The logical means for correcting this tendency, or at least keeping it in check, is to work on achieving empathy. This is accomplished through self-awareness (on the helper's part), through active listening, and the exploration fo the client's feelings.

Self-awareness is a prerequisite of our ability to explore, to understand, and to be helpful. When it is difficult to be tolerant or sympathetic with clients from a particular class or diagnostic category (e.g., neurotics, drug abusers, or demanding attention-seeking individuals) it may seem that most persons from this group are obstinate and uncooperative individuals who make your job more difficult than it should be. As a result of her impressions, the nurse may have come to expect the same kind of behaviour from everyone in that group. It is possible that she might respond to those persons in ways that actually cause them to confirm her expectations. The concept which describes this event is called self-fulfilling prophecy.

The nurse is only human; total and unflinching attention to the task at hand is an unattainable ideal. The helper may often experience prolonged periods of dissatisfaction and discomfort, and allow her mind to wander. This is particularly likely to happen when the client's story is confusing or repetitive. Difficulties surface in a variety of ways. Clients may exhibit sudden shifts of emotion, they may distort something they have said yesterday, often for unconscious reasons, or assign to the nurse trappings of omniscience. On the other hand the nurse may feel bored. The client may have difficulty in identifying emotions, express stress as somatic complaints, or focus on conversation fillers – such as a direct personal question about the helper. This may engender prolonged periods of puzzlement and impede the nurse's ability to examine the client's communication. It may appear that the client has a wish not to be understood.

All of this may prevent the nurse from focusing on the client's area of concern, and prevent the nurse from exploring feelings. Patterson (1974) described empathy as involving three aspects, or stages. First, the helper must be receptive to another's communications. Secondly the helper must understand the communication by putting herself in the other's place. Third, the helper must communicate that understanding to the client. Empathy can be blocked anywhere along the way from the communication to the sender to the perceptions of the receiver, to the receiver's communication back to the sender. Here, the focus is on the perceptions of the receiver.

When problems arise with our perception of the communication message, there is a need to examine our feelings with an associate, or competent supervisor. This may help to remove blocks and interferences to our understanding of the client's message. Additionally, there is a need to encourage our client to explore the feelings behind his words. At this phase of the relationship it should be possible to confront ambiguous communication by seeking clarification of the communicated message. The first step in responding to feelings is to explore and understand our client's feeling state.

Responding to feelings   Before we can respond to feelings, we must know what a feeling word is. Feeling words refer directly to feelings like happy, sad, or mad. Figure 7.2 provides a list of words that describe human feelings. The feeling categories are not exhaustive, but do cover many human feelings. You may feel that some words belong in different categories, and you may wish to add to the list. The important thing is that you have them at your command. By breaking the feelings into different categories you facilitate the appropriateness of your response. When you have feeling words available to you in different categories you can match them with the feelings expressed by your client. Thus the feeling category question would be: are they expressing happiness, sadness, anger, fear, confusion, weakness, or strength? You are now in a position to use a feeling word in your response to the client. Interventions should include the reflective format: 'You feel...'

Empathy is most effectively communicated when the helper's language and tone are synchronized with the language of her client. That is, your tone and choice of words should reflect that you have assumed the other person's frame of reference. Formal stilted language suggests detachment from the raw experience of the speaker, and so also does over-reliance on technical terms. For example:

Client   I don't know what I'm doing here. I was managing well enough at home. Anyway, here I am in this place – for what reason?
Nurse   I know it must seem pointless for you to follow a social therapy regime like this in this therapeutic milieu.

Apart from the unnecessary use of technical language, the nurse has personalized the message by using 'I know' and has failed to use the reflective formal, 'You feel'. It suggests that the nurse does not know, and is forced to use her frame of reference, rather than the client's.

Exploring personal meaning   The next step in exploring feelings is to assist the client to explore the personal meaning of feelings. Essentially, the nurse's role is to assist the client to recreate, as fully as possible, significant experiences that surface in his communication. Clients should be encouraged to give a detailed account of their problems and to anchor them in the evocative personal settings in which problems surface. In doing this the client moves away from the general to the particular, from the past to the here-and-now. The past is important only in terms of how it affects the client now.

In the case, for example, of a client who complains of recurrent depres-

Figure 7.2 Feeling words

Happy	Sad	Angry	Confused	Scared	Weak	Strong
aglow	apathetic	aggravated	abashed	afraid	confused	able
alive	bad	agitated	added	alarmed	deflated	active
amused	blue	critical	anxious	awed	defenceless	adequate
blissful	burdened	cutting	baffled	daunted	dull	confident
bubbly	deflated	disgruntled	bothered	frightened	exposed	determined
cheerful	despondent	enraged	confounded	harrassed	frail	firm
content	depressed	fed up	dazed	insecure	helpless	glorious
ecstatic	downhearted	irate	disconcerted	nervous	impotent	healthy
elated	dreary	irked	helpless	panicky	inadequate	invincible
excited	glum	hateful	hopeless	rattled	inferior	positive
gay	grave	hostile	mixed up	shaky	lifeless	robust
giddy	hopeless	indignant	muddled	terrified	powerless	solid
joyful	lonely	irritated	puzzled	timid	run down	super
jubilant	lost	livid	surprised	weary	sickly	vibrant
thrilled	miserable	mad	unsure	worried	submissive	
turned on	moody	miffed			unfit	
uplifted	morose	outraged				
wonderful	turned off					

sion (an abstract, non-specific term) the helper's aim should be to elicit the particular setting in which recent feelings of depression surfaced. For example, the nurse might facilitate exploration by saying: 'Tell me what happens when you feel depressed'.

In the case of a client who complains of being misunderstood or neglected, the nurse's aim should be to elicit the events associated with recently feeling misunderstood or neglected. The helper might say: 'What goes on when you feel neglected?' What might emerge is evidence of low self-esteem, a social skill, or a trust problem. That is what Peplau (1960) meant when she stated that there is a need to help clients to recreate the circumstances associated with their affective state. At the same time, the nurse should be mentally thinking about the feeling category being expressed, and considering words that fit that category. Feeling depressed could fit with sad, and under that category she might decide that her client feels disenchanted with treatment, and mistrustful of his helpers.

Exploring feelings and personal meaning enables the nurse to sit inside the client's world and sample the client's state of mind. From this position one is able to consider the relationship between many elements in the client's communication, for example, its general flow. The major function is that of matching themes that bring stories together. When that is matched with a new appreciation of the feelings behind the words, you are in a position to make a more detailed empathic response by responding to feeling and meaning.

Responding to feeling and meaning   Responding to how a person feels is critical but it is incomplete. To communicate a complete understanding of what clients are saying, helpers have to recognize the meaning of their statements, and communicate that to the client; meaning is the reason for the feeling. When responding to meaning, the nurse should not simply repeat what the client has said; rather she should try to capture and express the personal reason for the feeling. The client might say: 'I can't stand that treatment, I feel and look dreadful afterwards. I don't want to go back there anymore.' Here the response might be: 'You feel scared because your treatment might really harm you.' The 'might really harm you' part of that response supplied the client's reason for feeling scared. It summarizes the meaning in a personal way, rather than just repeating the content. Of course you might choose to substitute other words for scared – such as afraid, alarmed or uneasy. While your choice of words will be determined by your experiential knowledge of your client, the format: 'You feel... because...' enables the client to explore 'where they are'. At this point, by listening to the words, the tone, and observing other clues, such as a tear-streaked face, you are able to respond accurately to the client by using a vocabulary of feeling terms that he can recognize.

Providing your client with direction The ultimate objective of client-centred therapy is to assist the client to find solutions to personal problems. In order to learn new coping patterns, the client must first have the opportunity to explore current coping strategies. For example, you might choose to focus upon an ineffective coping strategy by asking: 'What would you like to happen at those times when you feel "mad"?', or 'How else can you get those people to do what you want?'

Once the nurse has helped the client to explore and evaluate potential coping strategies, she is in a good position to know where he (the client) wants to be. The key to a good clarification response is the inclusion of a specific client problem – and its simultaneous reflection of where the client wants to be. The following is an example of a response that is high in direction:

Client I've tried really hard, but reading this diabetic stuff is really hard for me.

Nurse You feel really bad because you can't understand the reading and you want to be able to stand on your own feet.

That response could be considered to be highly facilitative because it personalized where the client was and where he wanted to be. The second part of that response, 'and you want to be', provides the client with direction. An alternative format which may be used to provide direction could be: 'You want...and you would like to try...'. That response reflects the client's new solutions for problematic situations.

The termination phase of the relationship

The final phase of a relationship is termination. Termination is usually a gradual weaning off process where the amount of contact time with a helper is gradually reduced. Peplau (1957) refers to this final phase as resolution, where dependence is relinquished and the client resumes independence.

Ideally, termination should be done by mutual agreement when the client has demonstrated a greater level of independent functioning. In practice, it more often occurs with the client's abrupt departure or planned medical discharge. Particularly in nursing, premature discharge or transfer to another clinical area, of either the nurse or client, will often influence the rapidity with which termination occurs. As a consequence, nurses should anticipate and prepare the client for termination at a very early phase of the relationship.

The amount of time needed for a smooth and complete termination is dependent on the duration and intensity of the relationship. Generally, a long-established and intense relationship, such as may occur in chronic or long-term units, requires a longer time span before termination can be achieved. Conversely a brief, less intense relationship requires a shorter period.

Assuming that termination can be planned, there is no single criterion which in itself is sufficient to demonstrate readiness to terminate. However, Berger (1987) suggests that the following criteria are useful indicators.

1. An improved sense of autonomy (i.e., ability to be independent)
2. A reduced need to be defensive
3. The ability to use new-found insights to adaptively alter day-to-day functioning.

Problems associated with termination   Termination often engenders feelings of discomfort, pain and anger. The difficulties confronting the nurse are similar to those confronting the client. Nurses, too, need to overcome an unwillingness to separate, to give up exalted roles the client has assigned to them of idealized empathizer and omnipotent provider. Although the helping relationship ends with an expanded appreciation of the stories and convictions that motivate the client, in many respects it also ends on the same conflictual note on which it began – with expressions of ambivalence, and a recounting of successes and failures. The nurse may need to endorse sadness, the client's disappointment in them, and their own disappointment in themselves and the client.

In conclusion, the nurse must be alert to the surfacing of any behaviour on termination. Any of a number of client responses – repression, regression, anger, denial, sadness, acceptance and joy among others – may surface. When repressing, the client gives no evidence of emotional response. The nurse may respond by repeatedly observing that the client is not addressing the issue of impending separation, and may move to explore this avoidance. The client who reverts to a previously abandoned behaviour pattern with a message of 'I can't make it without you', or 'my life is now empty', demonstrates regression. The nurse may move to address possible underlying fears of abandonment while also stressing the reality of termination. A number of nurse authors have offered clinical examples of how to handle termination; these include Vennen (1970) and McCann (1979).

Preparing your client for termination   Vennen (1970) offers a humanistic approach to termination, viewing it as a separation of what was unique to the nurse and the client, and temporarily shared in the one-to-one relationship. It replicates some of the feelings of disconnectedness that follow bereavement. As I have stated it is a painful, difficult process characterized by depression, denial and, finally, solitary grief. In anticipation of termination problems, the nurse should prepare her client at a very early phase of the helping relationship for separation.

Summary of termination (resolution) phase

The following therapeutic tasks and nursing interventions should be considered:

1. Make a contract with your client which, among other things, clearly identifies the circumstances under which termination may occur. For example, you might say 'I have been assigned to this ward for ten weeks.'
2. Assist client evaluation of the therapeutic contract and of the psychotherapeutic experience in general. For example, encourage client's realistic appraisal of personal therapeutic goals and underline client's assets and therapeutic gains. This may include the development of new interests, such as hobbies, friendship relationships – or personal achievements such as walking unaided, or planning a household budget.
3. Encourage transference of dependence to alternative support systems. This may include reliance on spouse, relative, employer, neighbour, friend, or new therapist, for empathic emotional support.
4. As the client's independence from you grows, space contacts with the client further apart. Allow him time and space for interaction with other significant people in his life.
5. As the time for termination nears, focus increasingly on future orientated material. For example, continue to remind the client of impending termination, and be alert to surfacing of any behaviour arising on termination (repression, regression, acting out, anger, withdrawal, acceptance, etc).
6. Assist the client in working through feelings that are associated with these behaviours and anticipate your own reaction to separation. Share your feelings in a manner which does not burden the client. For example, foster feelings of guilt, or convey a sense of rejection.

The fate of empathy at termination   The therapeutic relationship never truly ends. In the minds of the participants, the dialogue continues for ever. They continue to mull over things they have said and done to each other, provided and failed to provide, or accomplished and failed to accomplish. As with all significant life events, over time, the therapeutic relationship is altered in memory and recreated anew, attaining the status of a new memorable story to add to all others. Similarly, the nurse helper becomes a new permanent transference figure for the client, receiving a place alongside parents, siblings, teachers and all others who have attained this status.

Clearly, the course of termination is influenced by the work that preceded it. The more that client and nurse discuss their successes and failures, their gratitudes and disappointments, the more the client will have benefited from the therapeutic experience.

Summary

The theory of client-centred therapy utilizes a number of concepts or constructs which have been extended to include a theory of personality and all interpersonal relationships. The basic philosophy of the counsellor is represented by an attitude of respect and neutrality towards the individual, and respect for the individual's capacity and right to self-direction and for the worth and significance of each other.

The emphasis is upon the relationship and climates required for self discovery and effective learning. The key helper behaviours, which facilitate the necessary conditions for client growth, are most usually described as empathy, warmth and genuineness. These qualities are said to be more important than the therapist's techniques, or ideological orientation towards psychotherapeutic work. Empathy has been found to be the primary ingredient in any helping relationship. Because nursing occurs within the context of a (sequential) relationship with the client, the conditions which facilitate a helping relationship are central to everything that the nurse does with her client.

References

Berger, D. (1987) *Clinical Empathy*, Jason Aronson, North Vale, NJ.

Boremand, W. (1979) Individual differences: correlates of accuracy in evaluating others performance effectiveness. *Appl. Psychol. Measurement*, **3**, 103–15.

Carkhuff, R. (1970) *Helping and Human Relations: a Primer for Lay and Professional Helpers*, Vol. 2, Rinehart and Winston, New York.

Cormack, D. (1983) *Psychiatric Nursing Described*, Churchill Livingstone, Edinburgh.

Cormack, D. (1985) The myths and realities of interpersonal skills use in nursing, in *Interpersonal Skills in Nursing: Research and Application* (ed. C. Kagan), Croom Helm, London.

Denny, E. and Denny, J. (1980) Broadening horizons: a cross-cultural clinical experience. *Nursing Times*, **76**, 1805–6.

Feitel, B. (1968) *Feeling Understood as a Function of a Variety of Therapist Activities*, unpublished doctoral dissertation, Teachers College, Columbia University.

Gerrard, B. (1978) *The Construction and Validation of a Behavioural Test for Interpersonal Skills for Health Professionals*, unpublished manuscript, Dept. Medicine, McMaster University.

Gurman, A. (1978) The patient's perception of the therapeutic relationship, in *Effective Psychotherapy: a Handbook of Research* (eds A. Gurman and A. Razin), Pergamon Press, Oxford.

Hogan, R. and Henley, A. (1970) *A Test of the Empathy-Effective Communication Hypothesis*, Center for the Study of Social Organisation of Schools Report, Johns Hopkin University, No. 84.

Hogan, R. and Manikan, W. (1970) Determinants of interpersonal attraction: a clarification. *Psychol. Rep.*, **26**, 235–8.

Kalish, B. (1971) An experiment in the development of empathy in nursing studies. *Nurs. Res*, **20**, 202–11.

Kalkman, M. (1967) *Psychiatric Nursing*, McGraw-Hill, New York.

Kendell, P. and Wilcox, L. (1980) Cognitive behavioural treatment for impulsivity: concrete vs self-controlled problem children. *J. Consul. Clin. Psychol.*, **48**, 80–91.

La Monica, E. (1981) Construct validity of an empathy instrument. *Res. Nurs. Health*, **4**, 389–400.

La Monica, E., Carew, D., Winder, A. *et al.* (1976) Empathy training as the major thrust of a staff development programme. *Nurs. Res.*, **25**, 447–51.

Lyons-Harlaris, A. (1979) *Relationship of Perceived Empathy to Nurses' Non-Verbal Communication*, unpublished Master's thesis, University of Illinois.

McCann, J. (1979) Termination of the psychotherapeutic relationship. *J. Psych. Nurs. Mental Health Serv.*, **17**, 45–56.

Miller, W. Hedrick, K, and Orlofsky, O. (1981) The Helpful Response Questionnaire. Unpuplished Paper. Psychology Dept, Univ. of New Mexico, Albuquergue.

Mitchell, K. and Berenson, B. (1970) Differential use of confrontation by high and low facilitative therapists. *J. Nerv. Mental Dis.*, **151**, 303–9.

Muldary, T. (1983) *Interpersonal Relations for Health Professionals: a Social Skills Approach*, MacMillan, New York.

Patterson, C. (1974) *Relationship Counselling and Psychotherapy*, Harper and Row, New York.

Peplau, H. (1957) What is experiential teaching? *Am. J. Nurs.*, **47**, 884–6.

Peplau, H. (1960) Talking with patients. *Am. J. Nurs.*, **60**, 964–6.

Peplau, H. (1962) Interpersonal techniques: the crux of psychiatric nursing. *Am. J. Nurs.*, **62**, 50–4.

Reynolds, W. (1986) *A Study of Empathy in Student Nurses*, MPhil thesis, Dundee College of Technology.

Reynolds, W. (1987) Empathy: we know what we mean, but what do we teach? *Nurs. Ed. Today*, **7**, 265–9.

Reynolds, W. and Cormack, D. (1987) Teaching psychiatric nursing: interpersonal skills, in *Nursing Education: Research and Developments* (ed. B. Davis), Croom Helm, London.

Reynolds, W. and Presly, A. (1988) A study of empathy in student nurses. *Nurs. Ed. Today*, **8**, 123–30.

Rogers, C. (1951) *Client-Centred Therapy*, Houghton Mifflin, New York.

Rogers, C. (1957) The necessary and sufficient conditions of therapeutic personality change. *J. Consult. Psychol.*, **21**, 95–103.

Rogers, C. (1960) *Self-Directed Education Change in Action. Epilogue in Freedom to Learn*, Merrill, Columbus, OH.

Rogers, C. (1961) *On Becoming a Person*, Houghton Mifflin, Boston, MA.

Rogers, C. (1975) Empathic: an unappreciated way of being. *Counsel. Psychol.*, **5**, 2–10.

Rogers, C. (1977) *Carl Rogers on Personal Power*, Delacorte, New York.

Rogers, C. and Truax, C. (1967) The therapeutic conditions antecedent to change: a theoretical view, in *The Therapeutic Relationship and its Impact: a Study of Psychotherapy with Schizophrenics* (ed. C. Rogers), University of Wisconsin Press, Madison, WI.

Rotheman, K. (1978) *Relationship of Empathic Disposition to Empathic Ability*, unpublished manuscript, San Francisco State University.

Siegel, C. (1972) Changes in play therapy behaviours over time as a function of differing levels of therapist-offered conditions. *J. Clin. Psychol.*, **28**, 235.

Stotland, E., Mathews, K., Sherman, S. *et al.* (1978) *Empathy: Fantasy and Helping*, Sage Publications, Beverly Hills, CA.

Truax, C. (1970) Effects of client-centred psychotherapy with schizophrenic patients: nine years pretherapy and nine years post therapy hospitalization. *J. Consult. Clin. Psychol.*, **35**, 417–22.

Truax, C. and Carkhuff, R. (1967) *Toward Effective Counselling and Psychotherapy: Training and Practice*, Alpine, Chicago.

Vennen, M. (1970) Notes on termination. *Perspect. Psych. Care*, **viii**, 211–18.

Zoske, J. and Pietrocarlo, D. (1983) Dialysis training exercise for improved staff awareness. *Am. Assoc. Nephro. Nurs. Techn. J.*, **10**, 19–39.

Chapter 8

Orem's self-care model: principles and general applications

P. R. UNDERWOOD

Introduction

Psychiatric nursing has traditionally used theory developed by other disciplines and, as a result, has focused on the same clinical problems and developed the same or similar interventions. We have expressed clinical problems in terms of disruptions in mental or psychological processes or behaviour and have focused on things such as self-esteem problems, affect problems, hostility problems, social skills problems, trust problems dependency problems, anxiety problems, reality orientation problems, thought process problems (e.g., delusions), or perception problems (e.g., hallucinations). Our interventions, like those of other mental health disciplines, have been aimed at reducing, correcting, or changing certain psychological problems to improve behaviour or psychological functioning. Our practice has tended to be more like that of other mental health disciplines than of other nurses. As a result we have often had difficulty explaining the unique contributions of nursing in psychiatric/mental health care and thus to justify either the need for education and experienced nurses or equitable participation on the interdisciplinary team.

The self-care model provides us with the opportunity to develop an independent practice of nursing that is grounded in and reflective of nursing rather than medicine or psychotherapy. We are then able to clearly identify our unique contribution to psychiatric/mental health care. However, it is often difficult to begin to practise from the self-care model because it does require that we change the definition of clinical problems, the focus of nursing interventions and the criteria for evaluation of nursing care. We must change the way we look at patients and nursing practice by shifting our focus from the individual's psychological problems, conditions, and symptoms to the individual's ability to meet self-care requisites.

When we use the self-care model the goal of the independent practice of nursing is to assist the individual to meet self-care demands and thus self-care requisites in living day-to-day. Clinical problems will be expressed as actual or potential self-care deficits such as inability to decide and/or to act to engage with others. Clinical problems are not expressed in terms of psychological problems such as low self-esteem, uncontrolled hostility, inappropriate dependency, or delusional thinking. Nurses will certainly need to recognize and understand psychological problems and psychiatric conditions but these problems are viewed as factors that affect the person's ability to meet self-care demands rather than clinical problems that require nursing care. The specific concern of nursing will be the person's self-care behaviour not the person's psychological problems or psychiatric symptoms. Nursing care is needed because an individual has a self-care deficit, not because an individual has a psychological problem or psychiatric condition.

This chapter will present Orem's self-care model through a discussion of the three component theories: self-care, self-care deficit, and nursing systems, and then present an application of that theory by examining how the nurse identifies clinical problems, plans interventions, and evaluates outcomes from the self-care model. The approach represents nursing care for any individual in whom affect, self-esteem, hostility, social skills, trust, dependency, anxiety, orientation and/or perception problems affect self-care ability.

Self-care model: principles

The deliberate action of self-care is essential for health and well being and when, due to health-related self-care limitations, individuals are unable to meet therapeutic self-care demands and experience self-care deficits, nurses are needed to assist persons to accomplish self-care. The nurse and patient meet in the helping situation where nurses design, manage, and maintain systems of care. These nursing systems include the social, inter-personal, and technological sub-systems and are designed to assist persons to meet self-care demands and thus to meet self-care requisites in living day-to-day. The self-care model guides the nurse to focus on the individual and his self-care behaviour in living day-to-day rather than on any specific psychological problem, symptom, or condition.

The theory of self-care

The theory of self-care explains why self-care activities are necessary to health and well being of the human being. The concepts of health and well being, deliberate action, basic conditioning factors, self-care requisites, and therapeutic self-care demands are central to the theory of self-care.

Self-care is defined as '. . . the practice of activities that individuals initiate and perform on their own behalf in maintaining life, health, and well being' (Orem, 1985, p. 86). Health and well being are closely related but separate states. Health describes structural and functional wholeness or integrity and is influenced by and influences physical, psychological, inter-personal and social aspects of living. Health is affected when there is change or disruption in the structural and functional wholeness or inte-grity (Orem, 1985 p. 173). Well being is associated with success in personal endeavours and sufficient resources as well as health; however, it is deter-mined by the individual's perception of condition of existence (Orem, 1985, p. 181). A sense of well-being depends on individual knowledge. Well-being, individual experiences of contentment, pleasure, and kinds of happiness develop in the process of becoming a person. In this process, the individual in interaction with his world seeks fulfilment of the ideal self to striving to '. . . perfect himself as a responsible human being who raises questions, seeks answers, reflects, and comes to awareness of the relation-ship between what he knows and what he does not know' (Orem, 1985, p. 180). Ideal self will, in large part, be determined by cultural and/or social values. In the American culture the highest values are put on the individ-ual and individual rights and responsibilities. This is reflected in Orem's theory in that the adult is a self-reliant and responsible individual and that includes responsibility for his own and his dependents' health and well-being. So within this culture a sense of well-being will include the ability to be responsible for one's dependents as well as one's own self.

Self-care is a human regulatory function and contributes in specific ways to structural and functional integrity and to growth and development. When self-care is not maintained, illness and/or disease and/or death will occur (Orem, 1985, pp. 85–87). It is required by every individual regardless of age, sex, culture, or health state. A number of variables including age, sex, developmental status, conditions of living, support systems including family, socio-cultural orientations, patterns of living, and health status called basic conditioning factors help us understand better the individual and the values he holds which influence his ability for self-care (Orem, 1985, pp. 220).

Self-care is learned, culturally linked, deliberate action. Deliberate action is purposeful, goal-directed, and result-seeking behaviour that includes all actions and activities that: (1) lead to a decision to act, and includes deciding what is to be done and for what purpose; and (2) follow the decision to act, including performance of the action. Even when self-care is performed largely out of habit, it is still a deliberate action (Orem, 1985, pp. 115–122).

Self-care is a response to the demand to attend to oneself. The purpose of the deliberate action called self-care is named self-care requisites. Orem identifies three types of self-care requisites: universal, developmental, and health deviation (see Fig. 8.1). The totality of action to be performed over time to attend to oneself is called therapeutic self-care demand. This term was devised to encompass all the actions required to meet self-care requi-sites. All self-care may not be therapeutic. Action is therapeutic to the degree it: (1) supports life processes and normal functioning; (2) maintains

Figure 8.1   Self-care requisites*

Universal: associated with maintaining general health and well being
1. maintain sufficient intake of air;
2. maintain sufficient intake of water;
3. maintain sufficient intake of food;
4. provide care associated with elimination;
5. maintain balance of activity and rest;
6. maintain balance of solitude and social interaction;
7. prevent hazards to life, function, and well being;
8. promote function and development in accord with genetic and constitutional characteristics and individual talents within social and cultural norms.

Developmental: associated with mental and physical development and events that adversely affect development
1. maintain conditions that promote normal resolution of developmental (age-related) crises across the life span;
2. prevent, mitigate, or overcome effects of situational (environmentally-related) crises across the life span.

Health-deviation: associated with management of the effects of illness and injury and diagnostic, therapeutic, and rehabilitative measures
1. seek appropriate health care;
2. be aware of and attend to, effects and results of pathological conditions;
3. carry out prescribed diagnostic, therapeutic, and rehabilitative measures;
4. be aware of, attend to, and/or regulate deleterious effects of diagnostic, therapeutic and rehabilitative measures;
5. modify self-concept in accord with changing health states and health care;
6. promote continued personal development in learning to live with effects of illness and injury and diagnostic, therapeutic and rehabilitative measures.

---

*Adapted from Orem (1985), pp. 90–9.

normal growth development and maturation; (3) prevents, cures, or controls disease process; (4) prevents or compensates for disability; and (5) promotes well-being (Orem, 1985, p. 89). The therapeutic self-care demands must be met if self-care requisites are to be met.

We usually speak of assisting persons to meet self-care demands rather then self-care requisites. Requisites are overall names for the purpose of self-care such as to maintain a balance of rest and activity, while demands represent the actual methods of accomplishing self-care, for example to decide to attend to the need for sleep and to act to obtain the required hours of sleep based on cultural, developmental and health conditions.

The theory of self-care deficits

The theory of self-care deficits explains when and why nursing is needed. Concepts central to the understanding of this theory are: self-care agency, self-care limitation, and self-care deficit.

Self-care agency is a human power and is defined as '...the complex acquired ability to meet one's requirements for care that regulate life processes, maintain or promote integrity of human structure and function, and develop and promote well being' (Orem, 1985, p. 105). Simply, self-care agency names the human capability to engage in self-care and is present and functioning when the individual can engage in deliberate action (deciding and doing) to meet therapeutic self-care demands. Agent denotes the person taking action. Self-care agent is self. Dependent care agent is other.

When an individual is restricted in providing self-care, there is a self-care limitation. Self-care limitations name the restriction. Orem identifies restrictions associated with: (1) knowing, (2) judgements and decision making, and (3) result-achieving actions (Orem, 1985, p. 125) (see Fig. 8.2).

Figure 8.2 Self-care limitations*

Knowing
Limitations related to knowing about one's own functioning, about needed self care and about operations to accomplish self care are associated with:
1. absence or lack of required knowledge;
2. disturbance in sensory, perceptual or cognitive functioning resulting in:
    (a) not being able to acquire or recall knowledge;
    (b) not knowing the environment or self in the environment;
3. Disturbance in sensory, perceptual or cognitive functioning resulting in:
    (a) not seeking knowledge;
    (b) not having knowledge that is basic to the doing aspect in result-achieving action.

Making judgements and decisions
Limitations related to one's view of oneself and one's pattern of decision making are associated with:
1. inadequate or inaccurate base of information, e.g., inability to seek or use rescoures appropriately;
2. reluctance or refusal to engage in decision making, e.g., inability to move from reflection to decision making.

Result-achieving actions
Limitations related to functional state and environmental conditions and circumstances are associated with:
1. Absence of conditions necessary for self-care:
    (a) lack of energy;
    (b) inability to attend to self to exercise self-care ability;
    (c) lack of interest in self-care.
2. Individual conditions of living:
    (a) deliberate interference in practice of self-care;
    (b) lack of social support necessary to sustain practice.

---

*Adapted from Orem (1985), pp. 125–8.

A self-care deficit is a function of the relationship between the therapeutic self-care demand and the individual's ability (self-care agency) to meet the demand. This relationship may be equal to, less than, or more than. When the relationship between the self-care agency and the therapeutic self-care demands of the individual, due to health related self-care limitations, results in ineffective or incomplete self-care, there is a self-care deficit (Orem, 1985, p. 34). Nursing is needed when individuals or groups with health-related self-care limitations have self-care deficits (Orem, 1985, p. 128). Not all people under medical care will need nursing care and not all people under nursing care will need medical care. The need for nursing is based on the individual's self-care deficit not on his medical diagnosis. When the self-care ability is less than the self-care demand and a deficit results, nursing care may be required. For example, the self-care demand may be to sleep a certain number of hours a night. However, as the result of psychosis, an individual may have a self-care limitation for engaging in results-achieving action. The person may be so pre-occupied with internal thoughts that he is not able to attend to the need for sleep. There is an imbalance between ability and demand and, therefore, the potential for a self-care deficit. Nursing is needed because the person is unable to meet the demand to engage in deciding and doing in such a way as to obtain needed sleep not because of the psychosis. The psychotic process may be central in producing the self-care deficit but it is the self-care deficit, not the psychosis, that requires nursing interventions.

The theory of nursing systems

The theory of nursing systems explains how persons are helped through nursing. The helping situation, helping methods, and social, interpersonal, and technological sub-systems and types of nursing systems are central to understanding nursing systems.

The nursing situation is a helping situation. A helping situation occurs when a person needing help interacts with a person able to provide that help. Ideally, the behaviour of the person needing help is complemented by the behaviour of the person providing help. In the complementary relationship the nurse acts in concert with the patient to provide self-care. The nurse either makes up the patient's lack of self-care capacity or assists the patient to maintain or increase his capacity for self-care (Orem, 1985, p. 59). The nurse uses the helping methods to assist the patient to meet his self-care demands and to assume responsibility for his own health-related self-care (see Fig. 8.3).

Nurses prescribe, design, manage, and maintain a system of care in which either the nurse or the patient, or the nurse and patient, act to meet the patient's self-care demands (Orem, 1985, p. 148). The three types of nursing systems: wholly compensatory, partly compensatory, and supportive–educative, each form a helping situation and reflects roles of nurse

Figure 8.3 Helping methods*

Doing and acting for:
Nurse: acts for patient
Patient: receives care.

Guiding and directing:
Nurse: provides necessary information to meet self-care requisites
Patient: uses information to meet self-care requisites.

Providing physical support:
Nurse: cooperates in meeting self-care demands
Patient: cooperates in meeting self-care demands.

Providing psychological support:
Nurse: provides empathetic listening and encouragement
Patient: may be able to cope with painful or unpleasant self-care situations.

Providing a therapeutic environment:
Nurse: provides environmental conditions that motivate the person to establish
         and meet appropriate goals for self-care
Patient: attempts to develop and meet appropriate goals for self-care.

Teaching:
Nurse: describes and explains self-care requisites and demands and identifies
         methods for calculating demands, compensating for limitations and
         managing self-care
Patient: develops knowledge and skill to meet, continuously and effectively,
         self-care requisites.

*Adapted from Orem (1985), p. 151.

and patient (see Fig. 8.4). Each type of nursing system includes the separate but interrelated social, interpersonal, and technological sub-systems. The sub-systems explain how nurses and patients relate. The social sub-system represents how nurses and patients are brought together. The need for nursing is determined by the society, and the nurse is empowered by the society to develop a relationship with the patient. This relationship is contractual in nature. This means that there is an agreement between the nurse and the patient as to what the nurse will do and what the patient will do (Orem, 1985, p. 213). The interpersonal sub-system represents the relationship between a particular patient and a particular nurse. This relationship is developed in order to provide the needed nursing care and to protect and foster the well-being of the patient. The relationship should allow the nurse and both patient and family to assume appropriate responsibility for health care and to participate positively in meeting present and future health goals (Orem, 1985, pp. 214–15). The technological sub-system represents the repertoire of nursing necessary to provide patient

Figure 8.4   Nursing systems*

Wholly compensatory system:
Nursing action: accomplishes self-care, compensates for inability for self-care,
                  supports and protects;
Patient action: receives care, support, and protection.

Partly compensatory system:
Nursing action: participates in decisions about self-care, performs some self-care,
                  compensates for limitations and assists;
Patient action: participates in decisions about self-care, performs some self-care,
                  accepts care and assistance.

Supportive–educative system:
Nursing action: participates in decisions about self-care and in the development of
                  self-care ability;
Patient action: participates in decisions about self-care and in the development of
                  self-care ability and accomplishes self-care.

---

*Adapted from Orem (1985), p. 153.

care. The nursing process organizes this repertoire. The technological sub-system is what we commonly think of when we say nursing practice (Orem, 1985, p. 200).

The theory of nursing systems explains how nurse and patients come together to accomplish the patient's self-care. Nursing systems include the social, interpersonal, and technological sub-systems and reflect the complementary nature of the helping situation in which nursing takes place.

Self-care model: application to psychiatric care

In addition to the self-care model the nurse must have knowledge about (1) human behaviour, both normal and disturbed, (2) the nursing process, and (3) the nurse–patient relationship. All of these areas are essential to the practice of nursing. The self-care model provides a focus for these knowledges and the skills developed from them that is unique to nursing. The model identifies the need for nursing when a person has an actual or potential self-care deficit and then assists the nurse to concentrate care in the most useful and productive way.

I will examine the use of the model with a psychiatric patient by discussing how we identify problems, focus intervention, and develop evaluation criteria. The following approach is used to determine whether the person needs nursing care, including psychiatric nursing care, and then to outline what that care will be and how it will be evaluated.

Identifying clinical problems

Psychiatric nurses can expect that individuals who come to our attention will have psychological problems, symptoms or conditions. However, in keeping with the self-care approach our concern will be with the individual's ability to meet self-care demands and thus self-care requisites. The nursing assessment is done to determine the presence of an actual or potential self-care deficit. To facilitate assessment, the writer developed a guide to potential deficits based on the general set of actions to meet eight universal self-care requisites developed by Orem. The original set was modified by integrating the requisites to promote normal functioning into all other areas, and by adding a requisite that focuses on personal hygiene. When dealing with adults, an assessment of developmental requisites is considered part of the developmental area of basic conditioning factors. The health deviation requisites and demands are included in the universal requisite affected. That is, the nurse asks what must the person do in each universal area to manage the effects of illness or treatment on this area. For example, if the person must learn to attend to external rather than internal stimuli in order to interact with others, that is included in the area of solitude and social interactions (see Fig. 8.5).

The nurse begins by assessing basic conditioning factors. This gives an idea who the person is, and what may have and will continue to influence his ability to meet self-care demands. Then, for each universal self-care requisite (Fig. 8.5), the nurse will ask the following questions. (1) What are all the behaviours usually necessary to meet this self-care requisite (therapeutic self-care demand)? (2) Was this person able to engage in all the behaviours in the past? (3) Does he have the potential to engage in the behaviours in the future? (4) Can the person presently engage in such behaviours? (5) What prevents him from engaging in the behaviours (self-care limitation)? (6) What specific behaviour is the patient unable to do (self-care deficit)?

The self-care model changes the definition of clinical problems by asking: 'Is there a self-care deficit', not 'Is there a psychological problem?' The presence of self-care deficits initiates the development of nursing intervention.

Identifying intervention

Changing the way nurses look at clinical problems changes the focus of interventions. Since clinical problems will be expressed in terms of self-care deficit, interventions will focus on self-care ability and therapeutic self-care demands, not on psychological problems. Nurses will ask: 'What type of nursing system, and what helping methods, are needed to meet the self-care demands?' The specific concern will be in assisting individuals to meet self-care demands, not in assisting individuals to overcome or

Figure 8.5   Self-care requisites and deficits*

General set of actions for meeting universal self-care requisites	*Potential for self-care deficits*
In accord with social, cultural developmental and functional norms individuals will:	Seriously mentally ill individuals have potential unmet demands and resulting deficits as follows:

1. Maintain sufficient intake of air/food/fluid

Taking in that quantity required for normal functioning with adjustments for internal and external factors that can affect the requirement, or, under conditions of scarcity, adjusting consumption to bring the most advantageous return to integrated functioning; preserving the integrity of associated anatomical structures and physiological processes, enjoying the pleasure of breathing, eating, and drinking without excess.	Unless there is a physical problem, most patients can meet demands associated with intake of air. The patient may have difficulty attending to intake of appropriate types and amounts of food or fluid. He may refuse to eat, or over-eat. He will most likely have limitations of judgement, decision making, and result-achieving actions. As symptoms subside, individuals can manage usual demands independently but will need assistance to learn to manage medication side-effects that affect intake.

2. Maintain care associated with elimination

Bringing about and maintaining internal and external conditions necessary for the regulation of processes of elimination (including protection of the structures and processes involved) and disposal of excrements; providing subsequent hygienic care of body surfaces and parts; caring for the environment as needed to maintain sanitary conditions.	The patient may not be able to attend to the impulse to eliminate or to control the impulse. As the acute symptoms subside he will be able to manage the usual demands but will need assistance to learn to manage medication side-effects that affect elimination.

3. Maintain body temperature and personal hygiene

Bring about and/or maintain internal and external conditions necessary for regulating body temperature processes; using personal capabilities and values as well as culturally prescribed norms as bases for maintaining personal hygiene; caring for environment to maintain a healthy living condition. (Developed and added by Underwood.)	The patient may not be able to attend to the environment and may not be able to meet demands associated with body temperature. The patient tends to have many deficits in personal hygiene, and suffers limitation in knowing, judgements and decision-making, and result-achieving actions. After symptoms subside he may continue to show deficits in this area and will need nursing assistance to meet and/or learn to meet self-care demands.

4. Maintain a balance between rest and activity

Selecting activities that stimulate, engage, and keep in balance physical movement, affective responses, intellectual effort, and social interaction; recognizing and attending to manifestations of needs for rest and activity; using personal capabilities, interest, and values as well as culturally prescribed norms as a basis for development of rest and activity patterns.

Patients are often unable to meet the demands associated with the balance of rest and activity. They are often unable to manage their day or to develop a regular pattern of rest/activity. They have limitations in judgement/decisions, knowing and result-achieving action. Patients continue to have these limitations after the acute phase and as a result deficits and problems in learning to select and/or participate in activities that stimulate, engage and balance one or more of the following: movement, affective response, intellectual effort or social interaction. Community-based services are most appropriate in providing the required nursing assistance.

5. Maintain a balance between solitude and social interaction

Maintain that quality and balance necessary for the development of personal autonomy and enduring social relations that foster effective functioning of individuals. Fostering bonds of affection, love, and friendship; effectively managing impulses to use others for selfish purposes, disregarding their individuality, integrity, and rights; providing conditions of social warmth and closeness essential for continuing development and adjustment; promoting individual autonomy as well as group membership.

Patients perhaps have the most difficulty meeting demands associated with this area. The person will most likely continue to have limitations in knowing, judgement and decisions, and result-achieving actions that produce deficits and problems in learning long after acute symptoms have passed, and will continue to need nursing help to meet and/or learn to meet these demands. Personal autonomy and enduring social relations are often demands that require life-long assistance. This assistance is best provided in a community-based service.

6. Prevent hazards to life, function, and well-being

Being alert to types of hazards that are likely to occur; taking action to prevent the occurrence of events that may lead to the development of hazardous situations; removing or protecting oneself from hazardous situations when a hazard cannot be eliminated; controlling hazardous situations to eliminate danger to life or well-being.

Patients will most likely not be able to meet demands due to limitation in knowing, judgement and decision making, and result-achieving actions. In addition, when acute symptoms are present the person may be of danger to themselves or others. The person will require on-going community-based assistance.

---

*The general set of actions in areas 1, 2, 4, 5 and 6 are quoted from Orem (1985), p. 92.

correct psychological problems. For example, nursing care can assist a person to meet the self-care requisite to maintain a balance of rest/activity by assisting the person to sleep by doing things such as creating an environment conducive to sleep, helping the individual develop a bedtime routine and/or teaching him relaxation exercises; in the process, the nurse will surely deal with anxiety or dependency, but interventions are focused on developing a rest/activity pattern, not on reducing or correcting psychological problems.

If the nurse must assume responsibility for the patient's self-care, a wholly compensatory system is needed, and acting and doing will be the primary helping method. If the patient can assume some responsibility, a partly compensatory system is needed and all helping methods may be appropriate. If the patient can meet self-care with education and/or support, a supportive–educative system is needed, and all helping methods except acting and doing may be appropriate. Interventions will identify both nurse's and patient's responsibilities.

Identifying evaluation criteria

As we change the way we define clinical problems and focus interventions we also change the expected outcomes of nursing care. Outcomes of nursing care will be measured by the individual's ability to meet therapeutic self-care demands so that self-care requisites are met to attain, maintain and/or regain health and/or well-being. Our specific contribution to the overall goal of health and well-being is to see that the self-care requisites are met. Nursing care may reduce, change, improve, or correct anxiety, dependency, hostility, or delusional thinking, however our interventions are developed and to meet self-care demands. Nursing care will be evaluated in terms of the person meeting self-care requisites, not in terms of the person resolving psychological problems. The outcomes or goals of nursing care are stated in terms of self-care requisites. When the self-care demand is met, and thus the self-care requisite met, then the nursing care is successful even if the patient continues to have psychological problems. The nurse's effectiveness is determined by how well the self-care requisites are met, not by the number or intensity of symptoms or the resolution of psychological problems. Nursing care is required when the person has an actual or potential self-care deficit, interventions are designed to assist patients to meet self-care demands and the expected outcome is that the self-care requisite is met.

Conclusion

The self-care model offers nurses the opportunity to develop an independent area of practice where clinical problems, interventions, and outcomes are reflective of nursing rather then medicine or psychotherapy. Many mental health disciplines, including nursing, are concerned with psychological problems, symptoms, or conditions, and their impact on health and well-being, but the specific concern of nursing is assisting the patient to meet self-care requisites in living day-to-day. When this is not the focus of nursing practice, patients are often deprived of nursing care and as a result may be unable to enjoy either health or well-being, because of self-care deficits. When nurses focus on assisting the patient to be self-reliant and responsible in meeting self-care requisites, we offer him the opportunity to enhance health and well-being, especially well-being. And in so doing, we make a meaningful and unique contribution to patient care and treatment.

Reference

Orem, D. (1985) *Nursing: Concepts of Practice*, 3rd edn, McGraw-Hill, New York.

Further Reading

Munley, M. and Sayers, P. (1984) *Self-care Deficit Theory of Nursing*, Personal and Family Health Associates, New Jersey.
The Nursing Development Conference Group (1979) *Concept Formalization in Nursing*, 2nd edn, Little, Brown, and Co., Boston.

Chapter 9

Roy's adaptation model: principles and general applications

K. DORSEY and S. PURCELL

The adaptation model by Sister Callista Roy was developed when, as a graduate student, she was challenged to develop a theory for nursing. During that time her studies were supervised by Dorothy Johnson at the University of California. Roy began by conceptualizing the goal of nursing as facilitating the adaptation of persons to their environment. Utilizing research literature dealing with stress and coping she provided the scientific basis for her ideas.

The model incorporates Selye's stress theory. Selye (1978) believes that the process of adaptation is the dynamic base of human life; existence itself is a continued game of coping with the environment and that the secret to life is successful adjustment to ever-changing stress. Selye states there are two roads to survival, flight and adaptation; most often adaptation is the more successful of the two.

Roy was one of the first theorists to use ideas that were well developed in other disciplines as a basis for theory building in nursing. The model was initially operationalized in a Baccalaureate nursing curriculum at Mt St Marys College at Los Angeles, California, and is now utilized in a variety of clinical and community settings throughout the world.

Since the initial development of the adaptation theory, Roy has continued to describe and clarify its components. Roy's model development has been influenced, Sato (1986) noted, by leaders in the field of adaptation, including Dohrenwend (1961), Helson (1964), Lazarus (1966), Mechanic (1970) and Selye (1978). Recently, Roy completed her post-doctoral education in the Robert Wood Johnson Clinical Nurse Scholars Program at the University of California in San Francisco.

Roy (1981) organized her model within three key concepts: 1. the first concept of man as the client and recipient of health care; 2. the second concept of the goal of nursing which is to promote adaptation through the client's individual adaptive processes; and 3. the third concept of nursing activities, including nursing assessments of client behaviours, causative factors, and nursing interventions which are based on the nursing process, incorporating nursing diagnosis. Basic assumptions of Roy's model include the description of man as a recipient of nursing care and the concepts of adaptation, health, stimuli, nursing intervention and goals.

Man as client and recipient of nursing care

Roy (1976) defines man the client as a bio-psycho-social being who is constantly interacting with the environment. Roy draws from the concept of Dunn (1971) that man can be compared to the dynamics of a cell unit whose parts have relationships which present an integrated whole. Like the cell, the constant interaction with internal and external environments requires matter, energy and information which result in continuous change. The constant responses enable man to maintain integrity or homeostasis throughout adaptation. Roy defines adaptation as man's positive or adaptive response to the environment.

Adaptation

Adaptation occurs through genetic, inherited responses or learned responses. The adaptation process can be considered as an open system involving input, feedback and output. The input consists of stimuli and the output consists of the adaptive or inadaptive responses.

Sub-systems of adaptation

Roy (1976) identified two sub-systems in the adaptive process: the regulator which is a genetic response and the cognator which is a learned or social response. The regulator and the cognator sub-systems comprise the feedback process within the system.

The regulator sub-system   The regulator sub-system involves mainly genetic responses. Neural, endocrine and perceptual motor pathways are utilized for transmission of stimuli.

Neural activities are the body's chemical responses which transduce or change energy into information that travels along intact nerve pathways. An example of a neural response is the neural activity occurring when a finger is accidentally burnt on the stove. The heat energy from the stove as it touches the finger is changed to information that travels along nerve pathways to the spine and eventually to the brain. Endocrine activities are automatic responses that increase heart rate when a person experiences injury. Under this sub-system both perceptual and/or motor activities occur through glandular and/or muscular activity as a result of the stimulation of the neural activity. Perceptual and/or motor activities are socially influenced; example: in some cultures one is expected to be quietly tolerant of the burned finger whereas in another the injured individual would be expected to cry out and express distress.

The cognator sub-system The cognator sub-system is comprised of four areas of activity: selective attention, learning, judgement and emotions. The cognator mechanism involves man's conscious perception of stimuli. The mechanism also involves the subconscious use of defence mechanisms.

Selective attention is the coding and memory activity which occurs in perceptual information processing. For example, an individual who inadvertently touched a finger on a hot stove will file the experience away. Storage of the memory and conditions such as personal readiness or unreadiness to cope are involved.

Learning will involve imitation and insight. When encountering a stimulus such as a burnt finger, one will refer to cultural standards of behaviour and react accordingly.

Judgement occurs through problem-solving and decision-making. How the burned finger should be treated will be based on the extent of injuries and availability of health care.

Emotions allow one to vent defences and to seek relief, to gain insight and to form attachments; crying, anger, seeking support and sympathy of others when unintentionally one's finger is burnt on a stove.

Man copes effectively with stimuli within an adaptation range which is shaped by an individual ability. Roy describes stimuli as anything which evokes response; she identifies three types of stimuli: focal, contextual and residual. Focal stimuli are those which demand most immediate responses. Contextual stimuli are all other stimuli occurring as the person copes with the focal stimuli. Residual stimuli are prior experiences expressed as beliefs and attitudes which are believed to impact on the individual's ability to cope. Focal and contextual stimuli influence behaviour and can be validated. However, the impact of residual stimuli on behaviour can only be presumed but not validated.

Adaptation level

The adaptation level is determined by focal, contextual and residual stimuli and by individual capacity to react in an adaptive manner. Roy proposes that adaptive behaviour maintains integrity whereas maladaptive behaviour disrupts integrity. Integrity is the sound or unimpaired function that may contribute to one's unity or completeness. Roy maintains that integrity is achieved through growth, reproduction, mastery and survival.

Adaptive modes

Roy views man as a bio-psycho-social being who copes with stimuli through four adaptive modes (ways): physiological, self-concept, role function and interdependence. Each mode meets a need which is essential for integrity. The responses result in behaviours which meet physiological, psychic and social needs.

In the physiological mode, behaviours meet physiological integrity needs. These needs include exercise and rest, nutrition, elimination, fluid and electrolytes, oxygen and circulation. Also included is regulation which involves temperature, the senses and the endocrine system functions.

In the self-concept mode, behaviours meet psychic energy needs. Self-concept is shaped by interaction with others. It includes one's view of self, and perception of how others react to one's actions. Physical sensations, body image and personal expectations also influence self-concept.

In role function and interdependence modes, behaviours meet social integrity needs. Role function is defined by tasks or behaviours based on one's varying positions in society. It includes considerations of the developmental level of the individual, age, group, sex, primary, secondary and tertiary roles. In the interdependence mode behaviours satisfy needs for love and support through interaction with others. Attention and gratification give meaning and purpose to life. Interdependence is a satisfactory balance between self reliance and relying on others.

The health—illness continuum

A basic assumption of the Roy adaptation model is that the health–illness continuum is a dimension of one's total life experience. Health is viewed as managing and coping with changing stimuli, resulting in integration and wholeness. Health is a dynamic process, utilizing positive adaptation to change. Roy has placed health and illness on a continuum that moves from death to peak wellness. Health is synonymous with function which promotes individual survival.

The grid in Fig. 9.1 illustrates the relationship between health levels and adaptive function levels. Good health results from behaviours at functional levels that maintain the individual. The person moves towards higher levels of wellness through increased adaptive capacity. When the individual moves towards poor health behaviours that hinder and can endanger survival, reduced adaptive capacity is evident.

Goal of nursing

The goal of nursing is to promote adaptation. The client can change from internal and external environments while maintaining personal growth and achievement. The nurse, after viewing the client at a specific point

Figure 9.1   Relationship between function and levels of wellness. (Source: death to peak wellness continuum, courtesy of Callista Roy. Functional continuum courtesy of authors.)

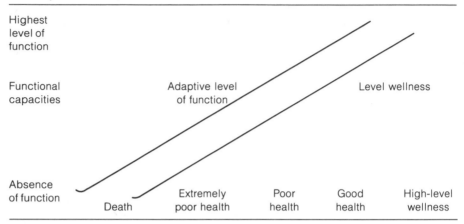

on a wellness–illness continuum, attempts to move the client toward maximum wellness. Nursing intervenes when stimuli fall outside the adaptive level and maladaptive behaviour occurs.

Nursing interventions involve altering the stimuli to fall within the client's range of effective coping. The nurse may select stimuli which may be changed to fall within the client's present range of adaptation. Stimuli may also be rejected as part of the nursing intervention.

Nursing activities

Nursing activity in Roy's model utilizes the nursing process including nursing diagnosis. The four activities of the nursing process are to assess, to plan, to implement and to evaluate.

Nursing assessment takes place on two levels as follows:

First level: The nurse observes and notes adaptive and maladaptive behaviours.

Second level: The nurse identifies and notes causative stimuli.

During the assessment phase, nursing diagnoses are selected which identify behaviours and stimuli. Each nursing diagnosis will become the focus of nursing interventions. As the nursing plan develops, specific goals are established that describe the expected client behaviours. Interventions developed by the nurse detail the plan for changing stimuli to promote adaptation.

Evaluation of the client's coping strategies or behavioural changes determine whether the goal of adaptation has been met. The entire process is repeated for each unmet goal. If the goal is not met, the process is still valuable, for it enables the client to utilize coping strategies in a healthier way. The model enables evaluation on several levels concurrently while promoting a holistic assessment.

Summary

The Roy adaptation model is clinically applicable because it provides a nursing framework to evaluate behaviour and structure appropriate intervention. Goal-setting is also facilitated.

The theory analysis identified by Dickoff and James (1968) provides a framework for analysis of the elements of Roy's adaptation model:

1. The goal is to assist man toward health by promoting and supporting his adaptive abilities.
2. The prescription involves manipulation of focal, contextual and residual stimuli.
3. The agency involves nurse–patient interaction. The patient must do the adapting. The nurse is the supporter and promoter of the adaptation.
4. Dynamics involve the patient, adaptive mechanisms and the nurses' problem-solving abilities.
5. Patency describes who is the recipient of the activity. Man is viewed as a bio-psycho-social being, in constant interaction with his environment on a particular point on the health–illness continuum.
6. The framework for the model is any setting, any time in which man is experiencing a relationship to a situation to health and wellness.
7. The terminus or completion of the nursing interaction is when the patient adapts to the stimuli placing unusual demands on him.

General application of the Roy adaptation model

The Roy model provides bio-psycho-social approaches associated with the client's mental health problems. Use of the Roy model in problems with low self-esteem is an illustration of implementation to promote adaptation using the nursing process.

Self-esteem has been described by Driever (1976) as the value the person holds of himself. Self-esteem is formed from the reaction of others which Driever terms self-definers. Driever postulates that adaptation through the self-concept model is facilitated by high self-esteem. Low self-esteem leads to less effective coping abilities. High self-esteem enhances effective adaptation.

Driever identified components within the self-concept mode describing social and physical behaviour. The four components of self-concept are:

1. physical self
2. moral–ethical self

3. self-consistency

4. self-ideal and expectancy

Physical self includes bodily sensations and self perception of body. Moral–ethical self describes a self-judgement of behaviour. Self-consistency describes the need to maintain a self-image that is consistent with self image. Any threat to self-consistency causes anxiety. Self-ideal and expectancy describes anticipation of future behaviour to achieve goals and to cope. Unmet goals result in powerlessness; met goals result in power and control.

Low self-esteem behaviours which have been identified by Driever (1976) are summarized in Fig. 9.2. Low self-esteem behaviour includes alterations in digestion, activity and rest patterns. Decreased concentration results in difficulty in initiating or completing tasks. Inappropriate social interactions include withdrawal, fear of criticism or arguing with others and isolation. Preoccupation with self and inner problems is evidenced in recurring somatic complaints. Nursing interventions presented in Fig. 9.3 are based on assessments detailed in Fig. 9.2. Together, information in Figs 9.2 and 9.3 comprise steps of the nursing process: assess, plan, implement and evaluate.

Figure 9.2   Low self-esteem behaviour assessment based on Roy adaptation model. (Adapted from Driever (1976), pp. 237–40.)

First level: behaviours	*Second level: stimuli*	*Nursing diagnosis*
Appetite changes – body weight more or less than required	*Focal* Event(s) that may threaten self-esteem	Actual deficit in self-esteem seen in behaviour changes in reaction to precipitating event
Bowel activity changes	*Contextual*	
Sleeping changes	Age	
Decreased motor activities	Sex Social values	
Decreased concentration	Personal values Cultural values	
Difficulty initiating and completing tasks	Growth/development/ situational crisis	
Withdrawal from others	*Residual*	
Fear of criticism or angering others	Prior life experiences Education	
Isolation	Occupation	
Inappropriate anger or hostility	Familial influences Religion Income	
Preoccupation with self		
Perception of self-worthlessness		

In Fig. 9.2 focal, contextual and residual stimuli are detailed. Focal stimuli are any events that threaten self-esteem. Contextual stimuli include age, sex, social, personal and cultural values. Illness, growth and development and situational crises are also considered contextual stimuli. Residual stimuli include social, familial and cultural experiences. Education and occupation may also may be considered residual stimuli.

Figure 9.3 presents a general application of nursing prescriptions focusing on low self-esteem. Interventions presented are applicable to both hospital and community settings, and are based on Driever's protocol for goals, intervention and evaluations. The goal is changed client behaviour indicative of higher self-esteem. The client collaborates with the nurse on goal setting.

Intervention focuses on changing or eliminating stimuli to facilitate client change. The nurse and client examine stimuli to identify factors that provide an opportunity for growth.

Contextual stimuli are reviewed to assist the client to identify self-definers and feelings. The client identifies stimuli that trigger low esteem. After exploring cultural values, the client makes choices about which

Figure 9.3 Nursing intervention for the client with low self-esteem based on the Roy adaptation model

Plan	Implement	Evaluate
1. Complete first- and second-level assessments and establish nursing diagnosis.	Nurse and client examine stimuli to identify opportunities for growth rather than to view it as a self-demeaning experience	Behaviour changes are examined by client with a predetermined time frame.
2. State nursing goal; client will demonstrate higher self-esteem through adaptive behaviour. Client and nurse collaborate on goals.	Client identifies self-definers, and increases understanding of own feelings.	Achieved goals are positive reinforcement. Unmet goals become basis for reassessment.
	Client explains how self values shape behaviour. Client explores prior life experiences to gain insight. Client will take charge of decision making process.	

stimuli will be accepted or rejected. Residual stimuli are examined to develop insight into the impact of prior life experiences.

Evaluation focuses on changed behaviour. The nurse gives positive reinforcement for met goals. Unmet goals are not seen as failures but provide the basis for reassessment. Although self-esteem behaviours may not change, the model provides a framework for bio-psycho-social assessment of the client's needs. The client–nurse relationship is essential to acquisition of valid data. The power of therapeutic communication can alter the client's perception of every aspect of life.

Summary of general application

In summary, Roy's adaptation model guides the nurse in the prescription of appropriate interventions through assessment of behaviour and altering stimuli to enhance coping capacity. Through utilization of the nursing process the nurse is able to assess and predict established outcomes. This strategy enables the client to regain mastery.

References

Dickoff, J. and James, P. (1968) Theory is a practice discipline. *Nurs. Res.*, **17**, 415–35.

Dohrenwend, B. P. (1961) The social psychological nature of stress: a framework for causal inquiry. *J. Abnorm. Social Psychol.*, **212**, 294–302.

Driever, M. (1976) Problem of self-esteem, in *Introduction to Nursing and Adaptation Model* (ed. C. Roy), Prentice Hall, Englewood Cliffs, NJ.

Dunn, H. (1971) *High Level Wellness*, R. W. Beatty, Arlington, VA.

Helson, H. (1964) *Adaptation Level Theory*, Harper and Row, New York.

Lazarus, R. S. (1966) *Psychological Stress and the Coping Process*, McGraw Hill, New York.

Mechanic, D. (1970) Some problems in developing a social psychology of adaptation to stress, in *Social and Psychological Factors in Stress* (ed. J. McGrath), Holt, Rinehart and Winston, New York.

Roy, C. (1976) *Introduction to Nursing: an Adaptation Model*, Prentice Hall, Englewood Cliffs, NJ.

Roy, C. (1981) *Theory Construction in Nursing: an Adaptation Model*, Appleton and Lange, USA.

Sato, M. (1986) The Roy adaptation model, in *Introduction to Nursing: An Adaptation Model in Case Studies in Nursing Theory* (ed. Winstead-Fry) National League for Nursing, New York.

Selye, H. (1978) *The Stress of Life*, McGraw Hill, New York.

Chapter 10

The eclectic approach: principles and general applications

P. SCHRODER and B. BENFER

Introduction

Psychiatric and mental health nursing practice by necessity is based upon the application of relevant theories, some drawn from nursing itself and others drawn from related fields of practice. There does not exist at this time one single theory that can encompass the broad scope of patients, ranging from personality disorders to major psychosis, to otherwise healthy individuals having difficulty in coping with either one specific aspect of their lives or one particular time when a crisis situation is encountered. Equally, psychiatric nursing spans a continuum of concepts, ranging from wellness and health, to severe illness. To further add to the knowledge-base required in psychiatric services, nurse's practise varies from out-patient settings where activities are directed toward prevention or practice in one of the therapies shared by several disciplines, to practice within an in-patient setting where the work is primarily within the hospital milieu, giving direct care and making interventions appropriate to individual patient needs.

The authors of this chapter contend that while many theoretical constructs apply to psychiatric nursing practice, there must be organization to the theories applied, with careful thought and attention to how the theories fit together. Certainly, two diametrically opposed theories cannot be used simultaneously by the nurse. Instead, one theory builds upon and augments another. In this chapter, the authors will set forth a combination of theoretical constructs that can serve as a basis for the practising psychiatric nurse.

Before a practitioner can develop a concept of illness, there must be a basis for normal growth and development, for understanding normal behaviour, and a theory of how or where problems begin that cause difficulty in later life. Psychoanalytic theory provides such a baseline, drawing on commonly held concepts of anxiety, defence mechanisms, and the unconscious as well as conscious aspects of personality or the development of the self. As a child develops, interactions with others, particularly parenting figures, shape future behaviour, and an interpersonal theory explains the impact of relationships between and among people, along with psycho-analytic theory of stages of development of individuals. Theories related to illness take into consideration the earlier experiences, the genetic predispositions, and current life situations. Ego psychology offers an overall view of human behaviour on a continuum, from areas of wellness to areas of weakness. Finally, theory related to the therapeutic use of self, as developed by Peplau (1952; 1965) gives the nurse tools by which intervention can be made, and concepts related to the milieu provide the nurse with an understanding of the environment in which change can take place.

Major structure of personality

Almost all theories used by nursing take into account the growth and development of the individual, with many having an origin in psycho-analytic concepts. While Freud (1917) was credited with the concept of persons having an id, ego, and superego, current psycho-analytic theory goes far beyond those original ideas.

Psycho-analytic theory is based on several assumptions, including the idea that all human behaviour is determined by antecedent life events, and that each person has a conscious, a pre-conscious, and an unconscious level of awareness. Personality development is seen in terms of three major structures: the id, ego, and superego; personality develops in stages, with crucial experiences or learning taking place at various stages. Within this premise, all human behaviour can be explained, and persons have flexibility which will permit change to take place, especially in those areas which are problematic for them (Johnson, 1986).

The id is seen as that part of the personality structure containing impulses and primitive instincts, and it is pleasure-seeking without inhibition. The id is present at birth, and continues throughout life, but it is contained or redirected by the ego and superego. Without the ego and superego, human behaviour would be impulsive, pleasure-seeking, unrelated to reality, and thus inappropriate much of the time.

The superego might best be thought of as the conscience of the person, that part which contains moral values, society's expectations, and beliefs of right or wrong which are learned from parenting figures. The superego has a primary role to play in the individual's conformity to laws, rules, and regulations, and the adoption of society's values as one's own. Unlike the id, which is present at birth, the superego is a result of the individual's interactions with important others, with a sense of right and wrong that is patterned after those of significant others. If the superego is too lax, or does not incorporate values in keeping with the society in which one lives, the individual is likely to operate more on id impulses, seeking gratification with little concern for others. On the other hand, if the individual develops too severe a superego, he/she is more likely to be inhibited and driven by guilt, with less ability to enjoy life's experiences.

The third component of the personality structure is the ego. This part of the personality makes up the larger part of what became known as the self system. The ego is generally the more rational and adaptive part of the personality, balancing the drives for pleasure of the id with the drives for conformity of the superego. The ego serves a regulatory function, not only keeping the id and superego in check, but simultaneously maintaining a balance with reality and new experiences.

Ego functions

In psychodynamic literature, the concept of the ego is further developed, with ego functions and ego defences identified. Bellak, Hurvich and Gediman (1973) formulated the ego functions into 12 components, each with the potential to foster general adaptation (ego strength) or to contribute to lack of adaptation (ego weakness).

Reality testing is one such function, representing the individual's ability to perceive accurately both internal and external events, and to distinguish between the two. Another ego function is judgement, representing the individual's ability to anticipate consequences of behaviour, as well as to use that information to determine behaviour, and how appropriate that behaviour is in relation to a given situation. Yet another ego function is sense of reality, or the degree to which there is clarification of boundaries between oneself and the world, including a sense of self-identity and self-esteem.

A fourth ego function encompasses regulation and control of drives, affects and impulses, or how drives are experienced in an adaptive way with neither over nor under control. Object relations as an ego function contributes to adaptation in terms of relations with others, particularly those which are significant to the individual. Thought processes is the ego function which includes the ability to conceptualize, to engage in abstract or concrete modes of thinking, and the extent to which language and communication reflect thought of a primary or secondary nature.

Adaptive regression in the service of the ego (ARISE) is the ability to be flexible in thinking, and to relax cognitive acuity; in other words, to be adaptive in approaches and ways of thinking. Yet another ego function, defensive functioning, is how effective the individual's ego defences are in maintaining the integrity of the self.

Stimulus barrier is an ego function that deals with tolerance for stimuli and effectiveness in dealing with excessive stimulus input. Autonomous functioning has to do with the degree to which there is intrusion of conflict, ideation, affect and/or impulses upon functioning in both basic functions and complex skills and habit as well as automatic behaviours.

Synthetic–integrative functioning is the degree to which there is integration or reconciliation of contradictory attitudes, values, feelings, behaviour, and roles, and how well the individual can handle more than one task or activity at a time. Last, mastery-competence is how well a person performs in relation to his capabilities, and to what extent he actively takes steps to master and affect his environment.

In addition to the three major structures of the personality (id, ego, and superego) and the ego functions to be carried out, an understanding of the personality must also include the three levels of awareness within which the personality functions. These include the conscious (what we are aware of), unconscious (that which is out of our awareness and which we cannot bring to the conscious level voluntarily), and the pre-conscious, (that which is outside awareness, but which when triggered to do so, we can recall). Many of the ego functions operate at an unconscious or preconscious level, as do ego defences.

Ego defences are mechanisms the ego pulls into operation to protect against anxiety or interpsychic conflict that creates internal tension. They are an attempt to cope by resorting to various forms of adaptation, including reverting to behaviour patterns that evolved during earlier stages of growth and development. Most of the ego defences operate on an unconscious level. The defences serve as a barrier to the unacceptable input from the environment or internal stimuli, or prevent threatening unconscious material from coming into the conscious awareness. Some of the most commonly used defence mechanisms are identified in Fig. 10.1. All persons use defence mechanisms to a greater or lesser degree. Healthy individuals most commonly use defences to cope with mild or moderate levels of anxiety so that the person is protected from feelings of inadequacy or from input which does not fit with their self-image. However, defences can be used to such a degree that ego disintegration occurs, creating instability in that person's ability to cope adequately or to maintain a hold on reality.

Developmental theory

Ego functions develop as ego strengths or weaknesses, and the selection of the ego defences an individual utilizes is based upon the experiences of the individual at different developmental stages starting at birth. Those experiences shape the self-image, or how the individual characterizes himself or herself, and influences how well he or she will relate to the world around them. Tasks to be accomplished, strengths to be developed, and areas which may later be problematic, have been understood through the work and writing of Erikson (1963), Sullivan (1953) and Mahler, Pine

Figure 10.1 Ego defence mechanisms

Defence mechanisms	Definition	Discussion/example
Denial	A mental mechanism whereby the person fails to acknowledge the existence of an affect, memory, or experience.	This defence mechanism helps the person get away from an unpleasant reality, such as a person with terminal illness enrolling in flying lessons.
Displacement	This is an unconscious transferring of emotions, feelings or ideas from its original object to a more acceptable or safer substitute.	For example, a person may wish to yell at his boss but that is not acceptable, so the yelling is at one's spouse or friends.
Identification	A person unconsciously takes on the characterist-ics or identifying traits of others. This contributes to ego development; however, it does not replace one's own ego identity.	Identification plays an important role in development of the superego and of acceptance of society's rules and standards.
Introjection	This is a form of identi-fication with another person or object which is taken in or incorporated into one's own ego.	Like identification, introjection plays an important part in superego development by incorporating parents' rewards and punishments.
Projection	The process of attributing emotionally unacceptable traits to another.	This mental mechanism is used normally in a variety of situations; however, it is used excessively by persons with paranoid thought patterns.
Rationalization	This is a defence mechanism in which the person attempts to make one's own behaviour appear to be the result of thinking rather than unconscious wishes or impulses. Everyone uses	This is a form of self-deception and is used unconsciously in order to tolerate certain logical feelings and behaviours that would otherwise be intolerable. For example, a student fails a course

Figure 10.1   (cont.)

Defence mechanisms	Definition	Discussion/example
	rationalization at one time or another. It is problematic only when used habitually so that harmful behaviour can be justified in one's mind.	but says the teacher is ineffective in teaching.
Reaction formation	A mental mechanism by which an individual expresses feelings and wishes that are directly opposite to unconscious feelings and wishes.	For instance, a teenager unconsciously wishes to be taken care of but, instead, is excessively independent in all actions.
Regression	A mental mechanism whereby a person returns to earlier behaviours in stages of development that were successful in order to resolve conflict and frustration.	Regression is normal, and everyone uses this mechanism at times when under stress. An example is the adult who utilizes temper tantrums when frustrated.
Repression	A defence mechanism by which a person unconsciously bars unacceptable thoughts, feelings, or impulses from consciousness.	A person using repression to relieve anxiety and mental conflict is unaware he is forgetting an unpleasant or painful situation.
Splitting	Separation of the perception of self or others into opposing polarities of all good or all bad, with vacillation between the extremes dependent on the affective response to the immediate situation.	The patient sees the nurse on days as being very helpful and understanding of his problems while the nurse on evenings has no understanding at all and never helps him but rather sets rules for him all the time.
Sublimation	Transformation of psychic energy from unwanted sexual thoughts or aggressive drives into socially acceptable pursuits.	A severely injured athlete becomes a successful artist.

| Substitution | A defence mechanism in which a person replaces an unacceptable need, attitude or emotion with a more acceptable one. | Example: young woman marries an older man who resembles her father. |

and Bergman (1975). Erikson (1963) has identified the eight stages of life, seeing development as a continuum from birth to death. During infancy, the development of trust (versus mistrust) is a major task to be accomplished, setting the stage for the individual to learn a sense of hope as well as trust. During early childhood, the task to be learned is autonomy (versus shame and doubt). During pre-school years, the child has the task of learning initiative (versus guilt), thereby gaining a sense of purpose to activities. During early school years, the task is to learn industry (versus inferiority), thus developing competence in tasks. In adolescence, the task is to develop a sense of identity (versus identity confusion); as a young adult the individual has the task of learning intimacy (versus being isolated) which is important in terms of learning how to love. In the mature stage of life, or adulthood, tasks continue, with the primary one being generativity (versus self-absorption), and in older years, learning integrity (versus despair and disgust at oneself and the world).

Sullivan (1953) frames developmental work in a parallel fashion, but with an emphasis upon interpersonal relationships and the way the individual functions within the social system. In his theory, the task for the infant is to learn to count on others to gratify wishes and needs; in childhood it is to learn to accept interference with one's wishes and to delay gratification. In the juvenile years, the task is to learn to form relationships with peers which are satisfactory; and during the teen years to learn to relate first to a friend of the same sex, to become more independent, and then to learn to develop heterosexual relationships which are enduring and intimate. Sullivanian or interpersonal theory purports that the individual's sense of self comes through the young child's experiences, developing a positive sense of self (good me) through the introjection, or taking on, of perceptions of a good mother, or a negative sense of self through the introjection of a bad mother (bad me), as well as not me, or that which is rejected as part of the self identity (Sullivan, 1964).

Mahler *et al.* (1975) are more contemporary psycho-analysts whose writings focus on the first six years of development. They view these as critical in shaping the child's adjustment or development of problems in future years. This theory has been quite useful in understanding the pathology of those individuals who develop personality disorders. Mahler *et al.* (1975) conceptualized the infant as starting out symbiosed with the mothering figure, encompassing the first months of life.

The next phase is that of separation–individuation, and it has four sub-phases; phase one is differentiation, and phase two is labelled practising. The differentiation phase is from approximately four months to 10 months; the practising sub-phase is from 10 months to approximately 18 months. Initially the infant is totally dependent, then he gradually perceives that the mothering figure is not part of himself, and as he moves into the differentiation sub-phase there is a decrease in bodily dependence upon the mothering figure, and a beginning sense of self as separate. During the practicing period, the child increases his motor skills, and begins to make tentative moves away from mother, but remaining attached and highly dependent for approval and affirmation as well as security. This marks the beginning of the child imitating autonomous ego functions of the parenting figures.

The third sub-phase of the separation–individuation period is called rapproachement, lasting into the third year of life. During this time, the child becomes more adept at walking, thus making him more mobile and able to actively pursue the distancing from the mothering figure. Concurrently there is maturation of mental abilities, and beginning ability to think cognitively, forming the nucleus of the ego, and the sense of self as different.

Rapprochement is followed by the fourth and final sub-phase described by Mahler *et al.* (1975): that of object constancy, wherein the child further refines ego functions such as memory, perception and reality testing, and is able to internalize experiences as memory. If the child perceives security and constancy during these phases, he will be able to move successfully from the symbiotic state with the mothering figure toward individuation and a sense of self that is separate. If, however, he perceives disapproval or rejection in his efforts to move away, he will be unable to complete the separation process, leading frequently to personality disorders in adolescence and young adulthood. Kernberg (1975) has described a comparable phenomenon as the ego defence of splitting, wherein the child retains the distinct images of good and bad for himself and for others.

Winnicott (1965) described the essential relationship in a child's development to be that which is established with the mothering figure, and coined the term 'good enough mothering'. By this term he was describing the phase-appropriate support that a child needs to mature optimally, recognizing that no parent can be perfect, but the good enough mother would respond appropriately often enough that the child would experience over time feelings of being held and supported, and develop an increasing capacity to be alone. In the beginning the child requires mother's presence much of the time, but as he internalizes her qualities, he can be apart and still maintain a sense of self and others.

From the theories which have evolved from the psychodynamic framework, there is the premise that in those instances where developmental phases are thwarted or the child is unable to master the tasks to be accomplished, problems of a psychiatric nature develop in later life. A characteristic of mental illness is the tendency for the person to repeat inappropriate or ineffective coping behaviour, resulting in dysfunctional interactions and interpersonal relationships with others. Peplau's (1952 and 1965) contributions to development of interpersonal theory is described elsewhere in this text, so will not be elaborated on here, except to note that she identified that the core of nursing is the interpersonal relationship between the nurse and the client, and that this relationship serves as the mechanism by which nurses perform therapeutic tasks (Peplau, 1965). Peplau added significantly to our framework for seeing nursing as an educative task, aimed at promoting movement of the personality in the direction of constructive and productive relationships. In Peplau's now classic work, *Interpersonal Relations in Nursing* (Peplau, 1952), she utilizes Sullivan's theory of interpersonal growth and development, and develops her interactive nursing interventions based on the belief that human behaviour is goal-directed, but with intense anxiety, over time disorganization occurs.

Nursing interventions require a working knowledge of the concept of anxiety and of human needs in order to assist the patient reach a state of equilibrium. Armed with her psychodynamic understanding of each individual's particular problems that necessitate seeking psychiatric help, the nurse can assess the patient's ego strengths and weaknesses as she develops a plan of care. According to Peplau, the nurse can utilize the milieu or environment in which the patient is housed, as a tool in working on recurring problematic behaviour patterns and disrupting them (Janosik and Davies, 1986).

Learning process

In developing an interpersonal relationship with patients, nurses need to have information about the patient in order to help them solve problems and develop more adaptive methods of coping. To acquire the needed information, a systematic method of data collection is required in the early states of the therapeutic relationship. Peplau (1963) has developed an operational definition of the concept of learning that provides such a method of collecting clinical data. This method further encourages the patient to learn and understand more about himself.

There are eight steps in Peplau's learning process. The first step is identified as observation; that is, the ability to notice what goes on around oneself. It stands to reason that the patient must first be aware, through observation, of his environment before he can take the subsequent steps. The second step is identified as helping the patient learn to describe. This is to encourage the patient to recall and give details of his experiences, or to give more substance to that which he observed in step one. The third step in the learning process is to analyse, which promotes the ability to go over the data presented in steps one and two, with another person, to make connections and associations with the data now recalled. The fourth step is to formulate, by restating in a clear, direct manner the connections made in step three, then to determine an alternative way of dealing with the problem or conflict. The fifth step is to validate, and it is accomplished by being able to check out with someone else the conclusions drawn in step four. In step six, testing, the patient is encouraged to try out the results of step four in situations in everyday living with others in order to determine how well the new behaviours work. Once the new behaviours or understandings are tried with success, then the seventh step is used; that is, to integrate. This requires the patient to be able to incorporate the new learning into the array of coping skills available to him. Finally, the eighth and last step is to utilize the new learned behaviours, using them both in adaptation as well as in being able to look ahead and know their likely response to stressful or conflictual situations that are similar.

In applying the steps of learning during interaction with patients, it is useful for the nurse to use structured questions to guide the learning process. Questions that suggest who, what, where and when help the patient focus on data that is recalled and discussed and aid in movement toward the next higher level step. By keeping the learning process in mind, the nurse can assess the patient's current ability to process data about themselves. Additionally, it will give the nurse direction in how to help the patient move to the next step.

Milieu

For the patient whose problems are of such magnitude that hospitalization is required, the milieu, or living environment, takes on special significance. Most of the patient's activities will revolve around the day-to-day life in the unit. Not only will eating, sleeping, and other activities of daily living take place, but it is in this arena that patients will have opportunity to work on their identity and ego weaknesses, to improve upon their interactions with others, and for their patterns of relating carried over from experiences prior to hospitalization to be observed, with the nurse having an active role in providing corrective experiences.

Within the hospital milieu, the re-enactment of past patterns will create situations where there is opportunity for learning new ways of relating as other patients represent siblings and staff members are viewed as parental figures, authority figures, or sources of potential nurturance. While the patients can at times mask their symptoms, in the unit the problems of any patient are likely to be seen in their most naked form, as the patient experiences episodes of panic, outbursts of anger and rage, or withdraws from interactions with others. The individual who engages in self-injury or self-mutilation will resort to those measures when overwhelmed by emotions.

The nurse must take into consideration that the milieu is not only made up of the patients housed there, but it also includes the physical environment and the treaters who participate in that milieu, as well as the interplay among the various components. The patient is influenced by factors such as personal space, amount of privacy, whether or not there is provision for the patient to keep personal items, and the subtle messages implied such as whether there is encouragement to interact with others or to learn new skills. One goal is for the unit to be safe, both in terms of personal protection, and also a safe arena to try new behaviours. However, the milieu should be such that it is not perceived as so safe and gratifying that the patient becomes unmotivated to leave it when his need for hospitalization is finished.

Sills (1976) and others have written much about nursing care within the therapeutic milieu over the years, and it has been a much-studied topic. However, careful definition has been difficult in that creating and maintaining a therapeutic environment or milieu is a process, and ever changing as a result of the actions and interactions of both staff and patients. Attitudes and expectations influence the milieu.

To be therapeutic, a milieu must be adaptable and constantly changing as the composite of the group and needs of individual patients change. A patient having difficulty with reality testing will need a different structure and different types of interactions than will another patient, and that same patient will need different stimuli from the milieu at different stages of recovery.

Not only can patterns of interaction and interpersonal relationships be improved within the milieu, but also it can be an arena in which the patient's ego strengths can be maximized, and improvement made in areas of ego weakness. To do so calls for a psychodynamic approach by the nurse. A psychodynamic approach embraces a theoretical assumption that current behaviours are influenced by past experiences (especially in the developmental phases but also by current experiences). It takes into account mental processes and affective components that influence human behaviours which have been previously discussed in the material on development.

To prevent chaos within the environment, organization within the unit is necessary. Both staff members and patients need to know what will take place, for whom, when, and where. Most hospitals are structured around those activities that are part of a daily routine: bathing, sleeping, meals, appointments and leisure. In spite of this, there is much variation among units, ranging from the highly structured unit to one where those within the milieu set much of the structure themselves. However, in any milieu, assessment of individual needs is important, as is the assessment of the patient's ability to take responsibility for his own activities, as well as to what degree it is therapeutic for him to do so.

In general, therapeutic aspects of the milieu fall into one of five major categories:

1. providing for the basic needs of patients, looking after their physical well being;
2. offering organization and structure, wherein boundaries are defined via schedules, limits, degree of supervision and assistance provided;
3. giving support and aiding intrapsychic growth such as interventions when spontaneous or unexpected crises occur, as well as ongoing supportive therapeutic relationships and a stable environment;
4. assisting the patient with interpersonal and interactional skills such as help in learning socialization skills, on-the-spot validation and feed-back, use of small informal groups and guidance; and
5. promoting coping skills in a teaching and learning environment, such as helping the patient learn decision making, participating in patient government, instruction on how to use leisure or to handle feelings, and creating an atmosphere where patients can practise new behaviours and new ways of relating (Benfer and Schroder, 1985).

Concurrent with understanding the unit environment in terms of the functions it serves, there is another framework used by nursing staff members when considering the psychodynamics of a given patient. The currently accepted concepts of ego psychology are readily embraced by the psychodynamically oriented hospital. Addressing ego strengths and weaknesses provides a common language among disciplines and be-comes a framework that each can relate to. As mentioned earlier, much of the nursing staff members' work with patients is focused upon under-standing the behavioural demonstration of internal conflicts and issues. Those activities associated with the static, or routine aspects of the milieu provide for indirect work with the ego deficits, that is, providing relief from anxiety-provoking situations, providing stability in the environment that gives the patient reality orientation, providing consistency through staff whom the patient can rely upon to be there and to give predictable re-sponses. In many respects, the hospital unit serves as an auxiliary ego for the patient at those times when his/her own sense of self and boundaries are lacking.

Symptoms of ego weakness have a behavioural manifestation, and, as a result, increased ego strength can be facilitated in the unit. Knowledge that this was so existed for some time; in fact, one can postulate that this was the premise upon which Dr William Menninger's *Guide to the Order Sheet* might have been based in the 1930s (see Menninger, 1982). That document provided guidelines for staff via a set of attitudes to be used with different patients. While that document and the concept did not become adopted nationally, the idea that there were reasons for approaching patients in certain ways had merit, and current knowledge of ego psychology as it is applied in psycho-analytically oriented hospital units can be seen as expansion upon the earlier idea. The ego strength and weakness scale developed by Bellak *et al.* (1973) has been found useful by nurses in linking what goes on within the unit milieu to the conceptual understanding of the patient. The scale offers a framework that nursing staff members can find useful in identifying what aspects of the milieu should be emphasized and what may not be helpful for a given patient, as summarized in Fig. 10.2. Much of the time, there are ego weaknesses in more than one area, and many of the interventions are by necessity multi-faceted. The intervention called for will vary with the degree of severity of the ego deficit.

Most patients admitted to the hospital have difficulty with reality testing to a greater or lesser degree, particularly in distortion of reality and in interpretation of events that occur. For example, Mr A, a 60-year-old schizophrenic, alternately identified one of the nurses as either his mother or sweetheart, often announcing to anyone that would listen that he was going to marry the nurse. Each time, the nurse would consistently tell him that this was incorrect; she was his coordinating nurse, she was neither his mother nor his girlfriend. Instead, there were specific tasks they needed to work on as part of his treatment, such as keeping to his defined structure and appointments for the day. This focus on day-to-day events is helpful in reality orientation as well as forming a basis for a clearly defined relationship. When patients struggle with increased disorganization, staff members find it helpful to direct the patient to concrete tasks such as straightening up their room, as a way of giving order to the patient's external world, thus aiding in giving order to the patient's internal world. Staff take the initiative and set the direction for the patient at such times, rather than offering choices. Choices call for selection between alternatives and accentuate the conflict, increasing the patient's sense of helplessness and lack of direction. For the patient with poor object relationships, the focus on staff members helping them with daily functions such as washing their clothing or cleaning their room, is more easily tolerated and less frightening than a sit down and talk experience.

For patients with less severe problems with reality testing and those with a higher level of functioning in other areas of ego strength, the task for nursing staff is to provide validation of correct perceptions via feedback or to give only the needed orientation to new or unfamiliar events in the patient's daily life. For still other patients, ego weakness may take more subtle forms, largely as projection of feelings onto others, distortion of reality in the form of hearing only messages they wish (or need) to hear, and shutting out reality or becoming more disorganized when highly anxious. The patient's defences take the form of attack on staff members

Figure 10.2 Selected nursing interventions responsive to the patient's ego strengths and weaknesses*

	Severe disturbance	Moderate disturbance	Minimal disturbance
Reality testing	Provide clear structure; give patient a schedule of when things are done, explaining any changes; provide consistent personnel and frequent reality orientation; increase one-on-one contacts; reduce group expectations, interactions, and stimuli; assist with activities of daily living; increase support when distortions are greatest.	Decrease structure; when distortions occur, correct them in an accepting manner; set up situations to try out new behaviours (increase emphasis on interpersonal relations, less on environmental factors). Provide structure with validation.	Encourage patient to apply new skills first in areas of relative comfort, then in areas of difficulty; increase group participation, independent actions, and self-responsibility.
Judgement	Provide safety from self via structure; give both physical and emotional protection (i.e., from actions that would be embarrassing later); select group interactions with staff members present.	Set limits only in those areas where judgement is poor; support those actions reflecting improved judgement; offer encouragement to continue new behaviours and look at alternatives; increase group interaction, especially in areas where patient can participate.	Encourage patient to test new behaviours in new situations as well as the outside world; validate actions.

Impulse control	Contain patient's impulses during times of loss of control; set goals in limited areas regarding most disruptive behaviours; use areas of strength; participate in highly structured groups.	Help patient to recognize signs of stress and to ask for help before loss of control; help patient explore alternative, using strengths.	Encourage more flexibility and less rigidity in expressing feelings.
Object relations	Provide continuity in contact by using one staff/shift with patient; be non-threatening and supportive; encourage one-on-one activities with staff and selected other patients; avoid intrusiveness or isolation; seek out for brief contact.	Encourage participation in rewarding activities (e.g., leisure with others); encourage expanding relationships from one to several; reinforce sharing.	Help patient look at remaining relationships that are perceived as problematic; encourage increased empathy for others.
Thought processes	Provide reality orientation; communicate clearly; help patient be clear; focus on messages to and from patient.	Re-affirm patient when he communicates clearly; encourage validation with other patients and staff members; use learning process to help patient begin to make connections.	Set goals with patient regarding areas of vague or unclear communication; set up situations to practise new skills.
Autonomous functions	Attend to stress or anxiety; decrease stimuli when there is evidence of overload; help with tasks one at a time; avoid group pressure or group expectations that patient cannot meet.	Give verbal support while encouraging patient to try new tasks; deal with change; reinforce what patient does well.	Explore areas where patient can perform at optimum potential.

Figure 10.2 (cont.)

	Severe disturbance	Moderate disturbance	Minimal disturbance
Synthetic–integrative functioning	Help with recognition of feelings; tie thoughts to actions through established relationships; validate when appropriate; communicate when what is said does not fit the situation; provide structure, with reminders.	Encourage patient to share feelings and thoughts with others, to be direct with others; help patients sort out feelings, thoughts, and actions and relate them.	Support patient when he is temporarily thrown by the unexpected; give positive feedback when patient handles situations well.
Mastery-competence	Encourage patient to do for himself what he can; assist him to do other things with help; start with simple tasks and goals.	Focus on areas patient can control; support his attempts to do so.	Encourage patient to take on leadership to make things change; help sort out appropriate ways to do so (e.g., patient government); encourage working with others toward shared goals.

*From Benfer and Schroder (1985), pp. 451–65, with permission of the publisher.

at times. When this occurs, it is extremely helpful for the staff member to validate with other members of the team or to use their individual supervision to understand the dynamics of the individual involved rather than perceiving the patient's projections as personal, or seeing the patient's behaviour as purposeful and manipulating. For example, the borderline patient often reacts to shortcomings in his/her own behaviour by projecting onto the staff: 'I cut myself because nursing staff members weren't paying enough attention to me', or 'I wouldn't have gone out to drink beer if the nursing staff had given me medication when I wanted it'. Nursing staff members recognize the importance of remaining consistent in their approach, calmly restating expectations rather than responding to the attacks. This procedure is repeated as often as necessary as the patient works within the various arenas of treatment to gain more understanding of his own behaviour and takes steps toward incorporating the external structure into his own internal world.

Ego weaknesses in the area of judgement run the gamut from acts which endanger the individual, such as violent or suicidal behaviour, to those that are less extreme, such as judgemental errors in forming relationships. When there is immediate danger to life, nursing staff members take immediate steps to provide safety for the patient. The immediate need for safety takes precedence for the time being over meeting all other psychological needs.

It is difficult for nursing staff to differentiate at times between actual suicide attempts and those acts that are self-injurious but where there is different motivation and desired outcome, for example, patients who cut themselves in an effort to express their degree of distress to others or to get others to respond to them with concern and caring. Unlike the schizophrenic patient who may be acting on his hallucinations, the judgemental errors of the self-mutilating patient demonstrate a regression to a less integrated way of experiencing events, with less logic, and more affective association to their actions. Nursing staff must move quickly to provide a safe environment for such patients, but it is equally important to help the patient return to his previous level of functioning before he/she becomes overly dependent upon the one-to-one supervision and protection. For example, a borderline female patient may make multiple cuts upon her body as an expression of her stress and anxiety and to negate positive gains recently made. In such instances, it is important to provide structure that conveys the message that 'we care and we will not allow you to hurt yourself'. Then, as soon as the patient is again able to use more adaptive defences, nursing staff members need to move with the patient to return some of the self-responsibility to the patient, encouraging her to use healthier coping mechanisms.

Poor judgement is frequently accompanied by poor impulse control and a volatile emotional state in individual patients. For example, a patient who fears he will not be allowed to go on a shopping trip may immediately become angry and destroy items in the unit, or he may abscond and engage in drinking or illegal drug use. Unless nursing staff members possess sufficient understanding of the relationship between the poor impulse control and the poor coping mechanisms as well as the primitive nature of the impulses being expressed, the unit can be ripe for strife and power struggles. Staff members may seek to control the patient in such instances, further threatening him and increasing rather than decreasing the anxiety.

Within the psychodynamically oriented unit, attempts are made to understand the patient well enough so that there is sensitivity to potential triggers for the patient's impulsivity, and activities are offered that can serve to sublimate the feelings involved. For instance, one of the exercise rooms may be offered to the patient likely to become physically assaultive, with verbal support being given at those times when the patient makes an effort to use more appropriate outlets for his impulses. At times, however, no amount of preventive efforts can circumvent a major episode of explosive behaviour. When this happens, staff members move quickly to contain the behaviour and remove the patient to an area of the unit where there are fewer stimuli. Structure and limit setting lessen the patients' fear of their own unleashed emotions and give them environmental cues that help them regain internal control as quickly as possible. Once the patient has calmed down, normal activities are resumed, emphasizing areas of strength rather than focusing on the maladaptive behaviour.

Many of the activities in the unit assume that the patient has at least a minimal ability to relate to others in the environment. At times, however, especially soon after admission to the hospital, the patient may be in a withdrawn state, fearful and distrusting of others. The process of forming a relationship becomes the first crucial task of nursing staff members, with the patient gaining enough trust that he can let others become part of his world. This is usually accomplished by the same nursing staff members who consistently work with the patient. With the patient having little ability to maintain object constancy, the trust that is often given to one or two staff members is not easily transferred to others. The patient has minimal tolerance of that staff member's absence on days off or vacation.

A dependent relationship quickly forms with nursing staff members, at times heavily influenced by the transference that occurs (Schroder, 1985). The nursing staff member is seen as a potential mothering figure, with symbiotic attachment. As staff members have an awareness of the dependency strivings as part of the dynamics of the individual patient, it is often useful to have more than one individual working with the patient; this encourages attachment to the group of nursing staff rather than to one individual. Since many of the patients have difficulty with separation/individuation, setting up situations where the patient can leave the unit but also return and find things unchanged is part of the planned programme. The overall goal for many patients is to combine a corrective experience for the patient with an understanding based upon knowledge of interpersonal and psychodynamic principles and conformity and uniformity are not sought, rather the approach is one of constant re-assessment of what is or is not useful for the patient.

The role of groups in the unit

Thus far in this chapter, attention has been given to the individual patient in the unit. However, many interactions and interventions take place within a group context, and the group is seen to be important in the psychodynamic setting. Interactions within a group that take place with staff and other patients serve to provide the treatment team with information helpful in understanding the dynamics of the individual being treated. Specific areas of ego weakness can be worked with within a group context; for example, within a community meeting, accuracy of perceptions can be checked with others, allowing the patient to see how others perceive events. Support is given the patients so that they do not feel devalued or threatened when they are not ready to accept a differing viewpoint. Such exchanges simultaneously allow the patient with stronger ego strengths to be helpful to others, thus improving that patient's self-esteem. Participation in group activities such as patient government can help the patient achieve a greater sense of mastery over his own life and environment.

Not all patients can benefit equally from group participation, and at times patients may need protection from both their own internal stimuli as well as the stimuli inherent in a group. This is particularly true for the schizophrenic patient who lacks the ego strength to participate meaningfully in groups. Forced participation in groups can further their poor reality testing, their disorganized thought process, reinforce a low self-esteem and highlight their poor social skills, particularly if the group scapegoats them or rejects them.

In other instances, however, groups are an important part of the in-patient treatment. The group can be an arena for the gradual integration of an individual into the social life of the unit; it can be a structured area where he/she may feel less likely to be rejected. For some who have felt an outsider to any close relationships, the group may pose less threat of closeness than does individual contact. As the patients listen to each other talk of issues, they begin to see options they may have for themselves. The borderline patient can borrow from the group's combined ego strengths and feel stronger himself. The higher functioning borderline patient does well within groups where there are peer expectations, and he can incorporate his peers' values into his own self-system. For some patients, groups may be frightening by virtue of size, and smaller groups may be more appropriate. Figure 10.3 outlines some of the risks and benefits to many of the various groups available in the unit.

Figure 10.3 Groups within the milieu*

Type of group	Purpose	Benefits	Risks
Community meeting: all patients and most staff members.	To discuss shared issues and concerns related to life in the unit, with input from both patients and staff members.	Patients gain support, learn from each other, identify with others in the hospital environment, and share in the solving of everyday non-personal problems.	Easily overwhelmed patients may find the group's size scary. Others may be overstimulated. It is difficult for staff members present to know how individual patients perceive events.
Teaching groups: one or two specific staff members.	To correct information deficits on specific topics (e.g., sexuality, medication, relaxation, assertiveness, CPR, drug abuse), using adult learning principles.	Patients gain new knowledge for use in other aspects of treatment, identify with others in the group, and gain increased self-esteem and a sense of control of their own lives.	Staff members may inadequately assess patients' readiness for subject material.
Task-specific groups: selected patients, by task and goal, and specific staff members.	To provide an arena for patients to learn about and have experiences in an area of identified deficits or interests (e.g., cooking, budget and money handling, discharge planning).	Patients identify with a group with specific, similar interests or needs.	Patients may feel forced to attend the group meetings if attendance is based solely on staff assessment (patients need choices).
Leisure groups: selected patient group, varying in size from two to all in the unit.	To give opportunities for using time on non-problem issues and to promote healthy, alternative emotional outlets and social interaction, including contact with the non-hospital community, either organized or spontaneous.	Patients gain new skills, feeling more at ease socially, and learn to initiate, participate, and share with others, and to identify with those of like interests. Staff members can be supportive, healthy role models.	Patients may be thrust into competitive activity when lacking skills and then be excluded in replay of earlier traumatic experiences. Staff members who compete with patients may create a sense of failure in them.

Type	Purpose	Benefits	Risks
Discussion groups: participants vary with topic, specific purpose, and philosophy of unit.	To provide opportunities for patients to discuss with peers a topic relevant to themselves, with staff members assuming the role of facilitator of the sharing process.	Patients learn to increase involvement with others, yet with safety of structure and time limit (half-hour or hour), and learn to integrate ideas into practical language.	If patients are too concrete, discussion may be disorganizing to them. The group may force too much closeness or stimulation.
Activity groups: participants usually determined by staff members.	To introduce unit-restricted or regressed patients to interaction with others in a low-demand, time-limited situation, with participation based on individual tolerance.	Patients increase involvement with others (as tolerated); and even less capable patients have their strengths reinforced without increasing their stress level.	Forced participation can arouse anxiety and anger. Low interest of staff members may promote further withdrawal or devaluation.
Multidisciplinary treatment groups: predetermined (i.e., by team) group of patients and staff members.	To provide a model of openness in dealing with problems, a data-gathering source unavailable one-on-one, a forum for feed-back to patients, and, in some cases, a way to handle patient requests.	Patients can see how others deal with similar problems, can negotiate requests, and can learn to be open.	Patients' privacy may be invaded. Patients (e.g., schizophrenic patients) may feel threatened by forced sharing and involvement.
Patient government: elected or appointed patients and staff adviser or facilitator	To provide patients with avenues for input on decisions about practices related to their environment. In some instances, to allow patients to monitor how their leisure budget is spent.	Patients can use areas of strength. Those elected gain increased self-esteem.	Patients may feel hopeless if unable to affect system and if unrecognized. They may replay prehospitalization events of competitive drive to excel.

*From Benfer and Schroder (1985), pp. 451–65, with permission of the publisher.

The role of nursing staff members in the unit

There is one additional element that needs to be addressed in order to have a complete picture of the events that occur in a psychodynamically oriented hospital unit: that is, the dynamics that go on with staff members in relation to the patient care that they provide. From the patient's point of view, there is the implication that nurses should fulfil all their needs, anticipate their needs in advance, and not make mistakes. Adding to the patients' expectations, nursing staff members themselves may get caught up in the struggle to be perfect, unless there is constant monitoring and effort by the nursing staff to understand their own transference and counter-transference feelings within the work setting. Main (1957) wrote a poignant article describing what went on with patients who were special, ones who made the nurse feel omnipotent and capable of giving better care than other nurses, but who ultimately left the nurse feeling drained. Staff members get caught up at times in trying unconsciously to be what the patient projects onto them. At those times, nursing staff members are vulnerable to the splitting defence of the patient, with staff divided at any given moment into the good and terrible staff. In between these extremes there is a point where the nursing care in the unit is not perfect but is good enough.

The concept of good enough originated with Winnicott (1965) who applied the term to the mother–child relationship of the borderline patient and the problems during the child's developmental years wherein the mother was perceived to be unable to respond adequately to the child, non-empathetic to the child's varying needs and demands. Winnicott (1965) describes good enough as providing enough that the child can grow and his needs are recognized, yet with allowance for the child to move away and become independent and for the mother to be real. The authors of this chapter conceptualize a similar dynamic that takes place in a psychodynamically oriented hospital between patients and nursing staff members. There needs to be conveyance of acceptance of the patient, assuring by attitude and actions that he is safe and won't be rejected, similar to that which a child needs from the mother. Using this concept, nursing staff members provide the patient with opportunities to correct earlier perceptions of self and the world around him, but like the good enough parent, the nursing staff members strike a balance between adequate and excessive caring. When the care given exceeds the desired level, the transference from the patient may include the fear that staff members will withdraw the caring and support in the same way the patient perceived the parent as doing if he dares to try to separate and be independent.

The good enough nurse is concerned with the model of healthy behaviour that he/she provides, demonstrating real behaviours and responses within limits. There is recognition by staff members that an image of themselves as always correct negatively sets up patients to strive for the same perceived perfection and increases their fear of making mistakes or trying new tasks or ways of relating. Trying to be perfect on the part of nursing staff also leads to fantasies by the patient that they have found the ideal parent. They believe that the nurse will leave her family and devote all her time to the patient, they may have rescue fantasies that the nursing staff member will take away all problems, and there can be blurring of the necessary patient–staff boundaries. Rather than trying to be all-providing, nursing staff members in a psychodynamically oriented hospital instead strive to be good enough – demonstrating empathy, understanding and support of the patient, yet with enough boundary setting and deprivation to help the patient grow. In other words, not doing for the patient what he can do for himself.

Within shared or individual supervision, nursing staff members use their own emotional reactions to the patient as a diagnostic tool. These human reactions allow staff to understand better the distorted interactions patients tend to activate in the unit as a re-creation of prior experiences. By sharing these collaboratively with other nursing staff members as well as with others on the team, a collective understanding of the various aspects of the split-off parts of the patient's intrapsychic life can be gained.

Summary

The authors of this chapter have described a theoretical base for psychiatric nursing practice, using a combination of psycho-analytic, psychodynamic, and interpersonal theories. A conceptual framework is presented for the nurse to use in the application of the nursing process, with description of ego structure, ego functioning, ego defences, and ego strengths and weaknesses. Developmental theory is provided that gives the framework from which to assess tasks that the individual may not have accomplished in earlier years.

Using the interpersonal relationship, the authors describe interventions that may be made within the therapeutic milieu, both individually and with groups. Finally, the role of the psychiatric nurse within the milieu is described. The authors emphasize that while the nurse needs to often use a combination of more than one theoretical framework, those theories used must fit together and compliment each other, so that the nurse has a clear integrated conceptual framework upon which to base psychiatric nursing practice.

References

Bellak, L., Hurvich, M. and Gediman, H. K. (1973) *Ego-Functions in Schizophrenics, Neurotics and Normals: a Systematic Study of Conceptual, Diagnostic, and Therapeutic*

Aspects, John Wiley, New York.
Benfer, B. and Schroder, P. (1985) Nursing in the therapeutic milieu. *Bull. Menninger Clinic*, **49**, 451–65.
Burd, S. and Marshall, M. (eds) (1963) *Some Clinical Approaches to Psychiatric Nursing*, Macmillan, New York. pp. 333–6.
Erikson, E. H. (1963) *Childhood and Society*, 2nd edn, Norton, New York.
Freud, S. (1917) *Mourning and Melancholia*, **14**, Hogarth, London.
Janosik, E. and Davies, J. (1986) *Psychiatric Mental Health Nursing*, Jones and Bartlett, Boston MA.
Johnson, B. S. (1986) *Psychiatric–Mental Health Nursing*, Lippincott Co., Philadelphia.
Kernberg, O. (1975) *Borderline Conditions and Pathological Narcissism*, Aronson, New York.
Mahler, M. S., Pine, S. F. and Bergman A. (1975) *The Psychological Birth of the Human Infant*, Basic Books, New York.
Main, T. F. (1957) The ailment. *Brit. J. Med. Psychol.*, **30**, 129–45.
Menninger, W. (1982) *The Menninger Hospital's Guide to the Order Sheet*, The Menninger Foundation, Topeka.
Peplau, H. E. (1952) *Interpersonal Relations in Nursing*, Putnam, New York.
Peplau, H. E. (1963) Process and concept of learning in *Some Clinical Approaches to Psychiatric Nursing* (eds Burd, S. and Marshall, M.), Macmillan, New York.
Peplau, H. E. (1965) The heart of nursing: interpersonal relationships. *Can. Nurse*, **61**, 273–5.
Schroder, P. J. (1985) Recognizing transference and countertransference. *J. Psychosoc. Nurs.*, **23**, 2–6.
Sills, G. (1976) Use of milieu therapy, psychiatric nursing 1946–1974: a report on the state of the art, *Am. J. Nurs.*, **76**, 23–5.
Sullivan, H. S. (1953) *The Interpersonal Theory of Psychiatry*, Norton, New York.
Sullivan, H. S. (1964) *Fusion of Psychiatry and Social Science*, Norton, New York.
Winnicott, D. W. (1965) *The Maturational Processes and the Facilitating Environment*, International Universities Press, New York.

Part Three

THEORETICAL MODELS SPECIFIC CLINICAL APPLICATIONS

The aim of this section is to demonstrate how the theoretical models presented in Part Two can be applied to specific clinical problems. All authors have utilized a model which they are using within their own teaching and clinical practices. We fully recognize the extent to which partial overlap exists between one or more of those models selected for inclusion in this book. Each author presents a brief case study and identifies specific client needs and problems. Examples include hallucinations, grief, lack of trust and low self-esteem. Each theoretical model is used to analyse the problem and to describe how the nurse may help the client to resolve or minimize the identified problems.

Authors have made reference to published research and other literature relating to their particular model. This section will enable readers to assess whether a particular model is a useful aid to clinical practice or whether it is as Luker (1988) described as pretentious theory. We are of the firm view that the authors of Part Three clearly illustrate the need for theoretical models and, more importantly, convincingly demonstrate how they can be applied to clinical practice.

Reference

Luker, K. (1988) Do models work? *Nursing Times*, **88**(5), 27–9.

Chapter 11

Cognitive therapy model: clinical applications

P. BARKER

Clinical example

Carol was a 26-year-old single parent. She lived with Amy, her daughter aged seven, in a tower block ten minutes' walk from her parents' home. Three months ago she returned home after a two-week stay in the psychiatric unit of the district general hospital. Carol had been receiving treatment from her general practitioner (GP) for anxiety and depression over the previous six months, the admission having been arranged by a social worker concerned for Amy's welfare. The history from the GP and social worker described the insidious development of the depression over the past two years. No obvious cause was apparent but a long history of poor relationships with her parents and failed relationships with men, including Amy's father, was noted. Carol was brighter than average at school, wanting to become a nurse, but at her parents' insistence left school early to train as a secretary. She had not worked for three years after being made redundant.

After a short period of assessment the unit staff discharged Carol to the care of a community psychiatric nurse based at Carol's health centre. The discharge plan proposed that the GP discontinue Carol's medication gradually and that formal psycho-social support be provided by the community nurse and social worker. Monthly appointments at the psychiatric out-patients department were also arranged. Arrangements were made for the community nurse to meet Carol in the ward the day before her discharge, where they arranged to meet at her home a few days later.

The assessment

Preliminaries

At the first meeting on the ward the community nurse (*J*) introduced herself, acknowledging that she had some information about Carol's situation, but indicating that she would prefer if Carol could outline her view of the key issues. Twenty minutes were spent discussing the precipitants of the admission, Carol's feelings of failure, and her worries for the immediate future. *J* summarized Carol's story briefly, checking her interpretation. Finally, *J* negotiated a time to visit Carol at home the day after her discharge. Carol had no questions at this stage. Before leaving, *J* asked Carol to complete two assessment scales, the anxiety status inventory (Zung, 1971) and the Beck depression inventory (Beck *et al.*, 1961). She had already used these scales, having completed them on her admission to the ward.

The objectives   The ward medical team had informed Carol of *J*'s future involvement. The meeting allowed her to put a face to the name. *J* had emphasized the need for Carol to define her situation. The existence of medical reports was acknowledged, but effectively relegated to a supportive position, in deference to Carol's information. *J*'s part in the subsequent conversation was facilitative rather than directive. She tried to show herself as a working listener: acknowledging key statements made, seeking clarification sensitively where events or feelings were unclear. She hoped her summary would convey attentiveness and, perhaps therefore, her genuine interest in Carol's welfare. The negotiation of the home visit showed her relative flexibility and acknowledgement of Carol's own needs. Finally, the scales would provide her with a general indication of levels of anxiety and depression, two of the life-problems noted by other professionals. These scores could be used to evaluate progress at a later stage.

The home visit

The setting: Carol showed *J* into her kitchenette when she called. She made coffee while *J* asked some general questions about the last few days. *J* suggested that they adjourn to the sitting room where she drew up a stool to face Carol sitting on the sofa a few feet from her. *J* tried to arrange the situation to express intimacy (closeness) and openness (face-to-face contact).

Preparation   *J* began by summarizing their first meeting, emphasizing the thoughts and feelings emphasized by Carol. She then asked Carol for her expectations of *J*. A few minutes were spent clarifying *J*'s own expectations for their working relationship: how she thought she might help Carol, and the part Carol could play in the whole process.

Establishing the base   *J* proceeded to outline her hopes for their working relationship. She suggested that Carol come to the health centre for all subsequent sessions. This would help her to feel that she was taking constructive steps to help herself. *J* suggested that, for the first few weeks,

Carol should come twice a week to establish a firm foundation for their work together. The most convenient times and days were negotiated and Carol was asked to make a note of these while *J* completed her own diary. Finally, *J* asked for a few minutes to outline how she hoped to structure the sessions. Here, the need to focus upon Carol's present problems was emphasized, taking account of how she felt about past events and other long-standing unresolved issues. An example of such an issue was selected from their first meeting where Carol had talked about her feelings towards her father. By asking Carol to re-create the incident in her mind, *J* tried to draw out the relationship between the feelings evoked by the memory and the thoughts which were present at the same time. Carol was invited to comment, and a few more minutes were spent clarifying the example and looking for the possible meaning of the situation. *J* gave Carol a copy of the self-help manual *Understanding your Feelings and Solving your Problems* (Barker, 1983) and asked her to read the opening section only before they next met. This summarized the role of thoughts in generating negative emotions.

The assignment *J* asked Carol if she could give some thought to the problems which they had discussed briefly at the first session. These had emphasized specific everyday problems involving Amy and her parents; both situations generating strong negative emotions. Carol agreed to make a note of these and, at *J*'s prompting, set aside time that evening and the following day to complete the exercise. Before concluding, *J* asked Carol to comment upon how she felt about what had been done so far. How did she feel about *J*'s role in their relationship? Was she clear as to what was expected of her? Did she have any suggestions or criticisms of *J*'s handling of the session? At this stage Carol had no comments and appeared a little embarrassed by the invitation. *J* thanked her for being open and helpful and clarified the details of their next meeting and the two assignments previously arranged.

Objectives *J* had five main objectives for this second meeting. These were as follows:

1. To clarify the nature of the therapeutic relationship. *J* had introduced the idea of a working alliance at the first meeting. Allowing for the novelty of this idea for Carol it was important to emphasize this further. At the same time as *J* tried to establish a positive relationship with Carol, emphasis was given to an open exchange of thoughts and feelings.
2. To give Carol an outline of the work they would undertake together. This preparation emphasized practical issues, with some time being devoted to clarifying further the content.
3. To provide Carol with a simple outline of the conceptual model. This

was done by a brief analysis of a recent event, supplemented by recommended reading.
4. To introduce Carol to the homework assignments. Her first task was
   to define, for herself, present life-problems. She would analyse these
   further with J's support at the next session.
5. To invite feedback from Carol on J's handling of the session.

Clarifying the goals

Interview 3   At the next session Carol summarized the past few days,
then described her experience of the assignments. J then focused on a
discussion of her presenting problems, encouraging her to read from her
notes adding any other comments as appropriate. Three main problems
were identified:

1. Carol felt that she could not trust anyone. Her childhood had been
   emotionally traumatic; her father having punished her indiscrimi-
   nately, her mother alternating between hostility and smothering affection. Although she had enjoyed good relations with many people
   in her teens and twenties, 'everyone' let her down. To protect herself
   and Amy she had decided to trust no one. She realized that this isolated
   her and made life difficult for Amy. She noted, however, that 'I can't
   help it, that's how I feel'.
2. Carol also reported feeling bad. Most often this involved a mix of emotions which swirled inside her. Sometimes these feelings followed
   specific events. At other times they appeared for no reason. As most of
   Carol's problems seemed to revolve around the unfairness of her past
   life and present situation, anger seemed to play a central role. Carol
   agreed that a chain of emotions was involved. She would begin feeling
   angry, then would feel sorry for herself, leading to hurt and later would
   feel helpless, ending up feeling depressed.
3. Carol's feelings about herself provided a backdrop to her everyday life.
   She reported feeling worthless and useless. When challenged to explain
   where her school record, secretarial training and good mothering of
   Amy fitted in, she dismissed these as unimportant. Her self-esteem
   appeared to be based wholly upon her parents' highly negative view of
   their daughter. Her father had made no secret of always wanting a son,
   and appeared to have vented his own frustrations incessantly upon his
   daughter. Her present status as a single parent, living on state benefits
   but still dependent for some practical support on her parents, were
   further indications of her failure. Carol had, by now, accepted these
   judgements as fact.

Self-monitoring

At the end of the third interview J reviewed the three target problems defined above, clarifying these in detail with Carol. Time was now allocated

	MONDAY	TUESDAY	WEDNESDAY	THURSDAY	FRIDAY	SATURDAY	SUNDAY
8-9	had breakfast	——	B/FAST				
9-10	Helped with dishes	9 AM DOCTOR	WENT TO O.T				
10-11	Talked with a	UPSET - spoke w B.	O.T.				
11-12	——	SLEPT	O.T				
12-1	LUNCH	LUNCH	LUNCH - NOT HUNGRY AT ALL.				
1-2	TEA + SMOKE	WENT FOR WALK	HAD TO TALK WITH JANICE				
2-3	PHONED J. HAD READ	WENT TO CANTEEN	COFFEE IN LITTLE ROOM				
3-4	READING	PHONED DEREK	'WINDOW - SHOPPING'				
4-5	TOOK A WALK	WALKING	BACK IN HOSPITAL				
5-6	TEA	TEA (NOT HUNGRY)	TEA.				
6-7	DID TEA DISHES	DISHES!!	WATCHED T.V. (BORING)				
7-8	WATCHED TV NEWS	READ PAPER					
8-9	SLEPT	LAY ON BED					
9-10							

Figure 11.1: Daily activity record

to a brief discussion of the next assignment. *J* reviewed Carol's positive response to the last assignment, reinforcing some of the comments she had made about the value of noting thoughts and feelings day-by-day. *J* now suggested taking this a stage further by keeping a slightly more detailed record of everyday life, she referred to this as self-monitoring. *J* gave Carol an example of a daily activity record (see Fig. 11.1) and invited Carol to keep a simple record of the major activities in which she was engaged, hour-by-hour, each day. The record could also be used to note any problems she experienced, or times she felt bad or had disturbing thoughts. If the situation was complex the event could be noted with an asterisk, and detailed on an accompanying sheet. The session concluded with Carol giving her personal view of the session overall, focusing upon *J*'s management of the time and the way she had handled Carol throughout.

New beginnings

Session 4 and 5 The next two sessions were devoted to reviewing Carol's daily activity record and negotiating assignments. Everyday life was complicated greatly by Carol's inability to trust people and by her feelings of low self-esteem. She avoided anything which would bring her into close interpersonal contact, and she chaperoned Amy wherever she went, not trusting anyone else to take care of her or, more importantly, to not abuse her as she had been abused. Amy's life, as a result, was severely restricted. Carol also avoided any activity which she thought might stretch her, intellectually or emotionally. She was anxious to avoid further failure. Nonetheless, she felt a failure for avoiding everyday challenges. *J* invited Carol to draw up a list of everyday situations which presented a challenge to her. J then discussed how Carol might judge the degree of difficulty involved in each challenge by using a simple rating scale.

J   Each of the situations on this list is difficult for you?

C   Yes, I can't handle this stuff (pointing to list) just now.

J   Let's imagine how you would feel if you *could* take on some of this stuff.

C   I just couldn't handle it. I told you.

J   (Pausing) Have you ever watched ice-skating on TV? Or maybe highboard diving, like at the Olympics? (Carol nods) How do you know who's done well or who's done badly?

C   The judges give a score, with cards and numbers.

J   Uh-huh. These scores are linked to degree of difficulty. The more difficult the dive or jump, the more points the person can get. Right? (Carol nods) Let's take one of your challenges as an example. What about this, phoning an old school friend. How difficult would that be? Give it marks out of (pause)...let's say marks out of 10. Ten means it is virtually impossible, one means it is dead easy. How would you judge this?

C   Oh, I dunno...it's about 7. But I would feel awful, I know I would, that's why I can't do it.

J   I understand. Maybe that's why you *won't* do it. (Pause) OK. let's imagine that you get yourself organized and you do call this old friend, how many points would you give yourself out of 10?

C   Oh, well...I probably would stutter or get embarrassed. Say, two or three.

J   If I said that phoning an old friend was difficult for me...and was about eight on the scale...but I went through with it...but I was really embarrassed, how many points would you give me?

C   Well...eight, I guess. You did it, that's the main thing. You responded to the challenge.

J   So what's so different about you? I get full marks for trying. You just get two or three.

C   I think I see what you're driving at.

Carol's assignments over these sessions involved selecting challenges from her list and integrating these into her daily plan. She was asked to record how much she felt she had achieved by tackling each of these challenges using the ten-point scale. If she failed to complete a challenge she should award herself a proportion of the points of difficulty involved. Using this approach even if she pulled out of a challenge she scored some points, at least, for beginning.

Objectives   Although these sessions involved Carol's actual and potential daily activity, the emphasis was upon her perception of the challenges.

J's use of the challenge-scaling, reversing roles at specific points to allow Carol to judge *J* rather than herself, helped her to be aware of her negative perception of challenging situations. By using the scaling method, judging her performance by the same standards as she might judge others, Carol gained a more objective view of her challenges and ultimately herself. The session had also alerted Carol to the difference between can't and won't statements. She was encouraged to be aware of related negative thoughts: situations where she told herself that she couldn't, didn't want to, or otherwise made negative predictions about what she was aiming to tackle. To help her handle these negative thought blocks *J* gave her a sheet of common negative thoughts and examples of how to answer them.

Example	Negative thought	Answer
	I can't do anything, there are too many problems.	There are problems in doing anything in life. How would other people deal with this? Is there anyone who could advise me.
	I don't want to.	I don't want to NOW. I did earlier on. Anyway, what I WANT isn't the point. I NEED to do this. Get on with it.

Catching negative thoughts

Session six Carol reported some satisfaction from her challenge assignment. About one half hour was spent reviewing her activities and associated feelings of achievement. She had undertaken a number of tasks which she had been putting off and felt good as a result. This success was noted and she was encouraged to develop this further over the coming weeks. Before concluding, *J* noted that Carol had not tackled any of the challenges which involved interaction with others, or which involved giving Amy any new experiences, or more freedom. Carol became visibly upset at this point. *J* gave her a few minutes to compose herself then proceeded.

J   Maybe we could talk for a moment about how you are feeling? Something is bothering you? (Carol nods) Something to do with this list?
C   Yes. I just can't go on with this. I mean...these things are OK. All this ordinary stuff. But going out...calling Janice...meeting people...letting go of Amy, I just can't handle that just now. I'm not ready for it. Never will be I sometimes think.
J   You think you can't handle them?
C   NO. I know I can't!
J   (Pausing) We've talked before about negative thoughts. You remember? (Carol nods) When we're upset we don't always think

straight. It's easy to be really negative about ourselves and our lives. Like thinking that you can't handle things, or that you'll never get any better. You don't have to try too hard to think those sort of thoughts, do you?

C I don't have to try at all.

J What do you mean? They just pop into your head, do they?

C Sort of. I don't think them up anyway.

J That's what I would call AUTOMATIC thoughts. They just happen without any effort on your part. (Pause) Do you think that these kind of thoughts are for real? Do they reflect things as they really are, or just how you see them?

C I don't know. Seem real enough to me!

J I understand. But maybe you won't know what you can handle until you've tried it. Maybe these thoughts bend the truth a little? I guess automatic thoughts are often DISTORTED. (Pause) Would you say that these thoughts are helpful?

C (Angrily) What do you mean...helpful! Course they're not helpful.

J Right. You're so right. Automatic thoughts are never helpful. They're downright UNHELPFUL. (Pause) But despite that, you accept them don't you? You never stop to ask if they're true or not? (Carol looks bemused) I mean...when you think to yourself 'I'm usless' or 'I'll never manage this', you don't ask yourself 'is this REALLY true?'

C No, I suppose I don't.

J Automatic thoughts can be very PLAUSIBLE. They seem genuine. It doesn't occur to you to question them. And it's difficult to switch them off, isn't it? (Carol nods) They are what I would call INVOL-UNTARY; as though you aren't in control? (Carol nods) So, at the end of the day negative thoughts just pop into your head, they distort the truth, they're very unhelpful because they make you feel bad, but you don't think to question them because they seem so plausible. Most of all they are damned difficult to switch off. They go on and on inside your head and you feel progressively worse.

C Well I certainly don't feel any better!

J then drew Carol's attention to a section in the manual which discussed handling negative thoughts. The four characteristics they had just discussed were noted in this section and advice was given about catching negative thoughts. Ten minutes were spent considering an example from the day before when Carol had knocked over a jar in a supermarket. A blank record sheet which described what had happened, how Carol felt and what she was thinking, was completed (see Fig. 11.2). Finally, Carol rated how bad she felt and how strongly she believed in the automatic thoughts. Using this example, J tried to reinforce the connection between Carol's thoughts and her feelings.

IDENTIFYING YOUR NEGATIVE AUTOMATIC THOUGHTS
We have discussed how the way you feel is influenced by the way you think. I want you now to practise finding out what sort of thoughts you have when you feel bad. Think about the last time you felt bad; you might have felt sad, or angry; guilty or frightened. Try to remember how you felt and what was happening around you, and answer the following questions.

Feelings
How did you feel? __Embarrassed__

How bad was the feeling – measure it by using a scale of 0–100 (100 is the very worst).

Score __60__

Situation
Where were you? __In supermarket__

What were you doing? __Shopping – knocked jar off shelf__

What was going on around you? __Assistant stopped to help.__

Were you thinking about anything in particular? __How can I pick this up__
__without dropping my basket?__

Automatic Thoughts

What thoughts just 'popped into your mind' at that time?	SCORE
She thinks I'm stupid	100
Why do I always drop things?	95
Now I look flustered	
I'm just hopeless	80

Did you believe these thoughts? Measure to what extent you believed them using a scale 0–100. (0 means you did not believe them at all; 100 means you believed them completely).

Figure 11.2 Questionnaire on negative automatic thoughts

J If I thought to myself...She thinks I'm stupid...now I look flustered...I'm just hopeless, how do you think I would feel?

C Well, not good I guess. I certainly felt embarrassed.

J I guess I would feel embarrassed too. Those are very embarrassing thoughts. They TELL me to feel embarrassed. I think that's the main function of negative automatic thoughts they make you feel bad, in all sorts of ways. They are the key to your feelings. I think that is just as true for me as it is for you. I don't want to make things

seem too simple but negative thoughts are the simplest way of explaining your negative feelings. This example here shows how
negative thoughts produce negative feelings. I would like you to
take ten or fifteen minutes each evening to try catching some negative thoughts from your day. Could you manage that? (Carol nods)
Use this format to recall any bad feeling from your day and see if
you can make connections between your negative thoughts and
negative feelings. Although this is difficult it will help you become
aware of the way that you think.

Objectives   The working alliance had been developing steadily over
the first five sessions. Although she found the assignments difficult, Carol
co-operated fully in their execution. In session six *J* narrowed the focus
of the working alliance, addressing Carol's primary problem, her dysfunctional thinking style. Using her avoidance of the everyday challenges
which reflected her three key problems, *J* teased out the underlying negative thoughts which supported Carol's avoidance. By careful questioning
she also helped Carol identify the four main characteristics of negative
thoughts and showed her how she could catch thoughts as part of her next
assignment. *J*'s main aims in this session were to help Carol become more
aware of the role played by her thoughts in stimulating negative emotions;
to recognize the key characteristics of negative thoughts and to learn how
to identify the negative thoughts associated with everyday upsets.

Evidence and alternatives

Over the next four sessions *J* focused attention on helping Carol to analyse
her thinking style, in an attempt to find other ways of construing everyday situations. Carol collected records of negative thoughts as part of her
homework assignments. Typically these reflected anxieties about Amy,
emotional upsets, especially involving anger, and feelings of depression
and despondency which appeared to be linked to her low self-esteem.
These records were used as the focus for the within-session analysis.

Facts and feelings   In session seven Carol was shown an example of a
completed record format which illustrated the challenging of negative
thoughts (see Fig. 11.3). She was encouraged to transfer one of her homework examples onto a similar five-column sheet. Carol then reviewed the
example, describing an incident when she had felt upset when someone
passed her in the street. *J* then asked her to present the evidence for the
thoughts which she had at that time.

J   Let's talk about the evidence for thinking the way that you do. Tell
    me what happened again.
C   I passed Sally in the street. I haven't seen her for ages. She just

DAILY RECORD OF NEGATIVE AUTOMATIC THOUGHTS					
DATE	EMOTION(S) What do you feel? How bad was it (0–100%)?	SITUATION What were you doing or thinking about?	AUTOMATIC THOUGHTS What exactly were your thoughts? How far did you believe each of them (0–100%)?	RATIONAL RESPONSE What are your rational answers to the automatic thoughts? How far do you believe each of them (0–100%)?	OUTCOME 1. How far do you now believe the thoughts? (0–100%)? 2. How do you feel? (0–100%)? 3. What can you do now?
Monday 15 Sept	Jealous, Angry (80)	Got a letter from my sister saying she has just got a new house	How come she has all the luck? My whole life has been a disaster! I'll never get out of the rut (95)	She is lucky to have a new house, but everyone can't be so fortunate. Some people are starving. Am I starving? Of course not. I just think my whole life is a mess. If I'm honest I haven't done so badly. (75)	1. My thoughts. ㊿ 2. My feelings. ㊵ 3. I could make a list of my recent successes. I could start putting away some money in my own bank account. I could make a list of things I would like to change.

Figure 11.3 Record of negative automatic thoughts

walked right past. Ignored me. I felt awful. I thought that I must
have upset her in some way.

J In what way?

C Well that's it...I don't know. But I must have, mustn't I?

J OK. Let's make a list of the things you have done to upset Sally?

C A list? Oh well alright.

J When did you last see Sally and what happened?

C That must have been last week. In the supermarket. I was talking to
her and her sister at the checkout.

J OK. And you said something to upset her then, right?

C No. She was fine. I was fine too.

J You're sure about that? (Carol nods) Maybe you've said something
to someone else then, since then. Something about Sally that's got
back to her?

C NO! (angrily) I don't talk about people behind their backs.

J So...you haven't said anything to Sally, or said anything about her.
So where's the evidence that you've upset her?

C (crying) I don't know. I just feel that I must have upset her. Why else
should she ignore me like that?

J Well what other reasons are there? (Carol is silent) Sally actually
looked right at you, looked right through you? (Carol shakes her
head) So if she didn't look at you how do you know she saw you?

C Well I don't know that for certain.

J Right. Can you think of any other reason why she didn't acknowledge
you?

C Well...maybe she was thinking about something...had something
on her mind.

J Right...now we're talking. First of all, maybe she didn't see you.
Sounds reasonable. Secondly, maybe she was preoccupied with
something else. That sounds reasonable too. Tell me, how many
people have you ignored recently?

C Why, none. I would never ignore anyone.

J You would NEVER ignore anyone? Well maybe not intentionally,
but how do you know that you don't pass people without seeing
them, or when you're wrapped up in yourself?

C Umm. Well I don't know that, do I? That might explain why Sally
passed me?

J Let's just review this for a moment. I ask you for some evidence,
right? (Carol nods) You say that you can't provide me with any hard
evidence to support the idea that Sally might think that you've upset
her. You don't recall upsetting her or saying anything to anyone else
that might have got back to her. So the evidence to support this
thought just isn't there, right? (Carol nods) But you *can* give me
some evidence that might explain why she didn't acknowledge you.

She wasn't actually looking at you at the time. That's a fact? (Carol nods) And you've also suggested that maybe she could have been thinking about something else. That's a possibility? (Carol nods) Maybe the first thing that you need to do when you get upset is to ask yourself 'what's the evidence for thinking the way I do?' Just because you believe something is true doesn't make it true. If you put your thoughts on trial, as we've done here, what would the verdict be? Would it stand up in court or would it be dismissed as irrelevant or circumstantial?

C It wouldn't really stand up.

J (Handing Carol a self-adhesive sticker) Maybe I could ask you to write 'am I confusing a thought with a face?' on this sticker? (Carol obliges) Maybe you could stick that where it can jog your memory, on your diary or even on the electric kettle. And what about a sticker with where's the evidence?'.

Objectives In this session Carol was introduced to challenging her negative thoughts through assessing the real, rather than emotional, evidence. J used Socratic irony to expose the weakness of Carol's argument, rather than try to convince her that she was wrong. The emphasis was placed upon working through one specific example, using this as the basis for teaching Carol one method of challenging her negative thoughts. Finally, Carol was asked to assess her belief in the thoughts and to rate the concurrent negative feelings: both showed a reduction.

Becoming more objective

In session eight Carol spent more time developing her skills in challenging negative thoughts. In addition to reviewing the evidence, she learned how to view situations from a different perspective. To achieve this J arranged a role-reversal, asking Carol to imagine that a similar (though not identical) set of events had occurred to a close friend, with similar emotional results. She was then asked to advise her friend, or to give her opinion of what was happening.

J So...your friend Janet has just had a row with her mother. They have never got on well together. This row is not unusual, pretty much par for the course. Janet confides in you and says she is feeling really bad about it all. She feels angry at her mother, but feels guilty at the same time. She tells you that although her mother frustrates her she shouldn't have shouted at her. This situation just shows what a bad person she is; fancy hating your own mother. OK. what do you say to her? You agree with her?

C Well no...I mean, Janet's only human. Her mother frustrates her and she gets angry, so what?

J So what? You mean it's OK for people to abuse their parents?

C She's hardly abusing them. She's 25-years-old after all. She's not a child. She's just sticking up for herself, that's nothing to feel guilty about.

J Right, let's turn this back to you. You had a similar experience last week with your mother. You felt guilty, right? (Carol nods) So you told yourself, 'I've nothing to feel guilty about. I'm hardly a child, I'm only sticking up for myself...etc., etc.?'

J went on to discuss the value of reviewing situations from an alternative perspective, emphasizing the value of switching places with others; seeing things the way they might see them. *J* noted that Carol was not keen to condemn her friend in the way she had condemned herself. Viewing her situation through the eyes of a friend helped Carol put some space between herself and her problems, helping her to be more objective.

Cause and effect

Carol's progress had been fairly dramatic during these eight sessions. She appeared to grasp the basic principles of the cognitive model and, after some initial hesitation, tackled her assignments with much commitment. She appeared to be buoyed up by feelings of achievement gained from dealing with challenges. At the ninth session, however, Carol was despondent. She had experienced several problems that week, with neighbours, her mother and Amy's teacher. Her thoughts in all three situations returned to her view of herself.

J Let's take this situation with Amy and her teacher. She appears to be finding it difficult to keep up with the class. What does that situation mean to you?

C Well, like I said...my whole life has been a complete disaster. I've ruined my own life, now I'm ruining Amy's.

J And that makes you feel...?

C (crying) Awful...simply hopeless, useless.

J OK. I hear what you are saying. You've had many difficult times in your own life. Perhaps you now see a similar situation happening to Amy. Tell me...when you think these kind of thoughts...does it help you feel better?

C No. Not at all. I just feel more hopeless.

J OK. It doesn't make you feel better. But does thinking about the past change the past?

C Certainly not. You can't rewrite history.

J I see. So what purpose does all this thinking serve?

C None, I suppose.

J You seem to be saying that thinking negative thoughts about yourself is AUTOMATIC. As soon as you encounter a problem, you start thinking negative thoughts. Blaming yourself. (Handing Carol a file card) Maybe you should make up a memory-aid right now, to help remind you what to do next time you think negative. What would you put on it. . .'brooding about the past makes me feel better?'

C No. Brooding about the past makes me feel more depressed.

J Well, maybe you should write that. And what about. . .'thinking about the past changes things?'

C No. . .what's done is done. . .there's no going back. . .there's no changing the past. . .it's all wishful thinking.

J Right, maybe you need to write that too. (Pause) Would you let me suggest one other thought? (Carol nods) Well, when you feel despondent and think 'I know that this has happened. . .and I know I don't like it. . .' you could ask yourself 'but what am I going to do NOW?'

Carol and J spent the rest of this session problem-solving the situation regarding Amy and her school work. This led to Carol planning to spend some time each night helping Amy with her lessons, and listening to her (in Carol's words) the way her mother never listened to *her*.

Cautionary tales

In the tenth session Carol and J reviewed progress and found that Carol's scores on the depression inventory and the anxiety scale had decreased markedly over the past month. Although this feedback cheered Carol greatly, J decided that now was the right time for a few words of caution. The session was devoted to reviewing briefly problems Carol had experienced at the beginning of the month, using these as illustrations of the need for persistence and caution.

1. Emphasis was given to the fact that challenging negative thoughts was an unusual practice: most people do not have to do this. J commented that people with emotional problems tend to have fairly equal numbers of positive and negative thoughts, whereas normal subjects have many more positive than negative thoughts (Schwartz and Gottman, 1976). J emphasized the need for consistent, regular practice, even when things were going well, in order to establish such a balance.

2. Sometimes Carol had reported that analysing situations on her own made her feel even more helpless. Sometimes she couldn't think of rational answers. J noted that at such times maybe the best thing to do was to do something else. Distraction, it was explained, is a way of taking the heat out of the situation. Once she was calmer maybe she could think straight, and could start challenging over again.

3. Often, Carol had been embarrassed about some of her answers. J reminded her that there are no RIGHT answers. Only ones which work for her.

4. When writing down her thoughts Carol had often felt silly. *J* reminded here that these were only further examples of negative thinking. Carol's negative thinking was the problem: not her intelligence.
5. Finally, *J* noted the progress made to date. By way of a word of caution she drew a parallel between negative thinking and smoking: both are easy to stop at the beginning. Negative thinking is a habit which needs persistent attention if it is to be broken. Carol was winning the battle so far, but now was the time to step up the pressure, not time to ease off just because she was feeling better.

J suggested finally several ways of maintaining her progress:

1. Carol was encouraged to practise *imagining* emotionally disturbing situations, whilst rehearsing in her mind the rational response which she had already worked out in session. She was encouraged to do this at least ten times a day, observing subtle changes in her emotional reactions (Maultsby and Ellis, 1974).
2. She was encouraged to prepare for difficult situations by rehearsing in imagination rational self-statements. Given that Carol found it difficult to visualize herself coping with specific situations (Lazarus, 1978) she was encouraged to practise the rehearsal several times before approaching the situation (Raimy, 1975).
3. She was encouraged to practise some of her new answers in a dramatic fashion: speaking her negative thoughts aloud in front of a mirror and shouting back her rational answers, or recording her debate on her tape recorder, playing back the recordings on her personal stereo. Burns (1980) has called this externalization of voices.
4. She was encouraged, finally, to set aside 15 minutes each day to worry. During this time she was to call to mind all the situations and personal defects which upset her. As soon as the time was up, she should return to her daily activity plan. This approach was based upon the habituation technique recommended by Lewinsohn *et al.* (1978).

Dealing with basic assumptions

In sessions 11 to 15 *J* continued to help Carol deal with her negative thinking; getting feedback on her homework, helping her identify and challenge negative thoughts she had during the week. Sometimes specific thinking errors seemed to be at work, as when Carol made negative predictions about specific events (crystal-ball gazing), or when she blamed herself inappropriately for events caused by others (personalization). *J* referred to the section in the manual dealing with thinking errors and helped Carol to identify the error she was making, checking that she had retained this at the end of the session, and at the next session. During these sessions Carol's basic assumptions were also revealed. *J* would invite Carol to explain what different negative thoughts meant to her, or would ask her to say why she thought certain events were so bad. Three basic dysfunctional assumptions, or beliefs, were identified and defined (Ellis, 1962):

> I am worthless unless I succeed (self-damnation).
> It is awful when people won't do what I want them to (awfulizing).
> People have let me down and I can't bear it (I-can't-stand-it-itis).

Carol was encouraged to appraise critically each belief as it arose in the session, describing associated values and disadvantages of the assumption. Again, a file card was used to summarize briefly that belief and to detail a more rational response and plan for change. Carol was encouraged to carry this flashcard with her, rehearsing the rational response at intervals throughout each day, and carrying out the various plans for change noted.

Fading involvement

A further 10 sessions were presented over a 38-week period: sessions 16–19 every two weeks, 20–23 at monthly intervals, and the final two sessions as two- and three-month follow-ups. The intervention spanned 50 weeks from assessment to termination. During the final sessions Carol developed new challenges, each of which stimulated new anxieties and became the focus for further testing of negative thoughts and dysfunctional assumptions. *J* could have withdrawn at the end of the fifteenth session, when Carol's mood had lifted and her anxiety levels had returned to within normal limits. However, she continued to work with Carol in an effort to prevent relapse and to prepare her to deal with life crises and other everyday obstacles which had contributed to her past difficulties. In this sense, the final sessions were in the form of a prophylactic.

Summary of the therapeutic process

The cognitive therapy intervention described above is a learning process in which the nurse progressively involves the patient in an examination and critical appraisal of her perception of herself and her world. The early emphasis was upon reducing emotional distress and establishing simple coping mechanisms. Gradually, this gave way to a clearer emphasis upon learning about the relationship between basic beliefs, negative thoughts and disturbing emotions. The approach relied heavily upon the nurse's therapeutic style and technique. The following points reflect the key considerations:

1. The nurse introduced the patient gradually into the working alliance, socializing her first and establishing significant goals for therapy.
2. She offered a simple rationale of the work they were doing at each strategic point in the programme.

3. She encouraged the patient to avoid having any hidden agendas, discussing emotions and thoughts openly and inviting critical feedback on her own performance.
4. She tried to be flexible, responding to the patient's needs within each session, rather than working strictly to plan.
5. She tried to focus attention upon hot cognitions (Zajonc, 1980) which underpinned Carol's key problems.

The emphasis of the overall intervention was to *challenge* dysfunctional thinking and belief systems which, it was hypothesized, supported or stimulated her distrust, her anger, anxiety and ultimate feelings of depression, and her feelings of low self-esteem. Although *J* acknowledged the importance of Carol's feelings, these were considered only as a function of her thinking and basic beliefs. Little time, if any, was allocated to straightforward emotional expression, as practised (for example) in some other humanistic therapies. At no point did *J* reassure Carol, or otherwise try to encourage her to think positively. Glass and Merluzzi (1981) question whether the acquisition of positive thoughts does anything to eliminate negative thoughts. For this reason the overall emphasis was placed upon helping Carol to challenge, for herself, the tenability or otherwise of her thinking style. Although the focus of the sessions was upon cognition, most of the assignments involved behavioural experiments, where Carol was obliged to put her thoughts and beliefs to the test. Indeed, it is doubtful whether any cognitive change would be maintained without the support of behavioural change. In this sense the cognitive therapy model and the behavioural techniques employed make for comfortable bedfellows (Salkovskis, 1986).

References

Barker, P. J. (1983) Understanding your feelings...and solving your problems, unpublished manuscript.

Beck, A. T., Ward, C. H., Mendelsohn, M. *et al*. (1961) An inventory for measuring depression. *Arch. Gen. Psych.*, **4**, 561–71.

Burns, D. (1980) *Feeling Good: the new mood therapy*, William Morrow, New York.

Ellis, A. (1962) *Reason and Emotion in Psychotherapy*, Lyle Stuart, New York.

Glass, C. R. and Merluzzi, T. V. (1981) Cognitive assessment of social–evaluative anxiety, *Cognitive Assessment* (eds T. V. Merluzzi, C. R. Glass and M. Genest), Guildford Press, New York.

Lazarus, A. A. (1978) *In the Mind's Eye*, Rawson, New York.

Lewinsohn, P. M., Munoz, R. F., Youngren, M. A. and Zeiss, A. M. (1978) *Control Your Depression*, Prentice Hall, Englewood Cliffs, NJ.

Maultsby, M. C. and Ellis, A. (1974) *Technique for Using Rational–Emotive Imagery*, Institute for Rational Living, New York.

Raimy, V. (1975) *Misunderstanding of the Self: Cognitive Psychotherapy and the Misconception Hypothesis*, Jossey-Bass, San Francisco.

Salkovskis, P. M. (1986) The cognitive revolution: new way forward, backward somersault or full circle? *Behav. Psychother.*, **14**, 278–82.

Schwartz, R. M. and Gottman, J. M. (1976) Towards a task analysis of assertive behaviour. *J. Consult. Clin. Psychol.*, **44**, 910–20.

Zajonc, R. B. (1980) Feeling and thinking: preferences need no inferences. *Am. Psychol.*, **35**, 151–75.

Zung, W. K. (1971) A rating instrument for anxiety disorders. *Psychosomatics*, **12**, 371–9.

Chapter 12

Behaviour therapy model: clinical applications[*]

A. HUME

Introduction

The collective aim of all psychotherapies is the amelioration of an individual's problems of living. The process by which this goal is achieved, however, will vary according to the particular orientation of the psychotherapeutic approach in question. The case illustrations presented in this chapter demonstrate the contribution of contemporary behaviour therapy to the resolution of three such problems of living, namely, auditory hallucinations, insomnia and grief. Fictitious names have been given to the clients, and the details of each case have been altered to maintain confidentiality. While aspects of assessment, intervention and evaluation will be described, it must be emphasized that the strategies employed throughout the therapeutic process were designed to meet an individual's requirements and circumstances; each intervention package has therefore been tailor-made to meet the needs of one particular person.

Case study 1: auditory hallucinations

Introduction

In Western cultures hallucinatory experiences have long been associated with dark and mysterious aberrations of the mind. While such experiences can indeed be symptomatic of psychopathology, the automatic assumption that they are indicative of mental ill health and thereby undesirable is questionable (Bauer, 1970; Andrade, Srinath and Andrade, 1988; Hume, 1988b). The word hallucination is derived from the Latin *alucinatio* which means to talk idly or to wander mentally. In the English language it has

*The author wishes to express her grateful appreciation to Doug Fraser, Principal Psychologist, for his encouragement and comments during the preparation of the chapter.

existed since the 16th century when hallucinations referred to 'ghostes and spirits walking by nyght' (Sarbin and Juhasz, 1975). Its clinical application, however, originated with Esquirol in 1837 (Esquirol, 1965).

Comparison of Western and non-Western cultural reactions to hallucinatory phenomena is of particular interest because of the widespread association in the West between hallucinations and psychiatric illness. Much emphasis in Western societies, for example, is placed on the precipitating conditions of hallucinations (Al-Issa, 1976) where the mere occurrence of the event is likely to prompt a pejorative response. In contrast, while non-Western societies need not welcome such experiences, their concern is generally focused on content and not on the occurrence of the phenomenon.

When hallucinations do present as a psychiatric symptom, they are often intensely debilitating and distressing intrusive experiences. While pharmacological intervention has proved useful in the reduction and control of dysfunctional hallucinatory behaviour, its success is limited and a proportion of patients remain handicapped by these disturbing private events.

As demonstrated by the paucity of publications in the nursing literature, the current state of the art in terms of nursing practices to ameliorate hallucinatory experiences, reflects stasis rather than evolution. However, researchers, particularly in the field of clinical psychology, have demonstrated the effectiveness of a number of therapeutic strategies. The origins of a significant proportion of these treatment techniques are to be found in the theoretical constructs of contemporary behaviour therapy. Commonly these methods focus upon anxiety reduction, re-adjustment of environmental contingencies and the manipulations of cognitive processes. While the research literature is by no means extensive and the results at times conflicting, there is a sufficient body of evidence to justify the consideration of behavioural intervention as an adjunct to medication (Alumbaugh, 1971; Slade, 1972; Samman, 1975; Ayllon and Kandel, 1976; Lamontagne and Parenteau, 1983; Glaister, 1985; Belcher, 1988.)

The client

Jean is a 57-year-old woman diagnosed as suffering from paranoid schizophrenia. Childhood memories for Jean are recalled with much pleasure and her school years are remembered as a time of achievement. During her final year at school however, Jean experienced what was to be the first of many breakdowns and numerous hospital admissions, which have always been precipitated by the occurrence of florid auditory hallucinations. The concomitant overt hallucinatory behaviour has frequently resulted in Jean being described as paranoid, grandiose and hostile. For the past five years Jean has been a resident in a long-stay psychiatric ward.

Assessment

As stated in the introduction to this chapter, only selected aspects of the therapeutic process which have particular relevance to each case will be described.

The broad aim of assessment is the identification and definition of the client's problem within the context of the whole person, the analysis of its nature, function and the production of a measure which will assist in the evaluation of change (Barker, 1985). This objective could not have been realized however if a therapeutic and empathic rapport had not been established. As Lazurus bluntly stated, 'If a person does not possess genuine compassion for the plight of his patients and have a strong desire to diminish their suffering, it would be a boon to psychotherapy if he would enter some other field of endeavour' (Lazurus, 1971). A complementary aspect of this fundamental rapport, and one which is often described as a characteristic of behavioural therapy, is the development of a collaborative relationship between client and therapist. From the outset therefore Jean actively participated in the selection of assessment methods, the setting of target goals and the subsequent treatment intervention.

Jean expressed her expectations in terms of volume control rather than the elimination of her auditory hallucinations. The problem, in Jean's view, was not the hallucinatory experience *per se*, but the loudness of the voices which disrupted her concentration, inhibited her ability to enjoy and take part in various social and recreational pursuits and precipitated periodic shouting and screaming episodes which invariably resulted in Jean being given a needle. If the auditory amplitude could be reduced, Jean felt that she would be able to ignore the hallucinatory vocalizations.

Jean described the voices as predominately male, frequently abusive and particularly distressing when they made sexually suggestive or disparaging remarks about herself or those with whom she had regular contact. The ward staff for example were accused of stealing her money, fellow patients were identified as nasty people and visitors to the ward as troublemakers.

According to Jean, the hallucinations occurred almost constantly throughout the day at low volume level. Intense episodes which resulted in Jean's overt verbal outbursts were reported by the ward staff as a common daily occurrence. A good day for Jean was one on which only two or three such episodes were recorded. While Jean's recollection of these events suggested a somewhat lower incidence, she questioned her ability to distinguish one incident from another due to the persistence of the hallucinations.

A precise assessment of Jean's auditory hallucinations involved a detailed functional analysis of the problem behaviour, (Kanfer and Saslow, 1969), direct observational assessment measures and self monitoring exercises. The key points which emerged from this comprehensive behavioural analysis included:

1. The significant role of anxiety in the precipitation of hallucinatory events.
2. Engaging the hallucinatory vocalization in an argumentative dialogue with increased volume intensity.
3. The existence of two self-control strategies, i.e., distraction and shouting.
4. The periodic and partial effectiveness of these self-control strategies in decreasing volume intensity, and in reducing the duration of the hallucinatory event.
5. The absence of clearly identifiable overt environmental determinants.

Baseline measurements

Baseline measurements established during a two-week pre-treatment period added further clarification and definition of the problem behaviour and treatment goals. These observations also contributed to the evaluation of treatment efficiency.

Initially, baseline observations included self monitoring of the frequency, duration and volume intensity of Jean's auditory hallucinations. Direct observation of Jean's overt hallucinatory behaviour involved the ward staff recording these episodes on a crisis incident format. Precision in the definition of the behaviour to be recorded was crucial, otherwise observations might have been made of behaviour unrelated to hallucinatory events. An average of three episodes per day was recorded on the incident format. As hallucinations are intrinsically private experiences, direct observational assessment methods have their obvious limitations. Jean was therefore asked to monitor aspects of her hallucinatory experiences. Self-monitoring exercises however, especially when observations are being made of high-frequency behaviour, can be demanding and must never be allowed to become yet another problem for the client. The appropriateness of self-monitoring methods must also be carefully evaluated as the act of self observation can produce a reactivity effect resulting in a transient increase or decrease of the observed behaviour. Jean agreed to monitor two aspects of her hallucinatory experiences – the frequency of the incidents and the approximate duration of each episode. The voices however instructed Jean to destroy the record sheet at the end of the first day. Jean had made valiant attempts to resist those commands but the volume of the auditions increased to such an intensity that she was forced to acquiesce. Surprisingly, Jean was neither discouraged nor unduly distressed by this experience and wished to try again. Her second attempt at self monitoring which solely involved observations of volume intensity did not precipitate these command hallucinations.

A simple numerical analogue scale which reflected Jean's ability to differentiate volume level was used to represent auditory amplitude at hourly intervals throughout the day (Fig. 12.1). Analysis of Jean's self-monitoring records indicated an average daily auditory volume of 3 on a scale of 1 to 4.

Figure 12.1   Scale for self-assessed
auditory amplitude of hallucinations

1	2	3	4
faint	clear	loud	shout

Two baseline measurements had therefore been established to assist in the evaluation of treatment efficiency – the crisis incident format maintained by the ward staff and the data provided by Jean's own observations regarding hallucinatory volume.

Treatment

No behavioural treatment approach is ever arbitrarily selected, or determined by a particular diagnosis. Intervention is designed on the basis of information obtained from assessment of the client's uniquely individual experience of a problem behaviour. In Jean's case, a number of factors were influential in the formulation of the treatment programme; the presence for example of an anxiety precipitant, the consequences of engaging hallucinatory vocalizations in an argumentative dialogue, and Jean's own attempts to control the intrusive auditions by distraction and shouting.

In an earlier discussion, Jean had mentioned how, as a child, she would alleviate the boredom of a school lesson by daydreaming. She had also demonstrated an ability to recall past events in considerable detail. When asked for her suggestion as to what would be helpful in reducing the discomfort of anxiety symptoms, Jean not unexpectedly replied that she could think of something nice. The experience recalled by Jean which subsequently was incorporated into an imaginal relaxation technique, occurred during a visit to the countryside. The vividness with which Jean remembered that particular incident was remarkable. With regard to inhibiting the development of an argumentative exchange with the hallucinatory auditions, Jean initially suggested engaging in an activity which would serve as a distraction. She acknowledged however that the initial alluring quality of the hallucinations would probably impede her ability to engage in an alternative activity. Her use of an expletive was, in her view, the most effective means of dismissing the auditory hallucinations. After a lengthy discussion, Jean agreed to a trial substitution of this rather colourful oath with the command 'stop'.

All Jean's suggestions were utilized in the design of the treatment strategy in which relaxation, thought-stopping and distraction were the primary components. On a card which Jean kept with her at all times, four words representing the treatment components, were printed in a colour associated with each technique. The first word, STOP, was for example written in red, followed by RELAX in yellow, COUNTRYSIDE in brown, and lastly ACTIVITY in green. Jean was instructed to look at the card immediately upon the onset of each hallucinatory episode, vigorously say the word 'stop', commence the relaxation exercise prompted by the words relax and countryside, and finally engage in a distraction activity from a pre-selected list. The verbal expression of the word 'stop' was subsequently faded into a covert utterance: Jean mentally said the word 'stop'.

Jean utilized this strategy with considerable success on a number of occasions. Analysis of the occasions on which the technique proved ineffective revealed a delayed implementation. Jean, in the belief that she could ignore the auditions, would postpone employing the treatment strategy. When she did so, the increased volume of the vocalizations rendered them less amenable to disruption. Re-emphasizing the importance of introducing the treatment procedure precisely at the onset of each hallucinatory episode proved an effective solution.

Treatment results

The results of the four-week cognitive self-management programme indicated a significant alteration in Jean's auditory hallucinations. Comparison of the pre- and post-baseline measurements provided statistical evidence of a 90% reduction in overt hallucinatory incidents and a similar decrease in audition volume intensity. Statistical evidence of treatment efficiency is however of little clinical value unless supported by a demonstrable improvement in the individual's quality of life. In this case, the therapeutic contribution of behavioural intervention was verified by Jean's own subjective evaluation of progress, by her substantially increased participation in social and recreational activities within and outwith the hospital, and by an improvement in concentration which resulted in uninterrupted viewing and enjoyment of her favourite TV soap operas. At one month follow-up progress had been maintained.

Discussion

The presenting problem was that of auditory hallucinations in a 57-year-old lady who achieved a significant reduction in her hallucinatory experiences by means of a cognitive self-management programme. The treatment package can be seen as an elaboration of Wolpe's thought-stopping technique which is consistent with the current emphasis on cognitive–mediational models of behaviour (Wolpe, 1973). As Barker (1982) stated, 'the golden rule is to select a treatment method to suit the patient and her problems rather than describe therapy for a particular diagnostic type.' Jean had indicated an ability to evoke vivid imagery, and assessment of her self-control potential revealed two major mechanisms. These factors were positively utilized in the construction of the treatment intervention. As a consistent pattern of dysfunctional cognitive activity had developed in response to the hallucinatory events, disruption of this sequence of events was essential, followed by a response incompatible with anxiety, in other words, relaxation. The implementation of an alternative cognitive activity, in this case visual imagery, provided an additional element of distraction. The attempt to control the disruptive intrusive experience may also have encouraged the development of adaptive attention control.

One of the common reasons for referring an individual to the psychiatric services is that the individual has reported a hallucinatory experience, or has engaged in behaviour which has led others to conclude that he or she has such experiences. Such a diagnosis, even if refined to conform with current psychiatric classification schemes, is often thought to preclude the application of behavioural treatments. It is to be hoped that this case study demonstrates that this is an unwarranted assumption.

Case study 2: insomnia

Introduction

That sleep is a universally valued human experience is unquestionable. It has inspired an elegance of expression from literary masters which is reflected in the verbal repertoire of the general populace, the majority of whom would, for example, have a passing acquaintance with the opening words of Hamlet's famous soliloquy: 'To be, or not to be...'. The significance attached to sleep is further demonstrated in the frequency of social exchanges which open with an enquiry regarding the quality of the previous night's sleep. The experience of sleep also serves as a performance projection of the day ahead, a lack of quantity or quality usually generates a prophesy of the debilitating consequences of a bad night. Its use by professionals and laymen alike to evaluate progress is equally familiar. While few details will be communicated by hospital staff to patients' relatives over the telephone, they will invariably be informed whether or not their spouse or child has slept well, and the degree of concern experienced by friends can be influenced by a comment on how poorly the person is sleeping. Disruption of sleep therefore, whatever the reason, has negative consequences ranging from annoyance to a pervasive deterioration in an individual's functional and affective state.

The prevalence of sleep difficulties reflects not only the cultural emphasis placed upon the importance of sleep, but also the increasing demands and pressures of living in a technological, achievement-orientated world. Surveys conducted in America reveal a substantial incidence of insomnia, demonstrated to a similar degree in Britain (Mellinger, Balter and Uhlenhuth, 1985; Espie, Lindsay and Brooks, 1988). The continued widespread use of sleep-promoting medication is extensively documented, (Kripke, 1983; Kripke *et al.*, 1983), as are the hazards of hypnotic drugs, in particular the dangers of dependency (Murray *et al.*,

1981; Hauri, 1982; Walsh, Sugarman and Chambers, 1986). Psychological alternatives to pharmacological intervention are therefore clearly desirable.

A number of behavioural strategies have been devised which have proved to be effective treatment approaches to persistent insomnia (Bootzin and Nicassio, 1978; Borkovec, 1982; van Oot, Lane and Borkovec, 1984; Lichstein and Fisher, 1985; Lacks, 1987). Perhaps the greatest measure of success has been achieved with the technique of stimulus control which was one of the strategies used to resolve the long-standing insomnia problem reported in this case study (Lacks *et al.*, 1983; Morin and Azrin, 1987).

The client

Marion is an energetic, fashion-conscious 67-year-old lady with a 23-year history of insomnia. For over a decade Marion has been an active member of a local charity organization with which her wide circle of friends are similarly involved and who regard Marion as the troubleshooter of their group. Marion once humorously remarked that survival was just possible without her moisturizing cream and filofax, but life without sleep was intolerable.

Assessment

The assessment tools used in this detailed problem analysis included the structured interview, psychological inventories and sleep diaries.

While Marion could not recall ever having been a good sleeper prior to a hysterectomy some 23 years ago, her inability to sleep for more than a few hours each night appeared to have few negative consequences. With the exception of periodic daytime tiredness, Marion viewed her limited sleep requirements as an advantage. It was following her discharge from hospital that sleep became a problem. Twenty-three years later Marion was, as she put it, now totally obsessed with her inability to sleep. Numerous hypnotic medications in maximum dosages had been prescribed over the years, none of which had been of any long-term value. Marion herself had tried various alternative remedies in an attempt to obtain a restorative and consistent sleep pattern, none of which had proved successful. She perceived her referral with considerable cynicism and some hostility generated by a belief that she was being labelled as a moaning neurotic and was now reduced to seeing a nurse rather than a doctor. Marion's initial aggressiveness rapidly diminished however following a comprehensive discussion of the nature of a collaborative therapeutic relationship and my open responses to her challenging questions.

Marion's experience of insomnia involved two common complaints: trouble falling asleep at the beginning of the night (sleep onset insomnia) and a disruption in sleep maintenance. Marion's frequent wakeful periods during the night were accompanied by difficulties in getting back to sleep.

Furthermore, an article in a woman's magazine some years ago had led Marion to believe that a healthy night's sleep could only be obtained if a person slept for a minimum of six hours with no wakeful periods, a misconception which dominated her perception of sleep requirements.

During the past year, the negative consequences of Marion's sleep difficulties had intensified. An increasing obsession with obtaining adequate sleep totally controlled her life. The constant worrying about the night ahead was significantly affecting the quality of her interpersonal relationships and her ability to derive enjoyment from previously pleasurable everyday activities.

To isolate factors which might be contributing to sleep disruption, Marion was asked to keep a diary of her daytime and pre-sleep routines including a record of usage of substances such as caffeine and nicotine, both of which are central nervous system stimulants (Edelstein, Keaton-Brasted and Burg, 1984; Kales *et al.*, 1984). Little of relevance was identified in Marion's daytime schedule with the exception of sleeping late into the morning and cat-napping after an unsettled night. Her bedtime routine however revealed an almost ritualistic sequence of activities over a specified period of time. This routine began at precisely 8.30 pm, involved 12 discrete behaviours which began with preparation for a shower and ended with Marion selecting the clothes to wear for the following day. Her diary further revealed an average caffeine intake of eight cups of coffee per day, the final cup being taken around 7 pm. She smoked about 10 cigarettes each day, but notably in the evenings. While Marion expressed an awareness of the arousal properties of caffeine, she assumed that not drinking coffee late in the evening would eliminate caffeine effects on her sleep pattern. Smoking was for Marion relaxing and not negotiable! Some time however after contact ceased, Marion sent me a postcard with the cryptic message 'I've stopped'!

A sleep diary maintained over a two-week pre-treatment baseline period identified a sleep onset latency averaging 95 minutes, frequent wakeful periods during the night, and a quantity of sleep totalling less than three hours. Marion described how she would lie in bed trying desperately hard to fall asleep. As the minutes ticked by, she would become increasingly tense, restlessly tossing to and fro and would switch on the lights every few minutes to check the time. More often than not she would read, knit, write letters or watch a late night programme on a small portable television which sat on her bedroom chest of drawers, while constantly worrying about her inability to sleep and the long wakeful night ahead.

Treatment

A sequential treatment plan was devised involving the following components:

1. sleep education;
2. reduction of caffeine intake;
3. alteration of pre-sleep routine;
4. imaginal relaxation;
5. stimulus control.

Throughout the treatment phase, Marion maintained her sleep diary.

An entire session was devoted to sleep education with the emphasis on the changing sleep pattern as an individual grows older. To complement relevant reading material which I provided to increase her awareness of sleep rhythms and requirements, Marion was asked to expand her knowledge further by carrying out her own research. In earlier discussions of Marion's commitment to a local charity group it became evident that her organization of various group activities was characterized by careful preparation and considerable attention to detail. These skills and attributes were utilized particularly during the treatment phase to encourage the adoption of a problem-solving approach to an aspect of Marion's life regarded by her as being beyond her control. Marion needed no suggestions from me as to how she might acquire additional information. If anything, her enthusiasm had to be curtailed otherwise every library and bookshop in the locality would have been visited. In addition to what Marion referred to as her fact-finding mission, she was encouraged to decrease her caffeine intake. Although these two strategies did not alter her sleep disturbance, they did resolve her previous misconceptions regarding sleep, provided an important sense of achievement which had been absent from this particular area of her life and reduced her sense of being overwhelmed by her sleep difficulties.

Flexibility in, rather than elimination of, pre-sleep activities was gradually introduced over a three-week period. During this time Marion was also taught an imaginal method of relaxation as an alternative response to somatic and cognitive arousal which intensified when she retired to bed. Imaginal relaxation, or guided imagery, involves the verbal construction of a scene in which emphasis is placed on the sensory stimuli of sight, sound, touch and smell, with the corresponding relaxation responses such as warmth, heaviness, muscular flaccidity, slow and regular breathing. Clients however are unlikely to engage successfully in this covert behaviour if they possess poor imaginal skills (Lang, 1977; Shielkh, 1983). The imaginal relaxation exercise set against a background of peaceful instrumental music was recorded on an audio cassette which Marion was instructed to play when she went to bed. While these latter strategies proved effective in decreasing sleep onset delay and in increasing sleep duration, further improvements were thought achievable by the introduction of a stimulus control procedure.

Stimulus control is derived from an operant conditioning theory of insomnia. A substantial proportion of behaviour is determined by environmental factors. For the majority of individuals, the bedroom is associated with sleep behaviour. The environment contains a number of cues, or stimuli which promote sleep – changing into night attire, getting into bed, arranging the pillow and bedcovers in a particular way are just a few examples of sleeping cues. The bedroom, or just thinking about sleep for others however, can become discriminative stimuli for not sleeping. As in Marion's case, the bed and bedroom had become associated with sleeplessness and sleep-incompatible behaviours such as letter writing and watching television while lying in bed. Perhaps the most significant sleep inhibitory behaviour for Marion was worrying – worrying about being unable to sleep and the long hours of anticipated wakefulness. Basically, stimulus control is all about re-associating the bed and bedroom with sleep, through the elimination of those sleep-incompatible behaviours and by the establishment of a consistent sleep pattern. After discussion and negotiation, Marion agreed to implement the following instructions:

1. go to bed only when extremely sleepy;
2. get up no later than 8.30 a.m. regardless of the quality and quantity of the previous night's sleep;
3. no activities while in bed other than sleep or listening to the relaxation tape;
4. no clock-watching;
5. if not asleep within 20 minutes, get out of bed, go into another room and select one of the following activities:
   (a) reading
   (b) listening to quiet music
   (c) knit
   (d) take a bath;
6. return to bed only when sleepy;
7. if not asleep fairly quickly, repeat 5 and 6;
8. no cat-naps during the day;
9. no smoking during or after pre-bedtime routine;
10. set aside a period in the early evening for charity-related tasks.

Treatment results

Three weeks later, Marion reported a reduction in sleep onset from forty-five mins to an acceptable 20 mins. She regulary slept for 4.5 hours without interruption and woke feeling refreshed. At three-month follow-up, Marion's improved sleep pattern had been maintained. A further three months later she contacted me to confirm her progress. Although she reported an occasional restless night, this was regarded as a normal experience and prompted no concern.

Conclusion

For over 20 years Marion had experienced significant sleep difficulties which had diminished her quality of life. A multicomponent behavioural treatment intervention effectively resolved Marion's chronic insomnia over a relatively short period of time. While further research is obviously necessary, this case study provides encouraging evidence to support the therapeutic effectiveness of a behavioural approach to insomnia. Psychological alternatives to medication, especially in respect to the treatment of the elderly (considering their vulnerability to toxicity), surely merits more serious consideration (Scharf and Brown, 1986). Despite an increased emphasis on the need for preventative health care and health awareness, today's society remains fundamentally pill-orientated, an orientation which is likely to continue in the absence of vigorous promotion of the viable alternatives.

Case study 3: grief

Introduction

Elizabeth Collick introduces a chapter in her book, *Through Grief*, with the following quotation from Edmund Burke: 'If the object of pleasure be totally lost, a passion arises which is called grief' (Collick, 1986). Grief, in varying degrees and modes of expression appears to be a universal human response to loss (Krupp and Kligfeld, 1962). The automatic association between grief or mourning and death is somewhat discriminatory, as loss comes in many forms: an amputation, hysterectomy, miscarriage or divorce may all involve the trauma of loss, the experience of grief and the need to mourn.

The manifestation of grief comprises a diffuse range of emotions and behaviour: crying, anger and aggression have been identified as universal transcultural responses to bereavement (Rosenblatt, Walsh and Jackson, 1976). A number of concomitant affective, somatic, cognitive and behavioural responses are similarly associated with acute grieving and occur with remarkable consistency across different populations and in different eras. Lindemann's classic study in 1944, for example, in which he describes the grief responses of those involved in the Coconut Grove disaster, echoes the more recent observations of Bowlby, Carlton and Raphael (Lindemann, 1944; Bowlby, 1973; Carlton, 1980; Raphael, 1981). The active nature of bereavement resolution was indicated in the early part of this century by Freud, and reiterated in the present by Worden, who refers to the four stages of mourning as tasks (Freud, 1917; Worden, 1983). The painful necessity of experiencing and working through the intense distress of significant loss is regarded as fundamental to adaptive grieving and mourning. However, bereavement, like any other normal process, can become obstructed and its natural conclusion prolonged or inhibited. A number of authors have identified specific factors which can be viewed as vulnerability predictors to the development of unresolved or pathological grief; loss of a highly dependent relationship (Horowitz, 1980), uncertainty of loss during for example, times of war when death may never be confirmed (Lazare, 1979), previous history of grieving difficulties (Simon, 1979), mode of death (Parkes, 1972), and the individual's distress tolerance level (Worden, 1983) are just a few examples of factors which can inhibit adaptive grieving.

Abnormal grief is defined by Horowitz (1980) as the intensification of grief to the level where the person is overwhelmed, resorts to maladaptive behaviour, or remains in the state of grief without progression of the mourning process towards completion. A classic case of pathological grief is demonstrated by the reaction of Queen Victoria to the death of her husband Prince Albert who in an attempt to deny the reality of her loss, insisted that the Prince's shaving gear be laid out every day (Worden, 1983).

Ramsay's proposition of a link between unresolved grief and phobic responses is fundamental to a behavioural approach to the resolution of maladaptive grief (Ramsay, 1976). Similarities are drawn between the avoidance response of phobic and bereaved individuals to anxiety- or distress-evoking stimuli. Resolution is therefore inhibited by the avoidance of the grief experience and results in bereavement stasis. Avoidance behaviour as a coping strategy for such painful psychological truama may be an extension of the numbness so often experienced after learning of the loss. As Worden (1983) suggests, the absence of feeling probably protects the individual from being overwhelmed by a deluge of bruising emotions. An essential component of behavioural-orientated grief therapy is therefore exposure to distress-evoking stimuli. While phobic responses can be effectively treated by a gradual confrontation of anxiety-provoking stimuli, for example by the techniques of systematic desensitization and graded exposure, there is unfortunately, as Ramsay states, 'no gentle equivalent' for unresolved grief. Consequently, therapy involves prolonged exposure to the traumatic event and the elicitation of the concomitant distressing emotional reactions which have previously been avoided. This approach should not be viewed as a resolution of grief but rather as a means of ungluing the person from the phase at which they are stuck. This facilitates progression through the bereavement process (Hodgkinson, 1980).

The client

Five years ago, Rebecca's husband who was returning from a business trip in Europe died in a car crash during the short journey between the airport and his home. As his injuries had been described as horrific, Rebecca was advised not to view David's body. David's father, a retired army officer, arranged a memorial service for his son during the week following the tragic accident. Rebecca was not considered well enough to attend.

Rebecca's and David's previous marriages had ended with much bitterness and acrimony, divorce had been a traumatic experience for both of them. Neither therefore had entered lightly into a second commitment, despite the encouragement of their friends who recognized the quality of their relationship and the profound happiness each gave to the other, a happiness which had not diminished over 10 years of marriage. David was 46 years old when he died, two years younger than Rebecca. There were no children. Friends visited Rebecca frequently during the months following David's death but, as their attempts to encourage Rebecca to pick up her life were being constantly rejected, their visits gradually decreased. Rebecca continued to live in the cottage which she and David had so carefully restored over the years, spending her days looking after a sizeable garden and occasionally getting involved in village community activities. She would not tolerate any mention or reference to David by anyone with the exception of her father-in-law who regularly spent the weekend at the cottage. During the past two years Rebecca had experienced increasingly intense anxiety symptoms. Occasions when she would cry uncontrollably for, as she put it, no particular reason were similarly occurring with greater frequency. Her general practitioner, in his referral letter, expressed the view that Rebecca's psychological problems were symptomatic of unresolved grief.

Assessment

During the initial session, I sought to establish an empathic rapport with Rebecca who was extremely defensive as she had anticipated being immediately quizzed about David. Discussions with her general practitioner had led to the realization, which she did not want to openly acknowledge because of the pain involved, that David's death had never been fully accepted or her loss resolved. Rebecca had 'braced' herself as she put it to reject any enquiries concerning David. She spoke rapidly emphasizing points with vigorous hand gestures. Periods when she would pause, as if struggling for control, would be followed by a flood of details about various aspects of gardening, after which she would again raise the issue of David's death. During this time, I limited my responses to largely non-verbal acknowledgements of whatever topic Rebecca raised, the garden, the church fete, the price of bulbs, her anxiety symptoms or references to David. Rebecca then suddenly fired a series of questions at me ranging from the innocuous to the personal, all of which were accepted and answered openly. Her enquiries stopped with the suddenness with which they had begun. During the short period of silence which followed, Rebecca was obviously formulating a further question which was not going to be lightly asked, a question concerning my own experience of loss. When faced with enquiries of a personal nature, clinicians must judge the therapeutic appropriateness of self disclosure (Jourard, 1971), a decision which can at times be difficult. On this occasion it was not difficult to make a judgement. Rebecca's questions were not asked out of idle curiosity. This client was in the process of deciding whether or not to take a risk and trust a person with the intimacy and acuteness of her pain. The therapist had to have substance and be prepared, as Rebecca later described it, to be real. Whatever the nature of the therapist's reality, it was acceptable to Rebecca. The following two sessions were devoted to preparation for the process of grief therapy. I described the rationale of the therapeutic process, explaining how avoidance behaviour had inhibited adaptive grief and mourning and the method by which the bereavement wheels could be set in motion, thus allowing for an eventual resolution to occur.

Rebecca was made aware of the intense level of distress which would be experienced during this process by, for example, the discussion of events relating to David's death by viewing and handling objects associated with him. My role would be to maintain the focus of attention on the distressing topic until the intensity of the emotional response had been exhausted. As this type of grief therapy will generate intense distress, careful consideration must be given to the organization of appointments. Rebecca agreed that her home, rather than the indifferent setting of a health centre clinic, would be more appropriate to the grief process. She also accepted that a break of two days between sessions would prevent her from becoming emotionally exhausted. The duration of each session would be determined by her level of distress, and I agreed to remain with her for as long as was necessary. The emotional arousal generated by this therapeutic process is intense. As Rebecca had already told her father-in-law of her decision to undergo therapy, a decision which he had encouraged, she welcomed the suggestion that he be invited to stay with her during what would be a painful and difficult time. Finally, as advised by Ramsay (1976), a contract was made and signed by both therapist and client which included the following agreements:

1. I will contact my therapist or my general practitioner if between sessions I experience extreme distress.
2. I will discuss with my father-in-law details of the sessions and accept his support and help.
3. If I experience any thoughts of suicide I will immediately contact my therapist or my general practitioner.
4. Only if my therapist concurs will I terminate therapy.

Rebecca's general practitioner was, of course, fully aware of and in agreement with the nature of grief therapy about to be undertaken.

Treatment

During the subsequent five sessions, some of which lasted for well over two hours, Rebecca discussed in detail her life before she met David, their joy at discovering one another, their 10 years of marriage, the circumstances of his death and her experience of such a significant loss. Initially

Rebecca attempted to avoid the distress which this entailed by reciting details in much the same way as she would describe items on a shopping list. Her body posture, facial expression and tone of voice reflected the effort involved in talking about David and the rigid control which she was finding increasingly difficult to maintain.

As I began to interrupt Rebecca's rapid litany of events by quietly reflecting back to her what she had previously said, her speech slowed and her rigid control gradually dissolved. During the periods of intense anguish which followed, I made no attempt to relieve this distress: Rebecca was gently but consistently encouraged to experience and express the pain of her grief. Mementoes of David and photograph albums which had been removed from the house by David's father after his son's death so that Rebecca would not be upset, were gradually returned and used during the sessions. Handling and viewing these objects provoked intense sobbing. Throughout these periods, while I would utter occasional words of encouragement, I chiefly maintained an active, empathic silence as she responded to her need for physical contact at moments when her grief became particularly difficult.

After the distress of each session had diminished, Rebecca expressed a sense of change which she described in terms of a lightening of a burden or weight. She also spoke of an increasing awareness of everyday things as if, she remarked on another occasion, she was becoming alive.

Towards the end of the third session, Rebecca expressed her regret at not being able to say goodbye to David. There were so many things she would have liked to have said to him; how much, for example, he had meant to her, the happiness he had brought into her life and her lack of apology when she had been at fault. She also wished that she had been more open with him, in acknowledging that he had irritating habits and in expressing her annoyance and disappointment when he bought, for a wedding anniversary present, a new cooker and not, as she had been expecting, a more personal gift.

The penultimate session therefore involved Rebecca in verbalizing these thoughts and feelings directly to a photograph of David using the present tense. Rebecca experienced a range of emotions from anger to sadness as she told David what she had not had the opportunity to say because of the suddenness of his death.

The final treatment session was held while walking along nearby country lanes, following David's favourite route. Here Rebecca said goodbye. She cried quietly but naturally and her tears were interspersed with happy recollections of their time together.

Treatment results

I met Rebecca on two subsequent occasions to review the course of therapy and to evaluate treatment efficacy which, in this case, was determined by Rebecca's own evaluation and the therapist's observations.

Rebecca no longer experienced excessive anxiety. She felt that a tremendous burden had been lifted from her shoulders, and while she experienced moments of sadness and tearfulness they were viewed by her as normal and natural. For the first time since David's death she had periods of happiness; she could enjoy her memories of David and share with her father-in-law recollections of their time together. Rebecca felt that she was becoming alive again in a way which did not minimize her loss or detract from her memory of David. Plans for the future were now being made; she had, for example, telephoned an old friend, accepted an invitation to visit, and arranged a holiday with her later in the year. A further area of improvement was demonstrated in her increased participation in village social activities and in her willingness to initiate social interaction.

My own observations confirmed Rebecca's evaluation of treatment effectiveness. In the house which had previously been devoid of any reminders of David, their wedding photograph was openly displayed on an occasional table in the lounge and Rebecca could speak of him without distress although, at times, with understandable sadness. She frequently smiled now and spoke of future plans with anticipation and modest enthusiasm. Rebecca had passed through a period of inhibited grief into one of adaptive mourning.

Contact was maintained by telephone over a three-month period during which time Rebecca continued to re-invest in the business of living without David.

Discussion

The similarities between phobic avoidance behaviour and the avoidance of bereavement cues in unresolved grief were suggested by Ramsay (1976). The exposure approach described in this case resembles flooding, one of the techniques employed in the treatment of phobias (Marks, 1977). The approach, also referred to as a guided mourning, has been used by Lieberman (1978), Mawson *et al.* (1981) and Sireling, Cohen and Marks (1988), with encouraging results. Behavioural literature on the subject of morbid grief is not however extensive, and caution must be exercised when evaluating the results of the studies which are available. The aim of therapy in this case is not to resolve grief, but rather to dissolve barriers so that progression through the grieving and mourning process can be continued.

References

Al-Issa, I. (1976) Behaviour therapy and hallucinations: a socio-cultural approach. *Psychother. Theory, Res. Practice*, **13**, 156–9.

Al-Issa, I. (1978). Socio-cultural factors in hallucinations. *Int. J. Soc. Psych.*, **24**, 167–76.

Alumbaugh, R. V. (1971) Use of behaviour modification techniques towards reduction of hallucinatory behaviour: a case study. *Psychol. Rec.*, **21**, 415–7.

Andrade, C., Srinath, S. and Andrade, A. (1988) True hallucinations as a culturally sanctioned experience. *Brit. J. Psych.*, **152**, 838–9.

Ayllon, T. and Kandel, H. (1976) I hear voices but there's no one there: a functional analysis of auditory hallucinations, in *Case Studies in Behaviour Theràpy* (ed. H. J. Eysenck), Routledge and Kegan Paul, London.

Barker, P. (1982) *Behaviour Therapy Nursing*, Croom Helm, London.

Barker, P. J. (1985) *Patient Assessment in Psychiatric Nursing*, Croom Helm, London.

Bauer, S. F. (1970) The function of hallucinations: an inquiry into the relationship of hallucinatory experiences to creative thought, in *Origins and mechanisms of Hallucinations* (ed. W. Kemp), Plenum Press, New York.

Belcher, T. L. (1988) Behaviour reduction of overt hallucinatory behaviour in a chronic schizophrenic. *J. Behav. Ther. Exp. Psych.*, **19**, 69–71.

Bootzin, R. R. and Nicassio, P. M. (1978) Behavioural treatments for insomnia, in *Progress in Behaviour Modification* (eds M. Merson, R. Eisler and P. Miller), Academic Press, New York.

Borkovec, T. D. (1982) Insomnia. *J. Consult. Clin. Psychol.*, **50**, 880–95.

Bowlby, J. (1973) *Attachment and Loss*, Vol. 2, In *Separation: Anxiety and Anger*, Hogarth Press, London.

Carlton, I. G. (1980) Early psychiatric intervention following a maritime disaster. *Milit. Med.*, **145**, 114–16.

Collick, E. (1986) *Through Grief: The bereavement journey*, Longman and Todd, London.

Edelstein, B. A., Keaton-Brasted, C. and Burg, M. M. (1984) Effects of caffeine withdrawal on nocturnal enuresis, insomnia and behaviour restraints. *J. Consult. Clin. Psychol.*, **52**, 857–62.

Espie, C. A., Lindsay, W. R. and Brooks, D. N. (1988) Substituting behavioural treatment for drugs in the treatment of insomnia: an explorative study. *J. Behav. Ther. Exp. Psych.*, **19**, 51–6.

Esquirol, J. E. D. (1965) *Mental Maladies*, Hafner Press, New York.

Freud, S. (1917) *Mourning and Melancholia*, Vol. 14, Hogarth, London.

Glaister, B. (1985) A case study of auditory hallucinations treated by satiation. *Behav. Res. Ther.*, **23**, 213–5.

Hauri, P. (1982) *The Sleep Disorders*, Upjohn, Kalamazoo, MI.

Hodgkinson, P. E. (1980) Treating abnormal grief in the bereaved. *Nursing Times*, January 17th, **76**, 126–8.

Horowitz, M. J. (1980) Pathological grief and the activation of latent self-images. *Am. J. Psych.*, **137**, 1157–62.

Hume, A. (1988a) Sound remedies. *Nurs. Times*, **84**, 42–4.

Hume, A. (1988b) Let me whisper in your ear. *Nurs. Times*, **84**, 39–41.

Jourard, S. M. (1971) *Self Disclosure: an experimental Analysis of the Transparent Self*, Wiley, New York.

Kales, J. D., Kales, A., Bixler, E. O. *et al.* (1984) Biopsycho-behavioural correlates of insomnia: clinical characteristics and behavioural correlates. *Am. J. Psych.*, **141**, 1371–6.

Kanfer, F. M. and Saslow, G. (1969) Behavioural diagnosis, in *Behaviour Therapy: Appraisal and Status* (ed. C. M. Franks), McGraw Hill, New York.

Kripke, D. F. (1983) Why we need tax on sleeping pills. *Southern Med. J.*, **76**, 632–6.

Kripke, D. F., Ancoli-Israel, S., Masson, W. and Messin, S. (1983) Sleep-related mortality and morbidity in the aged, in *Sleep Disorders: Basic and Clinical Research* (eds M. H. Chase and E. D. Weitzman), Spectrum, New York.

Krupp, G. R. and Kligfeld, B. (1962) The bereavement reaction: a cross-cultural evaluation. *J. Rel. Health*, **1**, 222–46.

Lacks, P. (1987) *Behavioural Treatment for Persistent Insomnia*, Pergamon Press, New York.

Lacks, P., Bertelson, A. D., Sugarman, J. L. and Kunkel, J. (1983) The treatment of sleep maintenance insomnia with stimulus control techniques. *Behav. Res. Ther.*, **21**, 291–5.

Lamontagne, Y. and Parenteau, P. (1983) Thought stopping for delusions and hallucinations: a Pilot Study. *Behav. Psychother.*, **7**, 177–84.

Lang, P. J. (1977) Imagery in therapy: an information processing analysis of fear. *Behav. Ther.*, **8**, 862–86.

Lazare, E. (1979) Unresolved grief, in *Outpatient Psychiatry: Diagnosis and Treatment* (ed. A. Lazare), Williams and Wilkins, Baltimore.

Lazurus, A. (1971) *Behaviour Therapy and Beyond*, McGraw-Hill, New York.

Lichstein, K. L. and Fisher, S. M. (1985) Insomnia, in *Handbook of Clinical Behaviour Therapy with Adults* (eds M. Herson and A. S. Bellack), Plenum Press, New York.

Lieberman, S. (1978) Nineteen cases of morbid grief. *Brit. J. Psych.*, **132**, 156–63.

Lindemann, E. (1944) Symptomatology and management of acute grief. *Am. J. Psych.*, **101**, 141–9.

Marks, J. M. (1977) Perspective on flooding. *Sem. Psych.*, **4**, 129–38.

Mawson, D., Marks, J., Ramm, E. and Stern, R. S. (1981) Guided mourning for morbid grief: a controlled study. *Brit. J. Psych.*, **138**, 185–93.

Mellinger, G. D., Balter, M. B. and Uhlenhuth, E. H. (1985) Insomnia and its treatment: prevalence and correlates. *Arch. Gen. Psych.*, **42**, 225–32.

Murray, R., Ghodse, H., Harris, C. *et al.* (1981) *The misuse of psychotropic drugs*, Gaskell, Royal College of Psychiatrists, London.

Morin, C. M. and Azrin, N. H. (1987) Stimulus control and imagery training in treating sleep maintenance insomnia. *J. Consult. Clin. Psychol.*, **55**, 260–2.

Parkes, C. M. (1972) *Bereavement: Studies in Grief in Adult Life*, Tavistock Publications, London.

Ramsay, R. W. (1976) Behavioural approaches to bereavement. *Behav. Res. Ther.*, **15**, 131–5.

Raphael, B. (1981) Personal disaster. *Aust. NZ. J. Psych.*, **15**, 183–98.

Rosenblatt, P. E., Walsh, R. P. and Jackson, D. A. (1976) *Grief and Mourning in Cross-Cultural Perspective*, HRAF Press, New Haven, CT.

Samman, M. (1975) Thought stopping and flooding in a case of hallucinations, obsessions and homicidal–suicidal behaviour. *J. Behav. Ther. Exp. Psych.*, **6**, 65–7.

Sarbin, T. R. and Juhasz, B. B. (1975) The social context of hallucinations, in *Hallucinations: Behaviour, Experience and Theory* (eds R. K. Seigal and L. J. West), John Wiley, New York.

Scharf, M. B. and Brown, L. (1986) Hypnotic drugs: use and abuse. *Clin. Psychol. Rev.*, **6**, 39–50.

Shielkh, A. A. (1983) *Imagery: Current theory, research and Application*, John Wiley, Somerset, NJ.

Simon, B. G. (1979) *A Time to Grieve*, Family Service Association, New York.

Sireling, L., Cohen, D. and Marks, I. (1988) Guided mourning for morbid grief: a controlled replication. *Behav. Ther.*, **19**, 121–32.

Slade, P. D. (1972) The effects of systematic desensitisation on auditory hallucinations. *Behav. Res. Ther.*, **10**, 85–91.

van Oot, P. H., Lane, T. W. and Borkovec, T. D. (1984) Sleep disturbances, in *Handbook of Psychopathology* (eds P. Sutker and H. Adams), Plenum Press, New York.

Walsh, J. K., Sugarman, J. L. and Chambers, G. W. (1986) Evaluation of insomnia. *Am. Fam. Physic.*, **33**, 185–94.

Wolfe, J. (1973) *Practice of Behaviour Therapy*, 2nd edn, Pergamon Press, Oxford.

Worden, J. W. (1983) *Grief Counselling and Grief Therapy*, Tavistock Publications, London.

Chapter 13

Peplau's interpersonal model: clinical applications

P. MARTIN

Peplau's (1952) interpersonal model provides a paradigm for nursing care. Peplau defines Man as an organism who strives in his own way to reduce the tension generated by needs. Health is defined as a word symbol that implies forward movement of personality and other ongoing human processes in the direction of creative, constructive, productive, personal and community living. She describes nursing as a significant therapeutic interpersonal process which focuses on both the nurse and patient. Four sequential phases in the interpersonal process are identified: orientation, identification, exploitation and resolution.

Orientation

The aim of orientation is to identify the dimensions of the client's difficulty, Peplau (1986). The nurse and patient meet as two strangers who are willing to learn about each other. Data collection begins and continues throughout the subsequent phases. The orientation phase of the nurse–patient relationship is of fundamental importance in setting the scene for the other successive phases. The nurse establishes rapport with the patient and ensures that he understands the purpose and boundaries of the nurse–patient relationship.

Identification

The second phase is reached when the nurse and patient are able to clarify each other's perceptions and expectations. Only the patient knows what his needs are and he is not always able to identify them; he only feels the tension generated by the needs. Therefore in formulating a plan of care the goals of the nurse and patient may not necessarily be the same. Peplau (1952) suggests that since nurses have professional knowledge and expertise the responsibility for specifying objectives for care lies with the nurse.

Exploitation

During exploitation interpersonal processes are fully utilized towards the reduction of anxiety and the promotion of growth. In this phase the patient derives full benefit from the nurse–patient relationship; other resources are utilized if necessary to meet the patient's needs.

Resolution

Resolution implies that the patient has overcome his health problems and is no longer in need of assistance from the nurse. The nurse–patient relationship is terminated and the patient assumes independence. Movement throughout the phases follows a developmental pattern and leads to personal growth for both nurse and patient. Throughout the four phases of the relationship the nurse adopts different and appropriate roles. The roles of stranger, counsellor, leader, surrogate, resource person, technical expert and other roles are used to facilitate personal growth processes.

Case study

Simon Manners, aged 49, first came to the attention of the psychiatric services some 10 years ago when he suffered from a depressive illness. He spent three weeks in hospital but then discharged himself against medical advice. Subsequently he agreed to be seen as an out-patient. He was admitted on two further occasions in 1981 and 1985, and following the last admission he attended the Day Hospital.

Simon married when he was in his twenties, but the marriage was short-lived and resulted in a divorce. Later he became friendly with a widow fifteen years older than himself. They lived together for six years. Their

Figure 13.1 Plan of care

Goals for patient	Goals of nurse
To interact with the nurse without resorting to hostile behaviour as a means of relieving anxiety.	To establish a relationship with the client.
To learn to trust.	To develop a basis for trust.
To share concerns.	To achieve professional closeness.
To reduce hostile behaviour which may be detrimental to health.	To identify problematic patterns in the client's behaviour.
To redirect energy consumed in maladaptive behaviours towards personal growth and maturity.	To identify those patterns more amenable to change and bring into awareness of the client.

relationship lasted until her death from cancer two years ago. Simon now lives alone in a semi-detached house in a pleasant semi-urban area. He has a half-sister who lives fairly near whom he sees quite often. His sister is also divorced. Prior to her divorce, Simon had very little to do with his sister and her husband as he disliked his brother-in-law.

Simon's early history was one of deprivation. His parents separated when he was five; both later remarried. His only brother went to live with their father in the North of England. At first, Simon joined them for his holidays, but distance and other factors meant that they gradually grew apart. Simon had a good education. Although his early school record was poor, he surprised his family by winning a scholarship to Grammar School. When he left school he joined a local firm as an office junior. He gradually worked his way up to a senior position in the company. He has never socialized with colleagues outside of the working environment and has more acquaintances than friends within the company. He is well thought of by his superiors. He runs an efficient office, even if his manner is rather brusque towards the staff in his department. His firm has been understanding about his illness, although the subject has never been broached other than at a very superficial level.

Simon Manners does not have a history of violent behaviour. His aggression is displayed passively. Previous records suggest that he relates better towards female rather than male nursing staff.

Introduction to Simon's nurse therapist

Susan Smith had only recently joined the Health Authority as a community psychiatric nurse (CPN) having moved from a similar post in another area. At the community liaison meeting, held once a month, Dr Kumar, a general practitioner (GP) asked if one of the CPNs would visit a patient – a Mr Simon Manners. Dr Kumar felt that Mr Manners could benefit from the support of a nurse. He was suffering from a mild depression and had been at home for two weeks. He wasn't, he added, an easy man to get to know. There was no immediate response to Dr Kumar's referral. Looking around her, Susan sensed a reluctance on the part of her colleagues to volunteer their services. Being relatively new to the district, and still building up a case load, she agreed to accept the patient. Later, when the meeting was finished, Susan found her colleagues only too willing to convey verbally and non-verbally information regarding Simon. He was known to both hospital and community staff; Susan noted that the words used to describe him included hostile, demanding, complaining and problem patient. One nurse remembered him as an in-patient, while another nurse had visited him when he was last discharged from hospital. One colleague who volunteered information about Simon had never actually met him, but knew him by reputation.

Susan Smith was an experienced psychiatric nurse with a sound theoretical background. She was familiar with much of the literature relating to the unpopular or non-compliant patient. She knew that a patient who fails to conform to the nurse's expectations of the patient role may well be labelled difficult (Armitage, 1980). Negative information about an individual is weighted more heavily and recalled more easily than positive information (Hamilton, 1979). Perhaps that was why Simon Manners was so well remembered.

Susan was an advocate of Peplau's (1952) developmental model, and she was determined not to allow negative evaluations to colour her perception of the client. Such perceptions would be detrimental to the establishment of a therapeutic relationship. Peplau (1960) emphasizes the importance of the nurse and patient viewing each other as strangers. If the nurse does not see the patient as a stranger about whom she knows nothing, but about whom she can learn much, then she will distort the facts of the situation.

Gallop (1988) warns that if the individuality of the patient is lost to a stereotype, and his behaviour is prejudged, then it is almost inevitable that the responses of both nurse and patient will follow a predictable nontherapeutic pattern. Furthermore, if a stereotypic category is stimulated before the nurse has met the patient, the nurse's expectation of the category may well ensure the consequence.

Orientation phase

When Susan Smith visited Simon for the first time his general demeanour and body language conveyed an attitude of forced politeness. Although Simon had agreed to Dr Kumar's suggestion that a community psychiatric nurse should call on him, he seemed inconvenienced by her visit. The nurse recognized these cues and suggested that she might call again but Simon muttered something about 'that won't be convenient...you'd better stay now...'. Simon led the nurse into his sitting room. He indicated an armchair where she might sit and then seated himself at the dining table, so that the table formed a physical barrier between them. Although these initial arrangements appeared to be unsatisfactory, Susan recognized the client's need for increased physical distance.

Assessment of a client's territoriality begins during a first encounter by observing how he uses body language to establish and maintain boundaries (Murphy, 1981). Anxiety is increased when a person perceives invasion of his personal space. Therefore, Susan did not attempt to reduce this space by moving closer to the client. The first meeting with a client is important in setting the climate for subsequent meetings. Susan used social reinforcers as a means of establishing rapport, but Simon responded little to her opening remarks. His general attitude was one of cool indifference. Susan realized the importance of giving him time and space until he was ready to respond. He expressed doubts about her ability to help and made it clear that from past experiences he held a poor view of nurses.

Despite Simon's perceptions, Susan described her role in helping and supporting him as he gained self-understanding. She acknowledged his feelings towards nurses and suggested that they might explore these feelings. Rather abruptly, Simon refused to consider this suggestion and Susan was left to cope with her own feelings of disappointment and rejection.

The manner in which the patient is approached is important. According to Green (1986), controlling personal reactive defensiveness is probably the most effective intervention against hostility. If the nurse reacts to the patient's hostility in a defensive manner, it will only serve to set up a pattern that escalates towards more anger and deeper resentment.

It is the nurse who, by virtue of her helping role, needs to consider her responsibilities to the patient and overcome the interpersonal impasse which lies between them (Schoen, 1967). A relationship which carries the capacity to maintain an interpersonal impasse will interfere with the patient's movements towards health, and limit the nurse's effectiveness in helping the patient reach his goals. The energies of both parties will be involved in protecting the self against anxiety (Schoen, 1967).

Research has shown that hostile therapists encourage patient hostility and then in turn tend to avoid patients who direct hostility towards them (Bandura *et al.*, 1960). Hostility cannot be a component of a trusting relationship, and the nurse had to develop approaches consistent with those approaches which assist in the development of trust; she had to continually demonstrate to the patient that she was a person who has a genuine interest in his welfare and who could be trusted.

Hostility is often one of the most difficult barriers for the nurse to overcome, and may be the result of a long and tangled sequence of experiences, of which only part is conscious and understood (Green, 1986). They hostile client engages in a self-defeating pattern of behaviour whereby he seeks help in a hostile manner, is rejected by the potential helpers and then feels justified in holding a negative view of the health care services (Stuart and Sundeen, 1983).

To develop a relationship with a patient who is less comfortable to be with, the nurse needs to begin with herself; she must acquire insight into her own feelings and ask herself why she feels as she does. If this search into the self does not take place the nurse will be blocked in her ability to understand the patient. She will be one of the professionals who will remain the same, she will grow older, but no more enlightened, awakened or accepting of human possibilities (Jourard, 1971).

Self-awareness is a gradual and continuous process of noticing and exploring aspects of the self; psychological, physical and behavioural aspects of the self are explored with the intention of developing personal and interpersonal understanding (Burnard, 1985).

Susan had to accept herself as a person with human frailties. She had to have realistic expectations of herself before she could have realistic expectations of others. Schoen (1967) suggests that nurses, like all human beings, have needs for recognition, acceptance and success in interpersonal relations. Instead of fulfilling these needs the hostile patient's behaviour nourishes feelings of doubt and insecurity. The professional nurse is offering a direct and specialized experience from which hopefully the patient will learn something of lasting personal value with regard to health (Peplau, 1960). The kind of person the nurse is will make a considerable difference to what the patient will learn (Peplau, 1952). The creation of a therapeutic environment in a patient's home doesn't just happen. It requires patience and tolerance, and a continuous interest and commitment on the part of the nurse before a patient will share his true feelings (Ruditis, 1979). Furthermore, the patient must know that what he reveals will be treated confidentially; otherwise he may be reticent about sharing private concerns. Susan indicated that she would want to discuss any important matters appertaining to Simon's health with his GP at this stage. Clarifying the nature and dimensions of confidentiality would hopefully prevent any misunderstanding later on.

Orientating the patient to what is involved in his problem is a complex task. Basically, the patient's needs are of a humane kind and can only be dealt with in a humane and understanding way (Yuen, 1986).

The chief complaint or presenting problem does not of course tell the whole story (Russell, 1983). When a nurse sets out to help a client change behaviour which interferes with growth and healthy living, it is the problematic pattern or patterns that should become the focus of change. In therapeutic work it may only be possible to focus on a sample of the client's problematic behaviours. This may be sufficient; if the client becomes aware of the patterns, as a basis for change, he may gain a method of further self-study (Peplau, 1987a).

The establishment of trust is basic to the nurse–patient relationship. If the patient is to feel able to take risks later on by revealing things which are important to him, then he must feel he is confiding in a person who is honest, genuine and trustworthy. Furthermore he must perceive the nurse as being credible and able to assimilate the knowledge gained in such a way as to be beneficial to the relationship. Trust has to be earned; to gain the patient's trust the nurse must show that she is worthy of that trust. Trust is not given freely by virtue of a person's professional position (Ruditis, 1979).

When a relationship has not reached a stage of mutual trust, more may be gained in the long term if the patient's state of readiness is respected (Collins, 1983). Pushing a patient into revealing what he is not ready to discuss can be harmful and result in an intensification of the anxiety that caused the problem in the first place (Kiening, 1978).

Susan had envisaged that the orientation period would be prolonged to enable her to gain Simon's trust.

Identification phase

Susan continued to visit Simon on a weekly basis. He seemed to feel a need to test her out: once by forgetting their appointment and on another occasion by belittling the value of her visits. Until such time that Simon felt safe in the relationship, Susan anticipated this might happen. Stuart and Sundeen (1983) suggest the need for testing behaviour declines as trust builds up.

Simon's behaviour towards the nurse fluctuated between a display of extreme politeness and courteousness and deliberate rudeness. Often a patient feels compelled to engage in certain behaviour without understanding why he is doing so; it may be his way of dealing with a lack of security or an attempt to gain mastery over himself and his environment. Mainly, the behaviour serves to relieve his anxiety. The more capable the nurse is of 'understanding and interpreting the meaning of the patient's behaviour the more likely she will be able to establish meaningful limits (Lyon, 1970).

Simon was informed that his rudeness was unacceptable and unnecessary; it made working with him difficult. Limit setting is an aspect of the nurse–patient relationship that helps a patient to reduce his anxiety, enabling him to establish himself at a more acceptable level. The need for limits is closely related to feelings of security and trust (Lyon, 1970).

Susan was aware that Simon's hostile behaviour was not necessarily directed at her personally. This made it easier for her to understand her client's position. The nurse is cast into surrogate roles more frequently than is perhaps realized. Surrogate roles are determined by psychological age factors that operate by reason of arrests in development, feelings that have been aroused by illness or demands made by individuals in a situation. Outside his awareness the patient views the nurse as someone else. Instead of relating to the nurse as he finds her he relates to her in terms of the older relationship. When past experiences have included intense hostility the patient is likely to re-activate such feelings and express them towards the nurse (Peplau, 1952). The degree to which the nurse is aware of her own hostile impulses and the behaviour patterns she has adopted to cope with them is a crucial factor in determining how effective nursing interventions will be when dealing with a patient's hostile behaviour. (Kiening, 1978).

Simon responded to the limit setting, although he required prompting and reminding from time to time that he had agreed to refrain from behaviour which interfered with the task in hand.

While Susan was assessing Simon she was also aware that he was assessing her. Susan continually monitored her own body language although she was careful not to over-use counselling techniques. Burnard (1987) emphasizes the importance of the nurse appearing spontaneous and natural. If too many techniques are used the counsellor may be perceived by the client as artificial, cold and even uncaring. Simon was still not ready to recognize or admit that he had problems. Susan's professional knowledge enabled her to observe and recognize her client's problematic patterns of behaviour and establish goals. Peplau (1987b) suggests that there is a tendency to try and correct separate acts of behaviour, instead of focusing on behavioural acts which manifest themselves in a pattern. These patterns focused mainly around his inability to trust and confide in others, and the hostility that acted as a relief-behaviour for his anxiety, and prevented others from knowing him. Simon didn't seem to be depressed and said he was his usual self. Susan discussed her observations and objectives with Dr Kumar. He was pleased to hear that she was still visiting Simon despite the difficulties she had encountered. When Simon returned to work Susan visited him in the evenings on a fortnightly basis. Susan also discussed Simon with her senior nurse manager. In giving support she needed to feel supported herself. She found that it helped her to keep things in perspective by confronting the realities of nursing practice. Additionally, it enabled her to consider different approaches and acquire new skills to enhance her own personal and professional development.

Exploitation phase

During the phase of exploitation, interpersonal processes were fully utilized to enable the nurse and patient to move forward towards defined goals.

When Simon began to verbalize his thoughts and concerns this demonstrated that he was beginning to experience feelings of trust towards Susan. He was encouraged to explore feelings and behaviour in an atmosphere in which she refrained from imposing her own value-judgements.

Throughout the relationship Susan remained sensitive to the cues Simon gave in terms of his readiness to move into a more mature relationship. Awareness of the current stage helps the nurse to avoid rushing into the next stage before tasks have been completed (Forchuk and Brown, 1987).

In the nurse–patient relationship social chit-chat is replaced by the responsible use of words. Words and sentences require organization of thought processes to enable the patient to focus his attention around a particular problem. Peplau (1960) suggests that there is a difference between a layman talking to a patient and a nurse talking to a patient. It is the nurse's responsible use of words which distinguishes her conversation from a layman's approach to the patient. Burnard (1987) identifies five aspects of a therapeutic conversation: an emphasis on the here and now; being non-prescriptive; ensuring the helpee remains the central feature of the conversation; and a focus on feelings and empathic understanding. The ability to empathize is a fundamental element of the helping relationship. It allows the nurse to view the patient from his own perspective. Burnard (1985) suggests that empathy is the basis for truly understanding another person. It involves the ability to fully focus one's senses on the other person and to resist the temptation to put a hasty interpretation upon what the other person says or does.

Empathic linkages are a major non-verbal communication category and focus on the ability to feel in oneself the feelings being experienced by another person (Peplau, 1986). Developing a relationship with Simon continued to be a slow process. Periodically he still expressed hostility towards her by using prolonged eye contact. Knapp (1980) suggests that a gaze lasting longer than ten seconds is likely to induce irritation or discomfort into a situation. Simon would also use prolonged silences or engage in conversation that avoided disclosing things about himself. Nelson-Jones (1983) refers to this as talking but remaining psychologically silent and suggests that these are ways of the client showing his hostility. Susan recognized her own discomfort in the situation, but she also recognized Simon's behaviour as a significant and powerful means of communication. She sensed that he was using silence as a means of expressing his anger and avoiding interaction.

Recognition that Simon seemed troubled was used to convey Susan's concern and willingness to help. Resentful silence had to be dealt with gently and directly, otherwise any meaningful nursing intervention could not take place. The ways in which a person acts out hostility may differ according to the circumstances in which he finds himself and the degree of stress which he is undergoing (Kiening, 1978). It is difficult for a nurse to accept a patient when hostility is constantly expressed, seemingly to sever the relationship. Nevertheless, however difficult the patient's behaviour is, it is still possible to convey respect without rejecting the whole person. Meaningful communication is a creative process, infusing knowledge, skill and feeling (Kingston, 1987).

In order to be helpful to the patient it is necessary to develop an understanding of how he perceives himself and the situation confronting him. Although the nurse may offer to assist the patient through the process of a helping relationship, not every patient can easily identify with those helping persons who offer to accept him. Often earlier interpersonal relationships have been so traumatic that it seems inconceivable to the patient that others can accept him as he is (Peplau, 1952). Gradually Simon began to be more open about his felt needs, which indicated to Susan that he was beginning to trust her. After a number of visits Simon began to accept and value the nurse's presence. Her presence indicated to him that he was perceived as a valued person. Gardener (1985) suggests that the nurse's presence is manifested in three dimensions: in the cognitive domain through verbal communication of empathy and understanding of a patient's experience; in the affective domain through the generation of positive regard, genuineness and trust; and in the behaviour domain by being physically available as a helper.

In her role as counsellor Susan helped Simon to understand what was happening to him so that his experiences could be integrated rather than dissociated from experiences in life. The process involved explaining experiences only dimly intelligible to Simon so that these experiences could be better understood by both of them. Peplau (1987a) suggests that it is very often the nurse who is able to use her professional knowledge to indicate new possibilities and steps for the actualization of these possibilities. Susan observed that Simon's concerns focused around experiences associated with his family and he referred to his experiences of hospitalization more than once. Gradually, the nurse was able to build up a clearer picture of how the patient perceived these experiences and the importance they held for him. Peplau (1960) emphasizes the importance of listening for themes, for variations and nuances of meaning that are conveyed indirectly.

Listening can be helpful when it enables a person to bring his feelings out into the open. It has been ranked as one of the most caring nursing interventions (Wolf, 1986; Burnard, 1987). If the nurse wishes to focus on the needs of the patient, then she must know how to listen and how to respond in ways which will further the patient's learning (Peplau, 1960). She cannot listen accurately if she is constantly judging or categorizing what she has heard. Burnard (1987) emphasizes the importance of learning to set aside one's own beliefs and values and to suspend judgement. A component of listening is to summarize the patient's dialogue; to mirror his thoughts back to him so that he can see himself, his attitudes and opinions, in a clearer light (Helms, 1985). Peplau (1986) suggests that messages conveyed by the body gesture of one person are inferred by the other often with amazing accuracy.

When the nurse observes inconsistences in the patient's verbal and non-verbal behaviours it can be useful to confront him. Confrontation attempts to focus his awareness on actions that are incongruent with his self-image and behaviour. However, when developing a relationship with a patient who is experiencing trust problems the nurse must bear in mind that trust is fragile and can easily be broken. The nurse–patient relationship is of prime importance, and it would be futile to risk destroying a relationship which has taken a great deal of time, effort and personal investment (Meize-Grochowski, 1984).

A judgement must be made regarding the patient's stage of readiness to respond to the sensitive use of confrontation. As a high-level communication skill, confrontation can be very effective in allowing the patient to explore feelings and behaviours of which he was previously unaware.

Simon was now expressing many feelings he had not expressed before, especially the ambivalent feelings he had towards his mother. He felt angry with his mother; even as a child he resented her remarrying and replacing his father. Now he felt guilty about possessing such thoughts, especially as his mother died several years ago. It wasn't something he had been able to talk about before. Bad feelings about a parent are not always easily verbalized. The nurse–patient relationship allowed him to explore feelings that a person's culture does not ordinarily approve of (Peplau, 1952). Nurses are frequently called upon to deal with the emotional problems of others. There is a positive correlation between the way in which a nurse handles her own emotion and the way in which she handles the emotions of others (Burnard, 1985). Nurses who pay attention to what they are feeling during a relationship with a client often gain invaluable empathized observations of feelings a patient is experiencing and has not yet noticed or talked about (Peplau, 1986).

Barber (1986) suggests that true care transcends instrumental activity and mere role performance. It requires the nurse to share aspects of her own humanity while staying alert and sensitive to the person before her.

The nurse may find it necessary to balance the roles she undertakes in order to have sufficient resources to meet the patient's needs (Hessler, 1980). She will need to perceive the role or roles in which she is cast by the client. The nurse may not necessarily make all her roles apparent to the client. Persistent hostility may act as a precipitation of physical health problems. The nurse may not necessarily make her role as a health educator explicit to the client, yet by helping him to verbalize his feelings of anger, and utilize energy productively, this may serve to promote his physical as well as his mental well-being. Suppressed anger may lead to psychosomatic illness and other self-destructive processes.

Through self-disclosure and within the context of the relationship the nurse revealed her own experiences and feelings. This provided Simon with a model or with evidence that his experiences were not outside the understanding of others. When self-disclosure is used thoughtfully, it can help the patient to view the nurse as a person who understands his problems and concerns. Self-disclosure is instrumental in reflecting the degree of trust and sense of security that a patient feels in a relationship (Collins, 1983).

Resolution phase

The stage of resolution implies a gradual freeing from identification with the helping person – Simon had been informed about the purpose of the nurse–patient relationship during initial meetings (he had devalued the relationship then). He understood that the relationship would end when he no longer needed the assistance of the nurse. If the terms and boundaries of the relationship are not made explicit to the patient, both nurse and patient may experience termination problems. The patient may try to prolong the relationship or the nurse may keep the patient on her books longer than necessary in order to fulfil her own needs and wishes. When the nurse and patient have developed a trusting relationship in which they have been able to share feelings, they may also benefit from sharing feelings about termination (Stankiewicz Sene, 1969).

Conclusion

For Susan, self-awareness was an ongoing phenomenon. In evaluating the personal growth which had occurred for both herself and her client, the benefits were mutual. She had met the client's needs for self-esteem, recognition and respect by accepting him as a person. Not only had working with Simon provided a challenge but the nurse's therapeutic skills had been tested fully. Over a period of 12 months the relationship between nurse and client had progressed along a continuum – from meeting as strangers to participants in a helping relationship. The phases of Peplau's development model had enabled the nurse to evaluate the progress being made as the relationship moved along the continuum. The flexible framework had enabled Susan to focus on her relationship with Simon, and on her own purposeful interventions.

Peplau (1965) suggests that there is no fixed formula for interpersonal relations. Interactions are dependent on the nurse's ability to recognize changes in the self and others. Peplau (1952) emphasizes the importance of the nurse and patient meeting as strangers. Susan had tried not to let any preconceived ideas influence her approach to the patient although it had not been easy to dismiss the evaluations of the patient which she had received from colleagues. Value-judgements are not conducive to a non-defensive atmosphere for communication where open two-way communication is possible.

Initially, the patient's hostility had been the most difficult barrier to overcome. Realizing that his hostility was not directed at her personally, but only towards the surrogate roles which he cast her into, made it easier to understand that the client's behaviour was a consequence of earlier unsatisfactory experiences.

Marson (1979) suggests that each person learns to be the kind of human being he becomes through interacting with fellow human beings who are his principal source of motivation, punishment and rewards. The quantity and quality of those relationships have the greatest influence on each person's unique personality development.

The hostility was sometimes direct but usually passive, and displayed in subtle ways, hidden behind a pleasant and helpful exterior. This type of hostility can be difficult to deal with. Simon had gained an understanding of his behaviour through the counselling process in which the nurse had been able to mirror back images of her client, so that he was able to perceive himself more realistically and learn how others see him. Simon admitted that Susan had given him food for thought. The outcome of this process was only partly satisfactory. Peplau (1987a) suggests that the nurse is not in a position to solve all the patient's singular problems. She can only identify the patterns of behaviour, and that they are manifested in a pattern theme by the client; and through sustained nursing intervention she may help the client to change these patterns.

All this time the most important nursing intervention was to accept the patient, but not his behaviour. Simon's deliberate rudeness and sarcasm were prohibitive to the development of a relationship and tested the nurse's endurance to the full. When building a relationship with a client the nurse may be afraid to impose limits on his behaviour in case this should spoil the relationship. However, there are times when the nurse must show the client that although she is willing to help in her professional capacity, she is also a person with feelings. She is not self-sacrificing; like the client she is also entitled to dignity and respect and cannot allow behaviour that is likely to be detrimental to the relationship.

It is possible that Simon projected his feelings of hostility towards others because he had never been able to own or talk about the feelings underlying his behaviour. Duldt (1981) describes two modes of anger: the maintenance mode and the destructive mode. In the maintenance mode the person describes his feelings of anger in relation to the here and now. He specifically identifies the need, threat or obstruction and theoretically the interpersonal climate could be supportive. In the destructive mode, the person avoids describing the source of his feelings; he denies responsibility for the anger by projecting the blame on others, generalizing or blaming past situations. As the stimulus for the anger is not identified, those nearest the angry person are unable to respond helpfully. Simon's relationship with the nurse had provided him with an opportunity to talk about thoughts and feelings he could not ordinarily share with others. Lego (1980) suggests that through the counselling process the nurse can help the patient to examine his current interpersonal experiences in order to improve them through the development of interpersonal competencies that had been lost or never learned.

Susan realized the importance of low-visibility nursing functions – (Brown and Fowler, 1971) – in helping Simon. Being there, being consistent, sincere and genuinely interested in him, and showing warmth in the face of hostility, had enabled Simon to experience personal growth. Through the process of accepting and providing support for the client, Susan had enabled him to recognize and utilize the more positive aspects of his personality, Many of Simon's feelings of anger and resentment related to events which had happened during his formative years. By talking about these feelings he was able to explore the underlying reasons for his anger. Painfully he recognized the effects of his behaviour on himself and others and he learned that the past cannot be changed. There had been changes for both nurse and patient during the course of their relationship. Krikorian and Paulanka (1982) hypothesize that two simultaneous critical processes occur in the dynamic helping relationship. As the person is

developing, the relationship is developing. As the relationship is developing, the person is developing. They suggest that the catalytic agent is the
self-awareness of the nurse. Vallot (1966) affirms that the committed nurse
gives self to others and through this giving grows personally. Throughout
the period in which Susan Smith had visited Simon, she had been able to
discuss his progress and some of the difficulties she encountered with her
peer group. Marriner (1983) suggests that this is important particularly for
nurses who work in isolation, otherwise they may develop habitual approaches to patient care which are not always the most effective way to
meet goals.

When Susan had originally accepted Simon as a client, she was made
aware of her colleagues' attitudes towards him. Indeed, Susan was no
different to her colleagues in as much as there were some patients she
liked more than others. Accepting Simon had made Susan think about the
matter a lot more. Since she did her basic training she had undertaken
further nursing studies. She was aware of the importance of reading nursing literature and using research findings. She knew that much of the
literature about problem patients pointed to a need for change in the
attitudes of the staff.

Stockwell's (1972) research highlighted the different behaviours that
nurses demonstrated towards popular and unpopular patients. Popular
patients were given more time, allowed a more personalized interaction,
allowed lapses in keeping the rules and called nurses by their Christian
names. Unpopular patients were ignored, their requests forgotten, gifts
and favours were refused, rules enforced and sarcasm used. When a patient is perceived as a problem, the term is frequently used to imply that it
is the patient who must change his behaviour, and yet the problem may re-
side in the nurse. May and Kelly (1982) suggest that therapeutic aspirations
are a central feature of the psychiatric nurse's image; problem patients may
be those who in one way or another deny the nurse's claims to therapeutic
competence. They suggest that nursing categorization of patients is constructed in a process of interaction in which the critical element is the
patient's willingness to legitimate the authority and competence of the
nurse.

Problem patients are therefore those who call to attention the fragility of
nursing authority by rejecting implicitly or explicitly the services that
psychiatric nurses provide. The readiness of psychiatric nurses to put
themselves at the disposal of patients is conditional on the patients being
perceived as in need of nursing care; the patient then legitimizes the
nurse's therapeutic aspirations. While nurses may be influenced by formal
medical diagnoses they are not dependent on them.

Furthermore, May and Kelly (1982) point out that much of the literature
written by or for nurses sounds of a high moral and prescriptive tone.
Where the existence of problem patients is acknowledged it is taken in the

final analysis as a manifestation of unfortunate and unprofessional attitudes on the part of the nursing staff, to be rooted out essentially by means of educational measures. These writers go on to say that few seem to consider the possibility that the reason why some patients are labelled as problems is precisely because they make life difficult for the nurses and undermine their claims to professional status.

Davis (1984) suggests that nurses' perceptions of patients and the labels provided by others, particularly senior health professionals, influence their behaviour towards them. He argues that although over the past few years trends have been directed towards planned individualized care, there is still much evidence to indicate that then, as well as now, nurses tend to deal with types of people, types of behaviour, and types of disease, rather than individuals.

Using research findings regarding unpopular patients may at first seem difficult for nurses, but as Doona (1979) suggests, it is difficult to accept that not all nurses are paragons of nursing excellence. Nurses and patients are moulded by their individual life experiences and both attempt to cope with problems in ways they find least threatening. All too often nurses allow themselves to develop myths and fantasies around the image of nursing practice, because in reality the truth is too painful (Pyne, 1983).

When a patient complains about something, the nurse must remember that whatever the cause of the complaint, he is only complaining because he knows some nursing situations can be improved or corrected. He is able to recognize factors which constitute poor care. He may be labelled as a problem patient merely because he has become an advocate – an advocate of quality nurse care for himself (Nicksic, 1981).

Simon Manners didn't conform to the descriptions of patients found in textbooks, which may in the past have caused management problems for nurses and contributed to the labelling process. Because he felt himself to be unpopular with nurses this had probably contributed towards his dysfunctional patterns of behaviour. Because Simon had been labelled as a difficult patient, nurses probably spent less time with him, and consequently the therapeutic impasse continued. A one-to-one relationship had enabled Susan to overcome this therapeutic impasse; she had got to know Simon as a person as well as a client. Susan liked Simon, she found he had some very admirable qualities. She hoped these qualities might become more apparent to others now. She knew that it is possible for nurses to change their opinions towards patients they disliked. In a study described by Roberts (1984) where nurses had changed their opinions about patients they disliked, the reason most frequently given was finding time to talk to the patient.

Earlier on, Simon had indicated that he was aware of his difficulties with nursing staff. It had caused him some concern. Skipper, Tagliacozzo and Mauksch (1964) found that patients expressed anxiety when they were rejected by hospital staff for not conforming to the role of the good patient. Simon had mentioned his experiences, and dislike of being an in-patient or day-patient. He said this was one of the reasons why he had agreed to see a community nurse. Susan had been able to empathize with him. Last year she had been in hospital for an operation. As Green (1986) suggests, it is not possible to emphathize without a background of similar experiences. 'Admission procedures and rituals assault the identity, treatments prod, hurt and invade and questions probe. The patient's role is typically one of vulnerability and powerlessness. If he doesn't take all this without complaint he is labelled.'

Towards the end of the termination process, Susan learned that Simon's friendship with a widow, fifteen years older than himself, had ended when she committed suicide. Simon had never talked about this before, and when Susan indicated that she was willing to listen, Simon declined to say any more because he found the subject too painful.

During a later visit he told Susan that Marianne had died from cancer. She never told him she had cancer and he only learned of this after her suicide. He was still shocked and hurt by her death and experienced feelings of intense guilt. She had not confided in Simon about her intentions to end life. The suicide note had been written to her mother.

Susan asked Simon if he would be prepared to see a counsellor – a person who specialized in bereavement counselling. After thinking it over for some time Simon agreed to this.

Susan was pleased that she had been able to act as a resource person enabling Simon to receive the expert help that he obviously needed. Furthermore she was pleased that he was willing to accept the help of another person. Through the nurse–patient relationship Susan had been able to facilitate experiences for Simon which led to the development of trust, and the reduction of anxiety.

One of the dangers in labelling recipients of health care as problem patients is that they may be denied or refuse to accept the health care services available to them. Of one thing Susan was certain: the labelling of a client as a problem does nothing to enhance the practice of nursing; it merely categorizes and negates the client and denies the nurse the privilege of knowing him.

References

Armitage, S. (1980) Non-compliant recipients of health care, occasional paper. *Nurs. Times*, **76**, 1–4.

Bandura *et al.* (1960) Cited by Duldt (see Duldt (1981)).

Barber, P. (1986) The psychiatric nurse's failure therapeutically to nurture. *Nurs. Pract.*, **1**, 138–41.

Brown, M. M. and Fowler, G. R. (1971) *Psychodynamic Nursing*, W. B. Saunders, Philadelphia.

Burnard, P. (1985) *Learning Human Skills*, Heinemann Medical Books, Oxford.
Burnard, P. (1987) Counselling: basic principles in nursing. *Prof. Nurse*, **6**, 278–80.
Collins, M. (1983) *Communication in Health Care*, Mosby, St Louis, MO.
Curtin, L. L. (1981) Privacy: belonging to oneself. *Persp. Psy. Care*, **XLX**, 112–5.
Davis, B. (1984) What is the nurse's perception of the patient? in *Understanding Nurses* (ed. S. Skevington), John Wiley, New York.
Doona, M. E. (1979) *Travelbee's Intervention in Psychiatric Nursing*, 2nd edn, F. A. Davis, Philadelphia.
Duldt, B. W. (1981) Anger: an occupational hazard for nurses. *Nurs. Outlook*, **29**, 510–8.
Forchuk, C. and Brown, B. (1987) Establishing a Nurse–Patient Relationship. Instrument Development (pamphlet), The Regional Municipality of Hamilton, Wentworth, Dept. of Health Services, PO Box 897, Hamilton, Ontario L8N 3P6.
Gallop, R. (1988) Escaping borderline stereotypes. *J. Psychosoc. Nurs. Ment. Health Serv.*, **26**, 16–20.
Gardener, D. L. (1985) Presence, in *Nursing Interventions* (eds. G. M. Bulechek and J. McCloskey), W. B. Saunders, New York.
Green, C. P. (1986) How to recognise hostility and what to do about it. *Am. J. Nurs.*, **86**, 1230–4.
Hamilton, D. (1979) Escaping borderline stereotypes. *J. Psychosoc. Nurs. Ment. Health Serv.*, **26**, 16–20 (Cited in Gallop, R. (1988).)
Helms, J. (1985) Active listening in *Nursing Intervention Treatment for Nursing Diagnosis* (eds G. M. Bulechek and J. C. McCloskey), W. B. Saunders, New York.
Hessler, I. (1980) Roles, status and relationships in psychiatric nursing. *Nurs. Times*, **76**, 508–9.
Jourard, S. M. (1971) *The Transparent Self*, van Nostrand Reinhold, New York.
Kiening, M. M. (1978) Hostility, in *Behavioural Concepts and Nursing Intervention* (eds C. E. Carlson and B. Blackwell), Lippincott, Philadelphia.
Kingston, B. (1987) *Psychological Approaches in Psychiatric Nursing*, Croom Helm, Beckenham, UK.
Knapp, M. L. (1980) *Essentials of Non-verbal Communication*, Holt, Rinehart and Winston, New York.
Krikorian, D. A. and Paulanka, B. (1982) Self-awareness – the key to a successful nurse–patient relationship. *J. Psych. Nurs. Ment. Health Serv.*, **20**, 19–21.
Lego, S. (1980) The one-to-one nurse–patient relationship. *Perspec. Psych. Care*, **18**, 67–89.
Lyon, G. G. (1970) Limit setting as a therapeutic tool. *J. Psych. Nurs. Ment. Health Nurs.*, **8**, 17–24.
Marriner, A. (1983) *The Nursing Process*, Mosby, St Louis, MO.
Marson, S. N. (1979) Nursing, a helping relationship? *Nurs. Times*, **75**, 541–4.
May, D. and Kelly, M. P. (1982) Chancers, pests and poor wee souls: problems of legitimation in psychiatric nursing. *Sociol. Health Illness*, **4**, 279–301.
Meize-Grochowski, R. (1984) An analysis of the concept of trust. *J. Adv. Nurs.*, **9**, 563–72.
Murphy, K. E. (1981) Use of territoriality in psychotherapy. *J. Psych. Nurs. Ment. Health Serv.*, **19**, 13–16.
Nelson-Jones, R. (1983) *Practical Counselling Skills*, Holt, Rinehart and Winston, Eastbourne, UK.
Nicksic, E. (1981) Problem patients or problem nurses? *Nurs. Outlook*, **29**, 317–9.
Peplau, H. E. (1952) *Interpersonal Relations in Nursing*, G. P. Putnam's Sons, New York.
Peplau, H. E. (1960) Talking with patients. *Am. J. Nur.*, **60**, 964–6.

Peplau, H. E. (1965) The heart of nursing: interpersonal relations. *Can. Nurse*, **61**, 273–5.

Peplau, H. E. (1986) Psychiatric nursing skills: today and tomorrow. A paper presented at the Third International Congress of Psychiatric Nursing, Imperial College, London.

Peplau, H. E. (1987a) Interpersonal constructs for nursing practice. *Nurs. Ed. Today*, **7**, 201–8.

Peplau, H. E. (1987b) Personal communication.

Pyne, R. (1983) Seeing reality through the myth. *Nurs. Mirror*, **157**, 35–6.

Roberts, D. (1984) Non-verbal communication, popular and unpopular patients, in *Communication – Recent Advances in Nursing Times* (ed. A. Faulkner), Churchill Livingstone, Edinburgh.

Ruditis, S. E. (1979) Developing trust in nursing interpersonal relationships. *J. Psych. Nurs. Ment. Health Serv.*, **17**, 20–23.

Russell, B. V. (1983) Is the chief complaint really the problem? *J. Psychosoc. Nurs.*, **21**, 24–8.

Schoen, E. A. (1967) Clinical problem: the demanding, complaining patient. *Nurs. Clin. N. Am.*, **2**, 715–24.

Skipper, J., Tagliacozzo, D. and Mauksch, H. (1964) What communication means to patients. *Am. J. Nurs.*, **64**, 101–3.

Stankiewicz Sene, B. (1969) Termination in the student–patient relationship. *Persp. Psych. Care*, **7**, 39–45.

Stockwell, F. (1972) The Unpopular Patient. Royal College of Nursing research project.

Stuart, G. W. and Sundeen, S. J. (1983) *Principles and Practice of Psychiatric Nursing*, Mosby, St Louis, MO.

Vallot, S. M. C. (1966) Existentialism: a philosophy of commitment. *Am. J. Nurs.*, **66**, 500–5.

Wolf, Z. R. (1986) The caring concept and nurse identified caring behaviours. *Top. Clin. Nurs.*, **8**, 84–93.

Yuen, F. K. H. (1986) The nurse–client relationship: a mutual learning experience. *J. Adv. Nurs.*, **11**, 529–33.

Chapter 14

General systems model: clinical applications[*]

S. A. SMOYAK

Overview

Ethnocentrism prevails for most of us – in our private and professional lives – unless we deliberately set out to discover and to understand how other folks live. The sights and sounds and smells of childhood produce a comfort and familiarity that follows us into adulthood. What feels right is what we knew – and continue to know – within our own families. 'Different', unfortunately, often carries the connotation of 'wrong'. Clinicians, in order to not assess others only within the measure of their own familiarity, need to engage in an ongoing pursuit for knowledge about the vast array of patterns and processes which guide the lives of family systems other than their own.

Because ethnocentrism affects all of us, that is what clinicians encounter in their first meeting with any family – normal or not, very disturbed or mildly troubled, seeking help because they think they need it or because they have been sent by courts, physicians or clergy. Any family feels that how it lives must be basically all right, because that is the sum total of the experience they've lived; this holds true even when there is incest, violence or serious mental illness within the family. Clinicians would do well to keep this basic fact in mind, and to realize that change, even when sought and valued, is accomplished only with great difficulty for most people. Further, clinicians should guard against making value judgements about families, and tending to assess them as abnormal, simply because their rules of organization differ from those of the majority, or from those of the clinician's own family.

*The author wishes to acknowledge the assistance of three Master's-prepared clinicians, in the writing of this chapter. Nora Albert contributed literature review data and clinical vignettes for the violence examples; Barbara Norman worked on the Scandinavian-American family section (work on normalizing) and Carolyn Whinery reviewed material on adolescent caretakers, and provided clinical data. Their own manuscripts are listed in the References.

As Froma Walsh (1987) has suggested, 'It has been said that the definition of a normal family is one that has not yet been clinically assessed.' The danger of overclassifying families as pathological stems from clinicians' ethnocentric tendencies and the fact that medical tradition, focused on psychopathology, is skewed toward seeing disorder, conflicts and deficits, rather than positive aspects and strengths. Clinicians primarily see troubled families, and are tempted to conclude that the trouble or disorder stems from, or is rooted in, particular family structures or patterns rather than biological factors or extrafamilial stressors. Not enough attention has been given to discovering the normal variants of family structures and patterns, where no pathology is present.

Walsh (1987) reports on a survey of family therapists who were asked about how they judged healthy family functioning. The methods varied widely, but the positive attributes correlated very highly with the attributes most valued by the therapists. For instance, psychodynamically-oriented therapists tended to value qualities such as empathic listening, trust and support, while structural family therapists rated parental leadership and strong generational boundaries as most important. Therapists tended to rate as normal those interactional styles that were either similar to or opposite from their own family experience. The latter may seem, at first, contradictory to expectations, until one considers the fact that therapists may see their own families as dysfunctional, and see an opposite case as the norm.

In this chapter, all of the families described are actual families, encountered either by me, in my private practice, or by my graduate students, placed in a variety of clinical agencies. The one exception is the family of the Greek Prime Minister. The clinical families are captured accurately in terms of their genograms, rules of organization, and maladaptations (violations of system rules), but their names (not their ethnicities or their religions) have been changed to assure anonymity.

Work as a normalizing dynamic

Families often view work as a normalizing dynamic. So long as a person works, their faults, shortcomings, or illnesses are handled and/or tolerated with less disruption than when the person does not, or cannot, go to work. Whether a mental illness prevents work, or whether not going to work precipitates a mental illness is a chicken and egg matter over which many families agonize. 'Is he lazy or is he sick?' is a question frequently asked of clinicians. For many families, struggling to live with a mentally ill family member in a home setting, the fact that the person does not work is frequently more distressing than their symptoms, even such bizarre ones as talking to voices, or strange gesturing and rituals.

Work is one of the crucial roles performed by people in any society.

Although the structure and nature of work vary immensely within and between societies over time, production through work remains central (Voydanhoff, 1984). Not only does work serve as a basic function of economic production, but in many societies, success and achievement in the occupational sphere are intertwined with indices of personal worth. Further, work often has religious and moral value.

Max Weber, creator of the concept of the Protestant work ethic, sees work as encompassing an entire philosophy of life, related to religious and economic values (Cherrington, 1980). The work ethic is comprised of beliefs that: (1) people have a moral and religious obligation to fill their lives with heavy, physical toil, (2) men and women are expected to spend long hours at work with limited time for leisure, (3) workers should be highly productive, and (4) workers should take pride in their work.

The Protestant work ethic and the Scandinavian–American family advocate similar values. The Johnsons (see Appendix A) are a two-generation, Norwegian/Swedish Methodist family. Dick and Doris, both 57 years old, share their household with Tim, a 28-year-old first-born son, diagnosed as having schizoaffective disorder five years ago. The younger sister, Sally, is married and has two small children. The Johnsons sought help from a Community Mental Health Center (CMHC) because of difficulty in handling Tim's behaviour at home.

Tim graduated from college, with a bachelor's degree, in 1983. After graduation he moved about 700 miles, taking a job in a research institute. Within six months, he had his first psychotic episode, which was associated with alcohol abuse. Tim has been hospitalized for short periods and referred to partial care. His attendance at the partial care programme is intermittent. Every few months he manages to find a job, works briefly, and then is fired or quits. At the present time he seems to be compliant with taking the antipsychotic medication, and attends Alcoholics Anonymous meetings twice weekly.

Tim's parents, Dick and Doris, are both employed; Dick as a construction worker and Doris as a secretary. They deny any problems at home, or within their marriage, and see Tim's illness caused entirely by his move away from home to Virginia. They believe that the move from an urban area to a rural one was not good for Tim, and verbalize this as the reason for his illness. Their voiced concerns are more about the fact that he cannot seem to hold a job than about this psychiatric symptoms. They focus on work as their chief concern, and seem unable to grasp the fact that their son has a chronic mental illness. They have shared, in family sessions, their belief that if a person works hard and goes to church, then one is doing everything that he or she can do. And, if one doesn't work, then one cannot lead a normal life.

The following is an excerpt from a tape-recorded dialogue during a family session:

Therapist Work seems important to you.
Father   It is. Tim with his problem holding a job... I've always felt
            that if a person stays away from work, they lose their desire to
            work... How's Tim going to make it in life if he doesn't work?
            You know, we're not going to be around forever.
Mother   I don't understand why this happened to Tim... He had a happy
            childhood. He was always a hard worker. He's been attending a
            programme here because they said they would find him a job
            (referring to the partial care programme).

For the Johnsons, work is a normalizing dynamic. Despite the fact that
Tim is delusional from time to time, they believe that he would be normal
if he would just get a job and stick with it. It is not quite accurate to view
the family as being in denial; rather, they seem unable to realize the implications of a mental illness diagnosis. So far, the therapist has not succeeded in getting them to consider an alternative explanation for his not
working. Tim's being at home again has drastically altered the life-style of
his parents; they are at a stale-mate in what some authors call the launch-
ing phase of their family development. With this family, since they insist
so strongly on focusing on Tim's employment, the degree to which other
family issues may or may not serve as stressors is unclear.

In another family, the Golds, American Jews, going to school (university/
college) is viewed in a similar, normalizing way, as going to work. Ruth, a
third-born, adopted girl, aged 11, has been diagnosed since early childhood as autistic, developmentally-delayed, schizoaffective, depressed and
with minimal brain damage. When the parents focus on the details of her
going to school, their affect and general demeanor are hopeful and positive. They resist efforts to turn the dialogue to considering future plans for
psychiatric care. She attends a school for emotionally-disturbed children,
which the parents see as necessary, but wish that the school were closer
to home. Including the long bus ride each day, she is away from home for
more than 12 hours.

The Folatys are a Ukrainian–American family (see Appendix B) also
struggling with the burden of trying to maintain a seriously mentally ill
member at home. Both parents are professionals; Steven is a physician,
and Anna is a music teacher. They had planned to retire within the next
five years, but now see that as impossible because of repeated hospitalizations of their son, John, in private settings where insurance no longer
covers the bill. Additional stressors in this family are the recent diagnosis
of Anna with cancer in her reproductive system and the impending divorce
of the older sister, Maria, who has temporarily moved home. The younger
sister, Rosa, also lives at home now because, she says, 'I'd feel guilty
ignoring this mess; I know I had better tune in and help out with all this
trouble.'

The Folatys value both work and education; work, in their family system, has to be of a professional nature. Maria is a graphic artist, with a dual degree in architectural design. Rosa is a musician, with a fine arts master's degree. The identified patient, John, diagnosed schizophrenic, earned a bachelor's degree, in political science, at a highly-respected university. Maria believes that her father's interference in the lives of his children is a considerable negative influence on all of them, but John particularly. Maria states, 'I guess I saw the trouble starting with John earlier than anybody. He began to be lazy – to space out, even without drugs – in his sophomore year. However, the trouble was that he was living at home and commuting, and my father would get on his case and keep at it until he turned in papers and did the work. My father earned that bachelor's degree, not my brother; the wrong name is on the diploma!'

By the time he had graduated, John was sleeping most of the day, avoiding family members, and listening to music in his room at night. He has not worked, other than at some temporary jobs which were below his status and embarrassing to the parents. When he occasionally gets violent, and pushes his mother about, the father takes steps to hospitalize him involuntarily, in private settings. The father, who is a general practitioner, is ambivalent about what his psychiatrist colleagues have told him. He says, 'I hear their words; I don't believe them. John needs reputable work. That would fix everything. I just don't know what went wrong. We are all hard-working, God-fearing, respectable people. I have no explanation for this. It doesn't make any sense.' Steven is able to state how schizophrenia is described in the Diagnostic Standard Manual, (DSM III-R), and acknowledges that John's symptoms match the descriptions, but then states, 'Show me the organism. Show me the damaged tissue. Show me something I can see with my own eyes, and I'll understand it.'

Anna, who has had surgery, and is undergoing continued treatment for her cancer, is very tearful whenever John is mentioned. Her view is that she failed as a mother because she didn't insist on his continuing to go to church when he started college. She says, 'I'm very worried about what God is going to do to me. Steven doesn't quite see it this way, but he's a scientist and I'm an artist. I know John's problem is that he forgot about God. Now he has nothing. If he got a job, maybe he'd return to church. I even asked our pastor to help. In the old days, they could get work for people, but times have changed.'

All three families, while they differ markedly in social class and ethnic/religious backgrounds, see work as normalizing, and are unable to see that mental illness prevents people from working. The belief that not working creates illness is embedded in belief systems. There has been some work in the field of psychology, attempting to understand how beliefs such as this, about health and illness, are formed, and how they can be modified (Leventhal, 1982).

In these families, the rule of organization placed work first as a normalizing, stabilizing focus. Maladaptation occurs when the ill member is unable to fulfil the expectations. Referring to the paradigm on exchanges in Chapter 6, what the parents and siblings want the identified patient to produce is not happening. Further, the patient wants to be left alone, and not be badgered about find.ng and keeping jobs. More stress occurs when family members differ in their opinions about how to manage the maladaptation. Continuing therapeutic dialogue is possible when the family is invited to see the issue as one of conflicting views and expectations, rather than as a right–wrong situation.

Families struggle with violence

In the wake of de-institutionalization, many families find themselves struggling to manage a seriously mentally ill individual at home. The family's coping strategies are challenged to the maximum when the mentally ill member is a young adult chronic person, who is very strong, very ill, and resists attempts at managing troublesome symptoms with psychopharmacological agents.

The process of public education has somewhat succeeded in changing people's minds about the mentally ill and their dangerousness. Yet, the fact of the matter is that untreated mental illness, especially in the community, is associated with increased episodes of violence. Lagos, Perlmutter and Saexinger (1977, p. 1136) conclude that: '...one need not fear the mentally ill *if* one learns to identify those whose condition leaves them vulnerable to outbursts, and *if* one learns how to handle that subgroup of vulnerable patients and *if* one can count on assistance in an emergency'. In relation to violence or threats of violence directed specifically at family members, Turkat and Buzzell (1983, p. 553) studied 49 individuals, average age 33, who had been hospitalized two or more times. They reported that 30% of all recidivist hospitalizations were a result of threats of violence against family members. They suggested that '... families need training in techniques for recognizing danger signals, diffusing patients' anger, protecting themselves from physical harm, and knowing when to seek shelter from neighbours and relatives'.

Families who care for their young, chronically mentally ill relatives at home feel ill-prepared to deal with the potential for violence. Creer and Wing (1974, p. 18) conducted two surveys of relatives who lived with or felt responsible for their schizophrenic family member in an effort to identify the problems encountered by this group. They interviewed 80 people and reported that 23% of them mentioned threats or violence occurring to a marked extent and that in some instances, '...the problem of violence could make life impossible in the household'. They also reported that relatives feared that the patients would harm themselves, as well as others. Although Creer and Wing made a point of mentioning that incidents of violence were uncommon, they also cautioned that the need for advice about managing disturbed behaviour in the home was a priority for the families

Other researchers, in Canada (Runions and Prudo, 1983) and in the United States, (Seymour and Dawson, 1986) have documented families' fears and reported distress with professionals failing to assist them in their home-care efforts. The term 'family burden' is commonly used in the literature. Themes of abandonment, helplessness and danger are recounted. With severe mental illness, not only is there maladaptation within the family system, but between the families and the professionals they consult for help. Too often the professionals fail to dispose what the families want to obtain, specifically, practical help with management of dangerous behaviours.

The Giovannis (see Appendix C) are an Italian–American family, with a mentally ill son living at home, where violent outbursts have become a frequent occurrence and a primary concern of the caregivers. The parents, John and Angie, are both retired, and are the caregivers for Eddie, their first-born son, who is 35 years old; Maria, the younger sister, recently divorced, also lives at home. Eddie's psychiatric history is fairly typical of the young, adult chronic population described in the literature. He began having overt behavioural problems in late adolescence, and was hospitalized numerous times at different public and private institutions. He has been diagnosed, over the years, as paranoid schizophrenia, anti-social personality, and recently, bipolar disorder with psychotic features. Eddie has always lived at home, and has never been able to maintain employment, other than for short periods. He frequently abuses drugs and alcohol and is non-compliant with his medications. Eddie refuses to attend family therapy sessions, but insists that his parents go. Excerpts from a family session capture the sense of the family's frustration:

Mother Eddie tells me how to manoeuvre. I want to be left alone to do what I want to do.

Father I feel threatened, intimidated by Eddie. I'm not the head of the household; he assumes the responsibility. I want to get to the source of our problems. I want to have the role of the father.

Sister Eddie is an alcoholic and a drug addict. I would like to make living normal and pleasant. Not like a nightmare. No more violence; there's been a lot of that. My parents can't handle him. When he acts up, they say, 'This is it!' and they take him back to the hospital.

The hospital stays, however, are short, and the family repeatedly have Eddie at home, with little change in his behaviour. Prior to one hospitalization, Eddie tried to choke his mother. Although his parents went to court, and a restraining order was served on Eddie, this was not enforced, and

Eddie returned home. He was furious at the court's intervention, and when his father asked him to leave the house he punched him in the eye, causing permanent loss of vision.

When Eddie is at home, the family has adapted to the fear of his outbursts by avoiding confrontations. Although Mr Giovanni is upset that his role as head of the household has been usurped by Eddie, he chooses most of the time to avoid head-on confrontations with him about power or authority. For instance, if Eddie is upset and demanding his mother's attention, even though it is dinner time, she pays attention to him and ignores her husband. Eddie stays in the kitchen with his mother, and Mr Giovanni eats alone, in the dining room. This is a particularly disturbing situation, since it is such a clear violation of the expected Gemeinschaft mode in an Italian household and it interrupts the solidarity of the marital dyad, leaving the possibility for continuing coalitions (of mother and son) across the generational boundary. Infants and children, because of their pressing physiological and psychosocial needs, have a built-in licence to engage in such interruptions. The expectation for older children, and certainly adult children, is that the marital dyad's needs are honoured.

At the moment that this chapter was being written, Eddie had again decompensated and was hospitalized involuntarily, after he threatened to ice (kill) his father. He was outraged at his family for their action, and voiced the belief that things that they had said about him in family therapy sessions had contributed to his involuntary status. The dilemma for families is how to take action for self-protection, while convincing the ill member that they are not doing so as an attack or an insult, but rather from fear.

The way in which families view the origin and the needed treatment of an illness may be in direct opposition to the way professional care-providers view the situation. Professionals often disagree about the most plausible explanation for behavioural events, as well as the most efficient course of action to bring the disturbance under control. For instance, some family theorists would view the organizational structure as creating the dilemma, while others would see the illness as creating anomalies in the family structure. In the United States, the National Alliance for the Mentally Ill, a voluntary group organized about a decade ago, challenges the four mental health professions (psychiatry, psychology, psychiatric nursing and social work) to justify their statements about the origins of illness and the best treatment available. They take particular issues with untested theories which implicate families as the causes of illness. Another position is that illness behaviour can most effectively be understood as a complex interaction of both biological or organic causes and organizational or structural variables.

It is particularly difficult to correct hierarchical maladies and put the parents back in charge of their family when there is a mentally ill adult child in the system, who frequently precipitates violent interchanges or threatens to do so. Clinicians, who in in-patient settings have available help, including chemical and physical restraints, with the manpower to execute the containment procedures, are sometimes at a loss to help families design strategies which will work in home settings. The police are often called upon in community settings to help get a family disturbance under control; for the most part, they are reluctant to do so, because they are ill-prepared to judge the nuances of the interchanges going on, and furthermore, no one then is willing to take the next step, and file a formal complaint. Police, refusing to respond to family violence calls, have said, 'We're enforcement officers, not social workers!' A police chief, asked to come to a Community Mental Health Center meeting to discuss plans for alternative strategies with family problems in an inner city area stated, 'Well, I see it as rather futile, family violence and the weather are the same: everybody talks about it, but nobody can change it'. Such demoralization unfortunately dampens the efforts to seek solutions to this pressing need.

Retirement plans derailed

The Flanagans (see Appendix D), Joe, 65, and Mary, 60, had been planning for many years for their retirement, looking forward to increased leisure and fulfillment of their travel dreams. Their four daughters, ranging in age from 35 to 25 years, had not been living at home for five years. Mary planned to retire at the age of 62. Joe had retired at 62 and was spending his time doing all the household repairs, which had been neglected, and watching Maura's pre-schoolers while she finished graduate school. Maura and John live ten miles from the Flanagans. The two younger daughters had moved to San Francisco, where they shared an apartment with two other young women. Their oldest, Sheila, was living in Washington, DC, with her political scientist husband, Michael, and three children.

As Mary describes their family: 'We were a typical family, fun-loving, family-centred Irish, happy. We were atypical only in that no one had any serious drinking problems. Then the bomb struck.'

The bomb was Sheila's telephone call, announcing that Michael had phoned her from Japan, and told her that he wasn't coming home from a business trip for 'a while' because he was in love with another woman, a Japanese business associate. He said that there was no need for hysteria, and that his mind was made up and settled. When Sheila consulted a lawyer and began to assess her financial status, she discovered that Michael had remortgaged their home, and that their second mortgage was three months in arrears. All of these bills were sent to his company, since their marital arrangement had been that he paid the household expenses and she paid the children's bills and her own expenses, from her salary earned as a junior level hospital administrator. Further, because of Michael's gambling, car payments were past due and both cars were in the process of being repossessed by the finance company. Sheila decided to ask her parents to allow her and the children to come home. Now Joe and Mary have a six-person household, together with Maura's two children, for most of the week.

There is maladaptation in:

1. Michael and Sheila's sub-system, with most communication managed by lawyers and long-distance telephone calls.
2. Joe and Mary's sub-system, with serious disagreement between the two of them concerning how long they should 'put up with' this new complexity.
3. Sheila's children, who are belligerent, tearful, and showing many other signs of distress, such as lying and stealing (Michael), bed-wetting (Bobby), and renewed thumb-sucking and frequent night awakening (Sarah).
4. Sheila and Maura, who are in conflict with each other, and in competition for their parents' resources (particularly around childcare).
5. Michael and John, who were college classmates and who now exchange heated, angry, international phone calls. John is convinced that if Michael went into treatment for his gambling, the old normative order of that nuclear family would be restored.

The family was referred for therapy when Michael, Jr, was caught with the money for the 4th grade class trip hidden in his school backpack. The family therapist, a Master's-prepared clinical specialist in psychiatric nursing, has engaged all of the family members on the genogram, including Sister Auntie (Mary's younger sister, a nun) in problem-defining and problem-solving sessions. Her work is primarily with Joe, Mary and Sheila; the focus is on the mutual expectations of each of the adults for one another.

In the intake session, when the third generation was present, the therapist asked Michael, Jr, if he had had a plan for the stolen money. He said he did, and that he had planned to send it to his dad in Japan, so he could 'pay all his debts and not be ashamed and be with us again.' He earned the designation, 'Signaller of System Distress', and when present at family sessions subsequently, often voiced what the adults were reluctant to mention. The adults in the family disagreed with the therapist's suggestion that they spend time grieving for the various losses (e.g., loss of husband, of marriage, of father, of cherished dreams). As Joe put it, 'Our dreams aren't dead yet – they just need a little resuscitation. When Sheila gets herself together, we'll be back to where we were, and we'll go on as we wanted to.' This view, of course, is debatable. Here is another instance where a family system's views and a clinician's views would not converge. Wallerstein and Blakeslee (1989) have documented the fact that divorce sends shock waves throughout the nuclear and extended family systems, sometimes for many years to come. To the degree that Michael, Jr, and all of the children are not assisted in their coming to grips with the loss of their father (and uncle), more acting out can be expected. The two younger sisters of Sheila may have reservations about making a commitment to a long-term relationship or a marriage. Joe and Mary may find that the increased physical demands on them exacerbate some physical symptoms, like Joe's hypertension, or Mary's arthritis.

Greek tragedy

In modern history, no Western head of state has ever deposed his First Lady. The rule of organization, honoured by first families, has been staying married, and usually living in such a way that marital fidelity also appears to be the case. Beginning in 1987, however, newspapers in Greece and abroad began to rumour that Prime Minister Andreas Papandreou was dissatisfied with the political activities of his wife, Margaret, and further, that he was in love with another woman and planning to divorce Margaret (see Appendix E). Ironically, since taking office in 1981, the Greek Prime Minister has introduced extensive social reforms, emphasizing family values. He also has publicly praised his wife's political accomplishments, such as her founding and becoming President of the Women's Union of Greece, an organization which champions world peace and women's movements. Margaret followed the script for a political wife – articulate, outgoing, a strong defender of her husband's policies (Cohen, 1989).

Extramarital affairs are semi-acknowledged among some European leaders, and tolerated in many Greek households. A divorce for a national leader, however, is decidedly a norm violation. Affairs are tolerated in Greek families so long as no one within the family – wife or children – is embarrassed. A modicum of secrecy and civility is supposed to prevail.

What made divorce thinkable, then, in this first family can be understood in the light of the earlier actions of both Margaret and Andreas. Margaret Chant, born in Illinois, met Andreas in 1948 when he was teaching economics at the University of Minnesota, having emigrated to America, studied at Harvard, and taken American citizenship. Margaret then headed a social issues public relations firm. Both Andreas and Margaret were married to others when they met. Each divorced their respective spouses, and married in 1951. Thus the couple had established a rule of organization for their own dyad – divorce was thinkable and hence, do-able.

From the various accounts of the life of the Papandreou family, in its within-family and political contexts, the following rules of organization can be extrapolated:

1. The marital couple's intimacy is solidified by public gestures of love (e.g., Margaret's visiting her political prisoner husband daily, for months, in the wake of a 1967 military coup).
2. Extramarital affairs, on the part of Andreas, (including fathering another woman's child) are tolerated to a degree; Margaret then confronts him and insists that the relationship end.
3. The career of the husband takes precedence over the career of the wife (e.g., the entire family returned to Greece, from America, so that Andreas could pursue his political career).
4. The career of the wife is tolerated so long as she does not outshine her husband.
5. Adult children may publicly comment about their father's political career and extramarital affairs. (They have begged him to resign as Prime Minister.)

As this chapter is being written, the Greek tragedy continues; readers will have to turn to the popular press for up-dates on how the family system decides to organize itself in the future. Andreas has made public statements that his new paramour, Dimitri Liani, aged 33, is the new 'First Lady'; she is a former airline stewardess on the Prime Minister's plane. The four Papandreou adult children range in age from 37 to 27. It is fairly common for families of divorce to have adult children struggling with the mechanics and new rules of trying to integrate the idea that one of their parents has married someone their own age. When families are in the light of the public press, this uncomfortable process becomes more so.

Adolescent caretaker sisters

Familial rules of organization about intergenerational obligations have many different variations. This section will describe one of them – when adolescent sisters become the caretakers of their younger female siblings, thus setting the pattern for later dysfunctional relationships among the grown women in the family. While the caretaking also goes on with the males in the family, the focus here will be the female relationships. The word caretaker is being used to connote that what is meant is a relationship in which reciprocity does not exist, and loyalty is one-way, from the caretaker to the recipient of care. This differs from caregiving, where both loyalty and reciprocity exist. This distinction is made by Bank and Kahn (1982).

The nature of the caretaker–care recipient relationship among siblings is one that is complex and qualitatively different from many other types of familial patterns. While dilemmas are frequently encountered by clinicians who work with families in which these patterns exist, there is relatively little in the literature to aid in conceptualizing or theorizing about its dimensions. Bank and Kahn (1982) are one exception to the minimal attention paid to the problem. The parental role is of such great significance and importance in the healthy development of children that researchers have focused almost exclusively on the multitude of functional, relational and organizational rules that parents transmit. Gilbert and Christensen (1988) maintain that families with a dysfunctional, unstable parent sub-system, which is unable effectively to negotiate and enforce parental roles, have increased difficulty in coping with developmental changes and life stresses. In dysfunctional, chaotic family systems, no one is clear about expectations; punishments for deviance come as a surprise, when the members are not clear about what the rules are, and thus these punishments are experienced as unjust and unfair.

In two cases, which will serve to illustrate this family problem, the parent was absent physically and/or emotionally, leaving a void in the parenting function. An older adolescent sister stepped in to carry out these parental functions, and had little support from any other adults as she carried out her tasks. Such role performance, then, tends to be inflexible and rigid, lacking warmth and care; the negativity resulting seems to have lasting effects.

The Daniels family (see Appendix F) is a three-generational, white, Anglo-Saxon system, with marked dysfunction in both men and women. Robin, now 76, has had three husbands, all alcoholics, and she is an alcoholic herself. Pat, the only child from her first union, was the adolescent caretaker sibling for Diane, now 35 and currently in treatment, and Diane's older brother, who died from a drug overdose. Pat is currently married to an alcoholic. As the adolescent caretaker, she was very autocratic in her disciplining and is described by Diane as somewhat erratic in her behaviour generally.

When Diane sought treatment, she presented herself as highly anxious, needy, disorganized and unsure of herself, with thoughts that were negative and obsessive in quality. Issues regarding differentiation from her family of origin, control, unresolved grief, guilt and failed role negotiations in her marriages were quickly apparent. She wanted first to address problems with her daughter, Robin, who witnessed much of the abuse that occurred of Diane by her first husband and Robin's father, Robert. Robin is vague and evasive when her father's drug abuse and death from AIDS, in 1987, is the focus of the session. Robin's childhood appears to have been as chaotic as her mother's; she was often the champion and protector of her mother against her father's abuse, but was never abused directly.

Robin first entered treatment at age seven, the same age that her mother was when Diane's biological father died, and Pat became the caretaker. Then, Diane expressed concern over her inability to sleep alone at night. She has sought treatment for her recently, this time with worries about her obsession with homework, her general negativity, her lack of friends, and arguments between mother and daughter. In the last year, Diane has married again, (within nine months of her husband's death from AIDS), moved to a new town, lost long-time family pets through death, and for Robin changed school systems. Both continue to express fear about the possible contagion from Robert's illness.

Diane's inability to sort out normal adolescent struggle from pathological levels of disturbance needing treatment, can be understood in the light of her own experience as an adolescent, with a harsh, unyielding caretaker sister. She both succumbs to Robin's demands and then erratically yields to them, accompanying her interactions with negativity and anger. Bank and Kahn (1982) assert that due to the inflexible and compulsive nature of the caretaker, who responds to non-compliance by inducing guilt and making threatening stances, the recipient often responds passively, but with underlying hostility and anger. The familiar pattern is being relived by Diane and her daughter. Limit-setting and warm expression of love both elude Diane as a mother.

The Shah family (see Appendix G) is a three-generational system of mixed cultures. Sam Shah, age 26, is the third son of Egyptian/Moslem parents who value education highly and themselves are white-collar professionals. Antoinette, age 29, is the fourth-born daughter of an Italian Roman Catholic family, whose parents were blue collar workers and did not finish high school. Antoinette's daughter, Grace, aged 9, was the product of a short-lived relationship. Sam is her first husband, but third relationship; they were married three years ago.

Antoinette's family of origin was highly chaotic, violent and dysfunctional. When she was seven, she witnessed the killing of her mother by her father, through multiple stabbings. Following the murder, she was raised by her second oldest sister, Theresa, then 17 years old. Theresa, although suffering from depression after the murder, became the caretaker because the oldest daughter had already married and left the home. Antoinette spent some time in a Catholic boarding school, but was expelled for arguing with the nuns. While living with Theresa and the other children, there was constant arguing and turmoil, mixed with severe disciplining on Theresa's part; Antoinette was occasionally thrown out of the house, and sent to live with other relatives. Antoinette over the years developed strong sibling bonds with her younger siblings, establishing loyalties with them, but continued animosity against Theresa.

Grace, aged nine, and the identified patient in this family system, is the only daughter of Antoinette. She was born when Antoinette was 19 years old. Grace never knew her biological father; he and Antoinette never married, and he departed shortly after Grace's birth. Grace has had multiple caretakers and has also served as a companion to her mother, helping her to struggle with loneliness and poor relationships with men. Grace becomes inappropriately demanding and controlling; Antoinette is ineffective as a parent and very inconsistent in attempts at limit-setting. Grace was referred for treatment by the school system, where counsellors expressed concern over her sexual acting out, provocative behaviour, and assertions of sexual abuse by a babysitter and her stepgrandfather from Egypt. The allegations of sexual abuse were investigated and not sustained.

Daughters are socialized to be women primarily by their mothers. When the primary socialization of the mother has been deficient or defective, there is a predictable inability to parent effectively, particularly with female children. When the mother, as a child, has experienced conflicting messages about femininity and expectations of women, and has had disturbing sexual experiences or poor role modelling from the same-sex parent or caretaker, she can hardly be expected to carry out mothering tasks normally. Frequently, when the parental dyad is dysfunctional, a child (often the oldest or most responsible female) emerges to function as protector of the dyad, by assuming childcare responsibilities. The unspoken hope is that by relieving the parents of some childcare tasks, they will be able to settle their problems and return to their normal tasks. Unfortunately, the hope is not fulfilled, particularly when the parents are abusing drugs and/or alcohol. Caretaker siblings not only do childcare tasks, but often care in parenting ways for the parents, such as preparing meals, rescuing them from drunken binges, lying to bill collectors, doing laundry and so on. The youngest caretaker sibling discovered by a university Community Mental Health Center in New Jersey was an eight-year-old boy, who successfully cared for six- four- and two-year-old siblings after his parents deserted the family. His caretaking went undiscovered for more than two months, and came to light when school officials investigated his absence from school more energetically. He had been feeding his family by going to fast-food places, and taking the discarded food, which was thrown out after each shift changed. His solution to running out of diapers was to toilet-train the two-year-old. The saddest part of this story was that this eight-year-old had a very difficult time returning to third grade, and being parented by foster parents. He felt almost depressed about having a very important and significant role taken away from him.

Clinicians have commented that caretaker siblings, grown into adulthood, seem continuously sad, if not clinically depressed. Having not experienced the joys of childhood, they seem unable to experience anything positive, let alone joyful, in adulthood. The outcomes of caretaker versus caregiver siblings have not been fully studied. There have been some preliminary studies of what happens in family systems to healthy siblings when there is a chronically-ill child. The social class of the families, and their available resources and support systems, seem to influence outcomes. For instance, the smaller the family, with few people to call upon for respite or simply lending a hand in a limited way, seems to result in more stress and disruption.

Multiple systems stresses

Rob and Lisa Smith (Appendix H), married for 22 years, have struggled to maintain a degree of family normality, avoiding serious discussion of differences, including Rob's war experiences in Vietnam, his many extra-marital affairs, alcohol problems in both families of origin, obesity in all four family members and life-threatening cardiac disease in Rob. One very problematic family rule is that Rob decides what he's willing to discuss and no one can persuade him to change his mind. Lisa complains that she is living with a changed person, that a different man came back from Vietnam, but she feels helpless to push past his no discussion rule. The family was referred for therapy, because Rob was a candidate for a heart transplant, but his serious obesity had resulted in his having a very low priority score in the donor review committee. They agreed to family sessions only with the understanding that this might improve Rob's chances of a transplant.

There are four generations alive in Rob's extended family. His maternal grandfather, 88, is thought to have Alzheimer's disease, and is cared for by his wife, 82. Rob's parents continue to endure a long-conflicted marriage, made more difficult by problem drinking and now a diagnosis of emphysema for Rob's father. His parents argue bitterly over whose responsibility the care of elders is, and what they owe Rob, who has many financial worries, besides the physical and emotional ones. Just as Rob lacked a role model, in his parents, of negotiating marital differences straightforwardly and respectfully, so did Lisa. Her father was an alcoholic, married to her mother, an asthmatic; Lisa's mother was an invalid throughout much of her life, yet controlled the family from her sick-bed. The caretaker adolescent in Lisa's family was the oldest sister. Patterns similar to those described in this chapter's section on adolescent caretakers existed through much of her growing up. Lisa fails to negotiate well with Rob, and does just as poorly with their daughter, Rita.

Over the years, Lisa has attempted to get Rob to accept the need for alcoholic counselling, marital counselling, or medical help for his obesity and heart disease. As she tearfully states, 'My life is just one long frustration; if I pushed too hard, he'd just walk out and leave – and have another affair. Then things would be no better, and usually just got worse.' She acknowledges her own obesity, but seems puzzled that clinicians list her children as obese (both are more than 60 pounds overweight). She says, 'Well, they just need to be more active. Exercise or work would help. But I guess they eat when they're troubled, just like I do.'

Current plans were under way to seek funding to admit the entire family into an in-patient setting, where a total family systems approach would be possible.

Working with families

In this chapter, several types of family problems have been illustrated, and the complexities and difficulties in working with such systems have been described. Many of the families could have very well been used to illustrate a family pattern other than the one under which they were grouped; the choice to place them in a particular section was made on the basis of the priority of the most compelling dynamic at the moment.

In clinical settings, a coordinator or supervisor would have carefully to assign clinicians with competence to intervene effectively and quickly; nurses who have earned a first degree for practice, such as the bachelor's degree (in the USA), could be assigned, for a delimited role, with someone who has more preparation and clinical skill. For instance, a first-level nurse might work with the Smiths on a weight-reduction regime, or with one of the identified patient children, on a behaviour modification programme, aimed at increasing self-esteem. First-level nurses also have shown that they can work very effectively as case managers, with the seriously mentally ill being cared for in communities, so long as they have access to clinical supports for themselves. They are particularly effective as case managers of community-based care because of their physical assessment skills, and ability to monitor drug therapy.

Maladapted families are usually so complex, and so difficult to treat, that a more experienced clinician is needed to design intervention strategies. Many agencies use a process of on-going clinical supervision, even for senior staff, to ensure that appropriate strategies are being implemented.

Hopefully, having read the intricacies of the family dynamics described in this chapter, nurses will have a new appreciation of the utility of thinking systems. Any one of the family members in this chapter could have been described as an individual, without the approach of the systems interchanges, but that presentation would fall far short of the actual lived experience of the person.

References

Albert, Nora (1989) Parents of the mentally ill: the impact of Violence (unpublished manuscript), Rutgers University, New Brunswick, NJ.

Bank, S. P. and Kahn, M. D. (1982) *The Sibling Bond*, Basic Books, New York.

Cherrigton, D. (1980) *The Work Ethic*, AMACOM, New York.

Cohen, M. (1989) When a First Lady's husband leaves her for a younger woman. *Good Housekeeping*, May, **135**, 82–6.

Creer, C. and Wing, J. (1974) *Schizophrenia at Home*, Institute of Psychiatry, London.

Gilbert, R. K. and Christensen, A. (1988) The assessment of family alliances, in *Advances in Behavioral Assessment of Children and Families*, Vol. 4 (ed. R. J. Prinz),

JAI Press, Greenwich, CT.

Lagos, J. M., Perlmutter, K. and Saexinger, H. (1977) Fear of the mentally ill: empirical support for the common man's response, *Am. J. Psych.*, **134**, 1134–7.

Leventhal, H. (1982) Wrongheaded ideas about illness. *Psychol. Today*, January, **73**, 48–55.

Norman, B. (1989) The Work Ethic in a Scandinavian–American Family (unpublished manuscript), Rutgers University, New Brunswick, NJ.

Runions, J. and Prudo, R. (1983) Problem behaviors encountered by families living with a schizophrenic member. *Can. J. Psych.*, **28**, 382–5.

Seymour, R.J. and Dawson, N.J. (1986) The schizophrenic at home. *J. of Psychosoc. Nurs. Ment. Health Serv.*, **26**, 28–30.

Turkat, D. and Buzzell, V. (1983) The relationship between family violence and hospital recidivism. *Hosp. Commun. Psych.*, **34**, 522–3.

Voydanhoff, P. (1984) *Work and the Family* Mayfield Publishing, Palo Alto.

Wallerstein, J. and Blakeslee, S. (1989) *Second Chances: Men, Women and Children a Decade After Divorce*, Bantam.

Walsh, F. (1987) Clinical utility of normal family research. *Psychother.*, **24**, **35**, 496–502.

Whinery, C. (1989) The Younger Female Sibling of the Adolescent Caretaker Sister: Roles, rules of organization and structure (unpublished manuscript), Rutgers University, New Brunswick, NJ.

Appendix A: the Johnson family

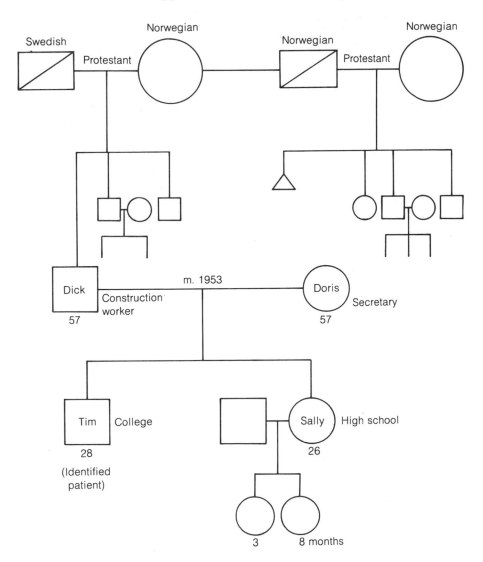

Appendix B: the Folaty family

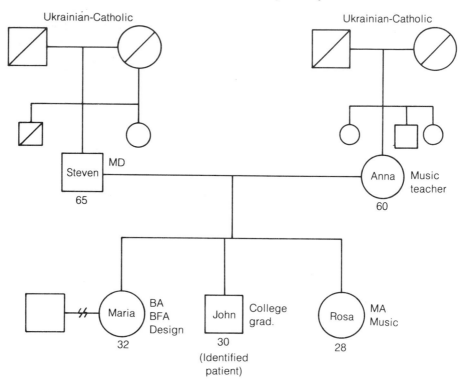

Appendix C: the Giovanni family

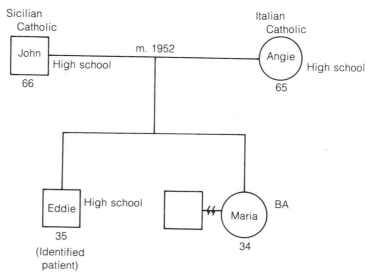

Appendix D: the Flanagan family

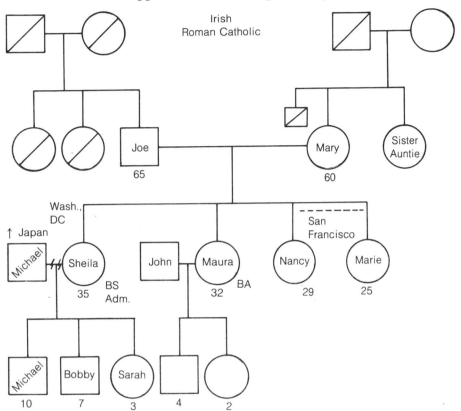

Appendix E: the Papandreou family

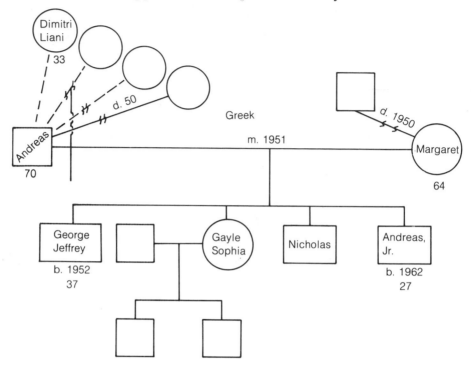

Appendix F: the Daniels family

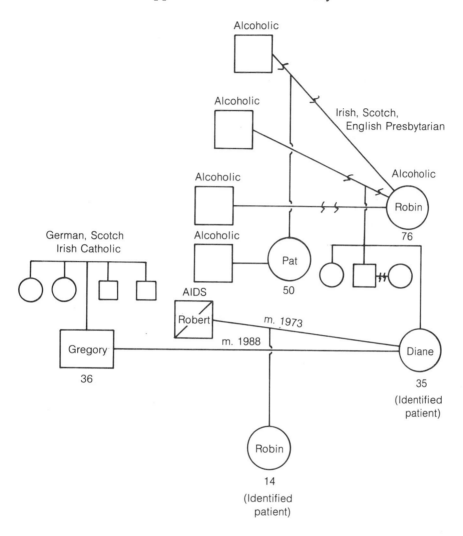

Appendix G: the Shah family

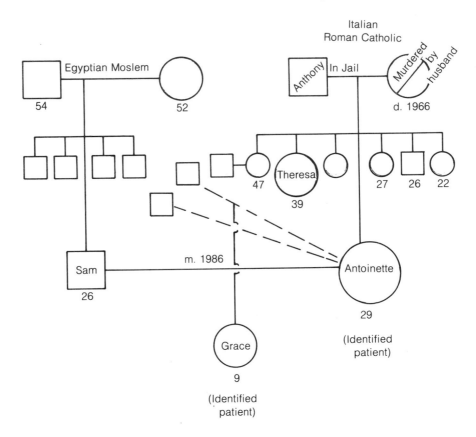

Appendix H: the Smith family

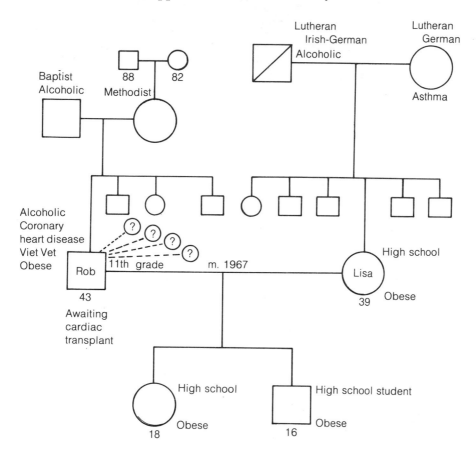

Chapter 15

The Rogerian client-centred model: clinical applications

D. A. BERTIN

Introduction

In this chapter I will discuss the clinical applications of the Rogerian client-centred model as applied to the psychiatric nursing setting. I will describe the psychiatric nursing intervention in the care of one particular in-patient during and after her stay in the acute admission unit of a psychiatric hospital. Discussing only one client has some obvious disadvantages: primarily a feeling that the model may be applicable only to this type of psychiatric client. However, in my opinion, it is essential (in a chapter of this sort) to give enough clinical information and verbatim nurse–client interactions for the reader to be in a position to ascertain the usefulness or otherwise of this model. I also intend to discuss the broad principles of its clinical applications.

Psychiatric nursing comprises various activities; in the course of one day nurses may find themselves dealing with the physical needs of their clients (food, warmth and shelter), the medical needs (medication, minor ailments etc) as well as activities that might be labelled psychotherapeutic. Indeed many people argue that they feel inadequate time is left for the psychotherapeutic side of their nursing. However, what is sometimes forgotten is that all of these activities are opportunities for achieving positive clinical changes. These very basic interactions are moments which are available for the therapeutic relationship to begin and to develop. All interactions between people, whether those people are labelled nurse and client, or teacher and student, are potentially therapeutic. In this way there are distinct advantages to the psychiatric nurse who has this regular, ongoing and varied contact with clients.

This raises the question as to what form these interactions should take; do we just talk to people, or is there some sort of style that may be of use? The Rogerian client-centred approach is ideally suited to psychiatric nursing as it can be used in all the types of situation that arise. Whether we are passing the time of day over a cup of tea or holding a more formal one-to-one session, the underlying principles of the model are usable and helpful. Talking to our clients is something we often do without considering the value or indeed the consequences of the content and manner of this interaction; paying more attention to this and basing our talking on a conceptual model will be of great value to our work and therefore ultimately to our clients.

The aim of all our nursing action should be to achieve positive therapeutic change; that is, the encouragement of growth and development, not just the amelioration of some disease process or troublesome behaviour pattern. Rogers (1986) stated: 'The person-centred approach, then, is primarily a way of being which finds its expression in attitudes and behaviours that create a growth-promoting climate. It is a basic philosophy rather than simply a technique or a method. When this philosophy is lived, it helps the person to expand the development of his or her own capacities. When it is lived, it also stimulates constructive change in others. It empowers the individual, and when this personal power is sensed, experience shows that it tends to be used for personal and social transformation.'

The fundamental aspect of such a process lies in the relationship between the helper and the one seeking that help; in a relationship that is not based on openness and trust, whatever effort is made, the therapeutic value will be severely diminished. What I will demonstrate in the case study is that the development of a relationship with a client is sometimes fraught with difficulty; that reciprocal trust is something that has to be developed. It is not enough for the client to develop trust in the nurse; the nurse has also to trust the client.

Client-centred therapy is based on several principles that have been outlined in Chapter 7. I do not intend to repeat them, but I will emphasize certain key elements. Rogers' concept of human beings is that we are basically rational, realistic, socialized and forward-moving. Also that we are generally cooperative, constructive and trustworthy when we are free of defensiveness. He rejected the idea of us being generally irrational, unsocialized and destructive. The prime aim is the development of a helping relationship, non-threatening in nature, to bring about the facilitative conditions for therapeutic change. The relationship is therefore not one of the expert nurse solving the problems of the unskilled client but rather the nurse acting as a mirror on which the client views his current dilemmas and gradually finds personal solutions. By using the concepts of empathy, warmth, and genuineness the nurse achieves a state of non-defensiveness in which the client can consider and experiment with alternative coping behaviours.

Different applications of the model

The Rogerian client-centred approach is not a rigid format; it is based on a set of principles which are applied with considerable flexibility. In psychiatric nursing we work with our clients in a wide variety of settings, and the flexibility inherent in this model is therefore one of the factors that enhances its applicability to our field.

An interactional skill

As already stated, psychiatric nurses spend a great deal of time talking and being with their clients. If we wish to make the greatest therapeutic use of this time we need to have some underlying rationale to guide our behaviour. Merely chatting to a client may be pleasant and may bring about some degree of temporary relief for the client but our aim should be higher than this. How many times have we all found ourselves wondering what to say to someone? We offer reassurance, information and comfort – valuable in their own way at the appropriate time but limited in therapeutic value. We also need to find the right words for many different clients with various needs and problems, a daunting task. This model has been found to be of value with a variety of diagnostic groupings both in and out of the psychiatric field (Truax, 1970). The key behaviours of the approach can be used equally as well in an informal setting as in the more formal. One could find oneself holding the same or similar interactions during a casual meeting in the ward corridor as in the interview room. It is not necessary, or indeed desirable, to announce that therapy is taking place! Neither is it the case that somehow therapy stops as the nurse and client leave the interview room; it is a process without boundaries that occurs whenever people get together to discuss a problem or dilemma. Therefore all the time spent with clients has the potential to be of therapeutic value; we should aim, therefore, to guide our time with an appropriate set of tools such as the ones offered by the Rogerian model.

Adjunct to another therapy

There are times when psychiatric disorders are such that no single therapy or treatment in its own right is adequate. An obvious example is that of the psychoses where medication plays an important role along with complementary and essential help such as social-skills training, self-care assistance and family therapy (Falloon, 1985). In other areas such as phobic anxiety and obsessional–compulsive problems, behavioural psychotherapy has an excellent track record (Barker, 1982). Obviously in these and many other situations we do our clients no favours by rigidly sticking to one set of rules and therefore denying access to appropriate help. Within the field of behavioural psychotherapy there has long been an argument as to the value of the relationship component of the treatment. Some behaviourists argue that the treatment package, for example graded exposure or applied relaxation, is the thing that brings about the clinical change, and that the relationship between the client and the helper is of limited significance or even of no importance at all. This rather extreme view is not held by many practitioners these days and it seems that there is a general move towards a more eclectic approach. In practice therefore we need to consider the right conceptual model or clinical technique (or combination) to suit both the personal needs of the client and the specific problem areas they have. However, I propose that the foundation of any therapy is based on the relationship between the helper and the client. Rogerian principles lend themselves ideally to this task and offer an appropriate basis for other approaches to proceed.

Therapy in its own right

The main purpose of this chapter is to illustrate the clinical application of the Rogerian client-centred model as used on its own. The case study is based on the care and treatment of one particular client whose main nursing intervention is based on this model. I say main because she was an in-patient in a mixed acute admission unit and therefore there were many people from a varied group of disciplines and it would be naive to assume that all staff were using the same principles. However, the nursing care was totally based on the Rogerian concepts detailed in the previous chapter. The following case study serves to demonstrate the benefits (and difficulties) of applying the model.

Case study

In this case study there were several therapists in that the case is set in an acute admission unit and therefore the client interacted with several nurses. There was, however, one main therapist who holds all the formal sessions and interacted more than any other nurse with the client. This was mainly because of the primary nursing philosophy that operated in this unit, but also because of the necessity (for the client) to develop a deep and trusting relationship with one person. The main items I will illustrate are the specific clinical behaviours and techniques used by the nursing staff. I have included several verbatim nurse–client interactions and have indicated the specific reason for the type of response given by the nurse. By doing this I will highlight the various component skills used in this model. I have also included some examples of the use of the clinical data collected during the sessions for care-plan development and nursing and multi-disciplinary discussions. The clinical data and nursing interventions described here are based on the care of an actual client, but certain information has been adapted in order to protect confidentiality.

Introduction to Sue

Sue has had several admissions to the unit over the last few years and has therefore become known to the staff, she has also become familiar with the ward and the system that operates within a psychiatric unit. The past is only important if it affects the here-and-now, so only a brief summary of these previous admissions is given below.

Life history

Sue was 26 years old, separated from her husband and unemployed. She lived in a small council housing scheme with her three-year-old daughter and had few friends and little social life. She described herself as difficult to get on with and too unsettled to ever keep a husband or a job. Her psychiatric history started when she was 17 when she took an overdose following a period of depression. There then followed a series of admissions for reasons such as drug overdoses, impulsive self-harm, problems with the police (alcohol abuse, civil disturbance, etc) as well as Sue's repeated statements of feeling fed up, miserable or depressed. The admissions were normally of short duration (two or three weeks) and no useful medical diagnosis was made apart from that of inadequate personality. The time in hospital was, generally, not felt to be of much use by either Sue or the staff. The main role of the admissions seemed to be to allow some heated situation to cool off and to give Sue a period of rest from the pressures of life. It also has to be said that she became a somewhat unpopular client and I think it is important to discuss here why this occurred and why Sue herself came to resent and doubt the value of these repeated stays in hospital.

When someone is admitted to a psychiatric unit it is essential that the nurse tries to plan and implement some form of meaningful intervention. The aim is to assist that person to cope more effectively with the problems that led to their admission, and where appropriate, to treat the underlying illness process. Our expectations may vary but we normally hope to achieve some degree of success or change. The client also has their own expectations and concept of the help they require. If the outcome is consistently negative the motivation of anyone to persist is limited, sometimes referred to as learned helplessness. For further discussion of this issue see Seligman (1975). Indeed in nursing we generally seek some form of excuse or reason for this failure, and it seems to be a common human failing that we tend to blame the other person. In this situation it seems that Sue blamed the staff for lack of achievement over the last few years; and the staff felt that it was Sue's lack of co-operation and effort that led to her repeated admissions. This theme is explored later in the chapter when some of the problems of relationship building and trust development are discussed.

Reason for admission

On this occasion Sue was admitted because several people (the general practitioner, the community psychiatric nurse and some friends) were concerned as to her safety. There had been a lengthy period of unsettled behaviour from Sue including alcohol abuse and noisy aggressive be-haviour towards several others. It was felt that, due to this and other behaviour, the safety of her three-year-old daughter was at risk, the child having been left alone on several occasions despite advice from several sources. Therefore the child had been taken into care, initially on a tem-porary order with a view to probable long-term care following a children's panel hearing. This was not the first time that this type of behaviour had occurred. Following the child being taken into care, Sue became sullen and uncommunicative and spoke in a very negative way about her future and herself. Although the community staff were in some ways used to seeing Sue like this, it seemed on this occasion to be more intense and distressing and therefore admission was suggested to her and she (rather reluctantly) agreed.

I will now discuss the various stages of the treatment of Sue and link this to the theoretical chapter that precedes this one. It should be made clear that the stages are in practice not so clear cut as in the theory. The helper often moves backwards and forward through them as the needs of the client and the situation changes. This also will be discussed as the case study develops.

The initial phase of therapy

The initial aim of therapy or the helping relationship should be to enable the nurse to understand the situation from the client's perspective. In this situation, Sue is in hospital again, having had several less than positive experiences in the past with her own opinions and feelings about the sys-tem in which she is a client. She had gone through a very traumatic experi-ence of having her child taken into care with a rather bleak outlook in terms of the child's return. It would be very easy therefore to make a whole number of assumptions about the way that Sue felt, such as it must be sad to have your child taken into care. This might lead to statements to her such as how terrible it must be for you to have your child taken away like that. On first impressions this may seem a very understanding thing to say, and it may be seen as a way of communicating our concern to the client. However what is that assumption based on? I would argue that it is based on our own value systems; not on the beliefs of the client that we are professing to understand. Therefore, the first stage of this approach is aimed at understanding this person's belief system from their perspective.

Aims of this stage
1. To clarify the purpose of these talking sessions (for the client).
2. To begin the procedure of developing the trust and openness essential to this approach by dealing with any barriers that may be present.
3. To begin the process of information or data collection needed for the accurate understanding of the client and of the nursing care required.

Key behaviours used during this stage
1. Allow time, giving a commitment (to the client).
2. The use of open-ended questions; no (or few) whys?
3. Focus on the non-verbal behaviour; commenting on any observed discrepancies between this and the verbal messages.
4. Allow silences, but use them at times to reflect on what they mean.

A number of things may happen at the beginning of this therapy: silence, hostility or a sudden outflow of mixed emotions and feelings. The nurse must therefore be prepared for whatever the client presents to them and should therefore be free of any preconceived notions of what the session will achieve. If one begins with the notion of wanting to collect a lot of background information, then the problem may be that the client will be silenced by a barrage of questions. She may also get the impression that you are not interested in her emotional side but rather are, in some way, just processing through the system. The overall aim is to convince this person that you are genuinely interested in her, her problems or dilemmas and what she wants to talk about. All of these items are essential in conveying empathy. It is important to remember that empathy is not only the accurate interpretation of someone's behaviour (verbal and non-verbal) but the communication of this back to the client. You may be the most understanding nurse in the hospital but if you are unable to demonstrate this then you are not truly empathic.

The sort of opening statement you make to the client at the outset of therapy begins this process. For example if one uses a directive question such as 'tell me why you drink too much' you have immediately set the tone of this, and future sessions. You have, in effect, taken control by deciding on the type of things that will be discussed and that you will ask questions that the client has to answer. In Rogerian therapy it is necessary to begin with less directive statements so that the client can talk about what he or she wishes. Examples of opening statements might be:

We have about forty-five minutes just now; what would you like to do with this time?
You have my full attention; it's over to you to talk about whatever you wish.
How can I be of use to you?

Let us now look at what happened at the start of the sessions with Sue.

Nurse Sue, I was wondering if we could spend some time just to talk privately? When would suit you?
Sue   Well, I don't know. Is there any point? I've told you it all before.
Nurse You feel it would be just repetition?
Sue   Maybe, will it help?
Nurse You sound doubtful?

Sue I've talked a lot, to various folk and here I am back in this place again.

Nurse It sounds like you feel that the previous admissions have not achieved anything?

Sue No...well yes; a bit I suppose. Maybe at the time, but the old feelings of despair just returned when I went home again.

Nurse That seems to have been a disappointment to you.

Sue Umm...yes (head is down and she becomes restless in seat).

Nurse I feel I've touched on something important; shall we talk more?

Notice in this example that the nurse generally reflected back to Sue the words and feelings that she expressed. Often this is as simple as merely rearranging the words into a different order, capturing the tone of voice that is used, or observing and commenting on the non-verbal behaviour. What is to be avoided is to reply to Sue's first statement with something like: 'Yes, of course there is a point; you must try to get over this.' In this reply you are falling into the trap of telling the client what is best and putting yourself in the role of expert and the client in the position of the recipient of your knowledge and wisdom. This is where we must start to trust the client and learn to take a passive role while the client does the exploring. Perhaps one of the hardest things to accept in this model is that our role is less controlling than in many other areas of nursing. At least now we have achieved the aim of getting Sue to begin the talking process. We must continue the development of the relationship by focusing on our empathic behaviours. The following extract is from the session that followed the previously described data.

Sue I guess that I should have known that things would still be difficult for me when I left here the last time. I just thought that it would somehow be OK.

Nurse But you found that it wasn't OK – it was just as bad or worse?

Sue Yes, worse. I never imagined it could of been worse; I just felt like the world was ganging up on me.

Nurse You felt alone and got at?

Sue Yes, as though no one cared or even noticed that I existed. I felt invisible . . . that's crazy, eh? (laughs gently).

Nurse Doesn't sound like you really feel it's funny....

Sue (starts to cry)

Nurse (gently puts his hand on Sue's shoulder and says nothing)

Here the nurse effectively used his silence and non-verbal behaviour to convey empathy. A gentle touch can convey more than words; but also the danger of a verbal response in this situation would have been that the words could have sounded hollow and phoney. The touch and the respectful silence were intended to show that the nurse was accurately picking up the client's feelings. Through similar sessions, during which the nurse used similar skills to develop this relationship, Sue began to become less defensive and to talk more freely than in the past. At this time however she still felt a great deal of anger and this sometimes was expressed towards staff in the ward. Two options presented themselves; one was to tell Sue that it was not acceptable to behave in this way, and the other was to attempt to understand Sue's reasons for this behaviour. The first option will convey to the client the message that you are only wanting to understand some of her behaviour and that anger is not acceptable. This I would argue is likely to harm the trust built up with her so far. Below is the way the nurse decided to tackle the problem following several angry exchanges.

Nurse I got the feeling that you were feeling rather angry yesterday. I was wondering if you wished to talk about it?

Sue Why don't you tell me why I was angry; you're the expert.

Nurse You think I know all the answers and you know nothing?

Sue You people are all the same; you expect me to do all the work, while you just sit there looking smug.

Nurse So you feel that I'm not helping you?

Sue Something like that... but admit it, you're not going to give me the answers are you?

Nurse No, probably not; but I look forward to the prospect of wrestling around with you to find some answers. I'm game to have a go if you are willing to take the risk.

Here I wish to point out that the final reply may be seen as rather harsh and unfeeling. However, what the nurse was doing was using another principle of Rogerian therapy called congruence. Congruence is the idea of being honest with yourself (and therefore the client) about the way that you feel inside. Mearns and Thorne (1988) defined it in the following manner: 'Congruence is the state of being of the counsellor when her outward responses to her client consistently match the inner feelings and sensations which she has in relation to the client.'

One of the fundamental principles of this model is that of genuineness; the nurse must be truly honest about his or her feelings. It should be noted that the nurse carefully stated his feelings in a manner that was both honest and useful.

One of the uses of such clinical interaction data is in discussing the nursing care required with colleagues. In this situation it proved of great use as it enabled consistency of care but also an understanding of the reasons behind Sue's anger and problematic behaviour. This proved to be a crucial turning point in the staff's attitudes towards her, moving from a somewhat negative standpoint to a truly empathic position.

By this stage it seemed that the staff and Sue had achieved a certain level of trust. She appreciated the commitment given and the honesty of the nurse in terms of his feelings; on one occasion she spontaneously commented on how she could respect someone who didn't pretend to be all sweetness and light as she knew that she was rude and inconsiderate a lot of the time. This is a very important statement as it highlights the clinical usefulness of being upfront and open with our clients.

The problem-solving phase

Now that a relationship had been set up and basic trust had been developed it was appropriate to move on in therapy. The second phase of this model is known as the problem-solving phase which accurately describes what is involved. It aims to check the understanding of the client's world and assist them in their own understanding. It also aims to pass beyond this into a deeper insightfulness and therefore to new solutions. This second phase is in many ways a continuation of the initial phase but is not so concerned with the development of trust, rather than with the deepening of our empathic perception of the client and the moving towards resolution of the difficulties.

Sue, as has been stated, had a number of problems relating to trust, both in trusting herself and others. Therefore it was a very significant step as she began to talk of some of the more hidden thoughts and emotions that she had. This is an incident that occurred after about a week in the unit.

Sue   When I'm at my lowest I go to a certain bit of the river near the house, then I do crazy things like picture myself being pulled out of the water by a policeman...dead. I then try and think who would bother if I wasn't here and I can't think of anybody...it's very odd.

Nurse   Odd? No, not to me; more like an important part of your life at the moment.

Sue   Yes, it is important; in a way its what keeps me sane. I was just so ashamed of it...I didn't intend to tell you, I don't know why I did.

Nurse   Yes...important and useful. I'm glad you told me and that you seem able to trust me; thank you.

Sue   (smiles and cries gently)

This is another example of honesty and congruence; here the feelings expressed by the nurse were positive, but sometimes professionals feel it is not quite right to say them out loud. If the nurse had *not* said this, an opportunity for a large step forward would have been lost. Through this type of sharing of feelings, and discovering that she was not rejected or laughed at, Sue began the process of rebuilding her self-esteem. In this example it is difficult to clearly relate it to one specific phase of therapy. The problem-solving phase has six components:

1. observing and listening;
2. exploring feelings;
3. responding to feelings;
4. exploring personal meaning;
5. responding to feeling and meaning;
6. providing your client with direction.

In practice the boundaries are vague and generally blurred. In the last transcript there were elements of the 'exploring feelings' and 'exploring personal meaning' phases. The key skills were, again, simple reflection of the client's words and feelings, though the nurse also attempted to pick up the strength of feelings being expressed and the meaning of the event to the client. Sometimes this is not always achieved first time but this does not matter as the following scenario illustrates.

> *Sue*   I was thinking about Ann (Sue's child) last night. I couldn't sleep.
> *Nurse*   You were upset by those thoughts?
> *Sue*   No...well, not really. Everyone seems to think I should miss her but I don't.
> *Nurse*   And that makes you feel...
> *Sue*   Sad...no, more guilty than anything.
> *Nurse*   Guilty for her being in care?
> *Sue*   Um...more for the way I treated her; I regret that but I think she is really better off without me.
> *Nurse*   So you feel guilty because you don't miss her?
> *Sue*   Yes, that's it.

In this example, note the use of understanding the meaning of the client's words and the nuances underlying the words. The nurse used the format of 'you feel...because' to test out their understanding of the client's meaning. The nurse was also helping the client to clarify her own understanding of the conflict and the mixed emotions within her. In this situation and many others, clients are often unsure of the nature of their emotional responses to the world around them; it is therefore the therapist's job in this model to 'bounce back' (reflect) the feelings and ideas picked up from the client. This enables the client to become aware of their own feelings by listening to the reflection of them from the therapist and, if required, to attempt to clarify or correct them. This example also shows that, by this stage of the therapy, Sue was beginning to trust the nurse with some deeper, more powerful thoughts; this is therefore a time for further exploration of these feelings.

However, it is not sufficient to merely discuss and clarify feelings; we must aim to move beyond that to assist with the resolution of the client's problems. Problem-solving though cannot be achieved until clients are in a state of mental readiness, in other words, until they feel clear about their feelings and accept their role as the major problem-solver. The nurse's role in this is certainly more directive than in the earlier stages of the therapy, but it is still the client who often has the solutions within them. The nurse's role therefore is to facilitate the verbalizing of these ideas.

Assisting with the clarifying of a client's feelings is achieved by the use of reflection and the 'you feel...because' technique. They enable the sorting out of often confused and contradictory thoughts to begin. This is how therapy progressed with Sue.

Sue   I was thinking about our last discussion. You know I said I felt guilty about not missing Ann.

Nurse Yes, are you not so certain now?

Sue   I'm not sure...I do miss her in some ways; you know, the nice times, like when she was a baby and was so dependent on me.

Nurse It was nice for you to be needed so much?

Sue   Yes, I suppose it was really; I don't think that anyone has ever needed me that much ever before; she also never doubted me, she trusted me...imagine that, trusting me!

Nurse You feel no one could ever trust you like that again?

Sue   No, why would they after all the things I've done. But Ann did trust me, and now....

Nurse And now...?

Sue   Now...there is no one to trust me but also no one to...

Nurse No one to need you in the way Ann needed you when she was a baby, is that it?

Sue   Yes, there is no one now. Just me.

Nurse And are you not important then?

Sue   Well that's the problem, I don't know.

Here the nurse is gaining access to areas of the client's feelings that have previously not been explored. Indeed the client herself is not clear about them, and therefore the benefit of this type of discussion is to clarify the precise nature and source of the emotions and thoughts within the person. This is achieved by the use of techniques such as reflection (once again), and congruence or honesty. The nurse, having by now established a trusting relationship with the client, is offering the means by which to explore the confusion of feelings and time in which to try and sort them out into a solvable state.

The final stages of the work with Sue were aimed at discussing the various avenues open to her in the forthcoming years. This was in many ways carried out in a fashion similar to the earlier stages of therapy. However, it was also essential now to begin to prepare Sue for the termination of therapy and to help her to work through the various feelings that might arise. We must remember that for Sue (and many clients) this may be the most satisfying and meaningful relationship that they have ever entered into. Moving on from it may bring on anxiety and even anger (at therapist) due to the feelings of isolation. Sometimes the client may feel that the therapist is rejecting them, leaving them alone to face the problems of the world. In many ways termination begins at the early stages, as it must be made clear that at some point the client will cease to be engaged in therapy.

This scenario is from a session held near to Sue's discharge back home following which the contact with the nurse would become less frequent and eventually cease.

Sue   I go home next Tuesday. Did you know?

Nurse Yes, I was wondering how you were feeling about it.

Sue   Were you? I sort of thought it would be a relief to you.

Nurse A relief?

Sue   Yes, come on, admit it. To be rid of this troublesome patient and get peace.

Nurse You feel that I'm not interested in you when you go home?

Sue   Well I...

Nurse You can't say, or do you not know?

Sue   Well I suppose it's hard for me to just accept that you seem to just take me as I am. It seems that you like me and that's hard to believe...sorry.

Nurse Why apologize? I always want you to tell me how you feel, even if it's not always nice.

Sue   It's funny. Knowing I'm going has brought back some of the old doubts and worries, I'd sort of hoped that they were gone for good.

Nurse So you had hoped to never feel sad again?

Sue   Yes, I suppose I had. (laughs quietly) That sounds rather silly doesn't it? I hadn't thought of it that way. Yes I did think that, and when the old feelings came back I blamed you for it as you were kicking me out!

Nurse And now...

Sue   Now...well, I've just to go home and get on with things, but I do feel more ready now. I understand myself better and I like myself now (or at least *some* of me!).

In conclusion, Sue certainly *said* that she benefited from the sessions and for the first time felt that her stay in hospital achieved more than just asylum from the world. She also maintained the sense of self-esteem she gained from the therapy and, although life was not always smooth for her, she felt she coped better than ever before. It could, of course, be said that she might have made these gains without the use of the Rogerian model. However, it must be remembered that she had previously been admitted on several occasions without any sense of achievement on either the staff or Sue's side. Perhaps the best way of concluding this case illustration is to let Sue speak for herself; when asked for her feelings on the sessions she said: 'I felt someone cared. Not because they were paid to or it was just part of their job but because they really wanted to see me sort out this mess. They seemed to believe in me, trust me, when I felt I didn't deserve any such trust. Gradually I started to trust myself like they trusted me.'

Summary

In this chapter I have illustrated the use of the Rogerian client-centred model by demonstrating its application to one particular client. Space does not allow for a complete and detailed analysis of every word or technique used in the therapy. What I hope to have done is give a flavour of the approach to link in with the preceding theoretical chapter. This has obviously meant that certain stages of the therapy have been somewhat scantily covered; I have, quite deliberately, concentrated on the 'relationship building' and 'exploration of feelings' stages for two main reasons. Firstly, I feel that these are the most powerful aspects of this approach, and secondly they were the ones that in Sue's case proved to bring about the most significant changes.

I feel that the type of problems dealt with in this case example did particularly lend themselves to the Rogerian approach. The anger and resentment felt by Sue, as well as the confused and unexplored feelings about her child, were issues that seemed essential to discuss for her to be able to move on in life. However, how could this have been explored without a deep and trusting relationship? Moreover, how could this type of relationship have been achieved without reference to the concepts of empathy, warmth and genuineness? It may be argued that just talking to people is all that we need to do and that the use of any philosophical model of man is just window-dressing. To take this attitude is to dismiss many years of research as not relevant. Most importantly, we are doing our clients a grave disservice by denying them approaches that can speed the resolution of their difficulties. I would also argue that, in most situations, these clients could not achieve this resolution without a model to guide our practice.

The Rogerian model can offer both the helper and the client a framework within which to work. It provides principles and techniques to assist with the development of a working relationship and to encourage a deepening of this relationship – and a format to encourage the formation of solutions to the problems faced by those who need our help.

References

Barker, P. (1982) *Behaviour Therapy Nursing*, Croom Helm, London.
Falloon, I. (1985) *Family Care in Schizophrenia*, Guildford Press, London.

Mearns, D. and Thorne, B. (1988) *Person-Centred Counselling in Action*, Sage Publications, London.

Seligman, M. E. P. (1975) *Helplessness (on Depression, Development and Death)*, Freeman, San Francisco, CA.

Truax, C. (1970) Effects of client-centred psychotherapy with schizophrenic patients: nine years pre-therapy and nine years post therapy hospitalization. *J. Consult. Clin. Psych.*, **35**, 417–22.

Rogers, C. R. (1986) A client-centred, person-centred approach to therapy, in *A Psychotherapists Casebook: Therapy and Technique in Practice* (eds L. K. Kutash and A. Wolf), Jossey-Boss, San Francisco, CA.

Chapter 16

Orem's self-care model: clinical applications

P. R. UNDERWOOD and S. MEUSER

Introduction

The seriously mentally ill adult presents many challenges to nursing because the condition is complex and complicated and often poorly understood. Serious mental illness produces disturbance in affect, perception, thought, and volition that result in a wide range of symptoms such as poor reality testing, loose association, hallucinations, delusions, isolation, poor interpersonal relations, lack of motivation, low self-esteem, and dependency. Symptoms fluctuate and present a remission exacerbation pattern and sometimes seem to appear and disappear on their own. Serious mental illness is most commonly associated with schizophrenic disorders, mood disorders (manic-depression, psychotic depression) and severe personality disorders (borderline). These disorders are usually considered to be chronic in nature and the patient can experience not only impairment, but disability and handicap as well (Farkas and Anthony, 1988).

Impairment is the disruption in structural and functional integrity caused by the disease process (Farkas and Anthony, 1988). Today it appears that genetic and/or neurological factors predispose some people to the disorders, especially the schizophrenic and mood disorders. There is good evidence that there is a biological or more specifically a neurochemical basis for the disease process and resulting impairment (Helzer and Guze, 1986; Freedman *et al.*, 1988). This does not rule out the influence of psychological or social factors but rather points out the biological vulnerability. Impairment is reflected in symptoms such as poor reality testing, hallucinations, and delusions and is most often the focus of psychiatric care.

Disability is the inability to perform activities within normal range (Farkas and Anthony, 1988). Disability is related to both the impairment (disease's progress) and the process of care and treatment. The process of care and treatment can produce disability when routine structure and control are used to create a care-giving environment that systematically dehumanizes an individual. Dehumanization includes denial of the right to self-care and self-determination in day-to-day living. Disability is a function of the interaction between the process of care and treatment and the impairment of the individual (Underwood, 1983). Some seriously mentally ill adults are so disabled that they cannot function independently. Disability is the focus of psycho-social rehabilitation.

In addition to impairment and disability, the individual may also experience handicap. This is a socially imposed disadvantage that limits the individual in fulfilment of normal roles related to age, sex, development, or culture. The seriously mentally ill are often handicapped in education or jobs or housing. Handicap is the focus of social rehabilitation (Farkas and Anthony, 1988).

At present it seems that seriously mentally ill adults require both treatment of impairment and rehabilitation for disability and handicap. Since we do not know the exact nature of the disruption in structural and functional integrity, we cannot ensure, even with the best treatment, that we can correct the impairment so that individuals may be completely symptom-free and able to enjoy mental health. However, if we provide rehabilitation, we can enhance well-being and quality of life.

The self-care model is particularly effective with this patient population because it offers a nursing approach that focuses on not only impairment but on ability as well. When we focus primarily on impairment and identify clinical problems as psychological symptoms, problems, or conditions and develop interventions to change, improve, or correct these things, nursing care is often seen as ineffective, frustrating, and difficult. When using the self-care model with the seriously mentally ill, the nurse considers impairment as factors that affect the person; however, the nurse is specifically concerned with the person and his ability to meet self-care requisites in living day-to-day. We can and do enhance well-being by assisting individuals to be self-reliant and responsible for meeting self-care requisites in living day-to-day so that they can function as independently as possible in a community with other people, wherever that may be. In practice we have found that nursing care based on self-care is not only effective with patients but rewarding for nursing staff as well.

We will demonstrate this approach by presenting a brief psychiatric history of a person with serious mental illness and then by identifying clinical problems, interventions, and outcomes based on self-care.

The patient and his mental health problems

History of the present problem

John, a 25-year-old single unemployed male, was readmitted to the psychiatric unit of a large county hospital after being discharged for one day. He was first admitted after police picked him up on the highway. He was incoherent and mumbling something about walking to a distant city to get out of his mother's house. During his first admission, he licked the floor and walls, gestured obscenely, and issued sexual remarks to males and females. He was treated with fluphenazine and in five weeks his symptoms had improved significantly. He refused further treatment or rehabilitation and was discharged and went to his mother's home. At discharge he still required a partly compensatory nursing system for all self-care areas. A week later he had had several episodes of obscene gestures and speech and frequent jerking of his head and neck, and he was returned to the hospital. In addition, he was in a near-vegetative state, preferring to sleep night and day, not eating or drinking unless prompted, complaining of constipation, not attending to hygiene, and feeling sad and hopeless about his disease and present condition.

He was re-evaluated and his medications changed to haloperidol (20 mg by mouth in the morning and 30 mg by mouth at bedtime) and benztropine (2 mg by mouth twice a day).

(a) Developmental, family, and social history John is the second of four sons born to the same mother from two fathers. Pregnancy and delivery were normal, and developmental milestones were accomplished on time. John's mother is a high-school graduate who works as a nursing aide in a convalescent home. She has never married. The mother denies psychiatric illness in her family. The history of John's father is unknown; he left home before John was born. The father of the youngest son has never lived in the home. The oldest son is 27 and in jail for burglary. The third son is 24 and has had multiple admissions to psychiatric facilities and is presently diagnosed as schizophrenic and residing in a long-term care facility. The youngest son is 10 and lives at home with his mother.

One of the mother's relatives (aunts, mother, cousins) took care of the boys until they started school. John is characterized by his mother as a shy child, and he reports never having any close friends and knew primarily the street people he hung around with. He has had sexual relationships with a girl but has never had a girlfriend. John reports that he never liked school and dropped out in the ninth grade. Except for five months with the Conservation Corps, he has been unemployed. He lived at home until his first admission. His mother is his primary source of emotional and financial support.

(b) Medical history Medical history and examination unremarkable. John does admit to poly-drug use since the age of 12, including marijuana, alcohol, and crack cocaine. He currently smokes one pack of cigarettes a day.

(c) Mental status exam John, a thin young man dressed appropriately for his age, is oriented to time, place, person, and situation. His recent and remote memory seems intact but he is vague about the exact sequence of events just prior to and after each admission. He appears apathetic, has a flat affect, little eye contact, and says he feels sad and hopeless. He often looks away and smiles inappropriately. He is able to answer simple questions in a logical, organized, but concrete manner. However, interactions are frequently interrupted with unrelated obscene words and gestures. John reports that he hears voices unpredictably that tell him to speak and gesture. He thinks the jerking of his head and neck is somehow related but he can't say how. Intellectual functioning seems appropriate to age and education; judgement and insight poor. He wants discharge immediately. He then plans to walk to a distant town because his mother's house is too crowded and makes him nervous.

DSM III-R diagnoses
Axis I: 295.93 Schizophrenia, disorganized, subchronic with acute exacerbation
Axis II: Deferred
Axis III: None noted
Axis IV: Psycho-social stressors: exacerbation of symptoms, inadequate finances, limited social support (predominantly enduring factors)
          Severity: moderate
Axis V: Current GAF: 25
          Highest GAF past year: 55

Identifying clinical problems: self-care assessment

Ideally, a particular nurse would be assigned to John's care and would use the above information as well as the self-care assessment tool (see Appendix A) to collect data from which to make an assessment and to identify clinical problems (see Chapter 8, Fig. 8.5).

Basic conditioning factors

John is a 25-year-old male who has lived at home, primarily with his mother and brothers, all his life in a lower socio-economic neighbourhood in a large metropolitan area. His family is characterized by poverty and a fragmented male presence. His primary source of emotional and financial support is his mother. John appears to be of at least average intelligence but has had little formal education or vocational training. He has no significant work history. His general health is good at present. He has no history of untreated or chronic problems outside his mental illness. He is diagnosed as schizophrenic.

(a) Past ability to meet self-care demands and pre-existing self-care deficits   Up to six months ago, according to John and his mother, he had no deficits in air/food/fluid, elimination, or personal hygiene. He took all meals at home, had no bowel or bladder problems, and had a regular hygiene routine, including caring for his own personal belongings and living space. He helped his mother with house-work and stayed with his younger brother when his mother was at work. However, it would appear that he has had difficulty with rest/activity and solitude and social inter-action for some time prior to the onset of acute symptoms. He did not en-gage in any regular way in any of the actions necessary to meet demands associated with rest/activity. He hung around on the street and slept ex-cessively. This may be reflective of the socio-cultural factors of unemploy-ment, poverty, and family expectations as well as his illness. John has never engaged in actions to meet self-care demands associated with soli-tude and social interaction. John reports always being shy and suspicious of people. He never had a close friend or belonged to any group except the loose collection of boys on the street. He has not really been able to develop individual autonomy or group membership. He cannot meet demands associated with prevention of hazards as evidenced by drug and alcohol abuse.

(b) Potential for developing ability to meet self-care requisites indepen-dently   John's strengths are his physical health, intelligence, and his concerned and supportive mother. However, he will need long-term treat-ment and rehabilitation if he is to have any sort of future other than the extremely bleak one that he sees at present. John would benefit from a case manager approach that would include a two or more year's supportive relationship with an individual who would help him navigate the mental health system, organize rehabilitation efforts, and link with the community where he will eventually return. The fact that John decompensated so rapidly (1 week) after his first hospitalization is an indication that he is at high risk of being labelled a treatment failure if he does not have ongoing management and rehabilitation. The rehabilitation process can start in the hospital by assisting John to become independent in self-care associated with maintaining intake of air/food/fluid, elimination, and personal hygiene and begin to develop skills needed to maintain balance of rest/activity and solitude/social interaction. Since there are pre-existing deficits in the last two areas, we cannot expect to see independent functioning in these areas during hospitalization.

Present ability to meet self-care demands and present self-care deficits

Air/food and fluid   John cannot decide to act to meet self-care demands associated with intake. He does not drink fluids unless offered or reminded and does not eat unless reminded and encouraged. He is unable to sit for any period of time at meals in the dining room.

Elimination   John is unable to decide and act to meet demands associated with elimination. Due to his deficit in intake as well as his medication, he has constipation and requires laxatives for regular elimination.

Personal hygiene   John cannot decide to act to meet self-care demands associated with personal hygiene. Without specific direction and supervision he will not bath, brush his teeth, change his clothes or take care of his personal belongings.

Rest/activity   John cannot decide or act to meet self-care demands associated with rest/activity. He stays in his room on his bed and reads his Bible or sleeps. With encouragement and direction, he will attend unit activities such as visits to the patio.

Solitude/social interaction   John cannot decide or act to meet self-care demands associated with solitude/social interaction. He attends to internal stimuli (voices telling him to act), which increase in situations calling for social interaction. He is able to spend time with his mother when she visits.

Prevention of hazards   John cannot decide or act and must be protected.

Identifying nursing intervention: self-care planning

Due to limitation in knowing, judgement and decision-making, and result-achieving actions, John has deficits in all self-care areas. At present his self-care deficits in all areas require a wholly compensatory nursing system (level I in Appendix A). While he may be able to perform some actions, he will require almost constant direction and supervision. The nurse must protect the patient and accept responsibility for seeing that self-care demands are met. She will use the helping methods of acting and doing for, providing guidance and support and a therapeutic environment.

Setting goals

Goal-setting includes the participation of both patient and nurse. Long-term goals address needs over time and cannot always be met during hospitalization. They may require months or years to accomplish. During hospitalization, patients often do not have or cannot articulate long-term goals.

John's long-term goals   None at present
Nurses' long-term goals John will be able to meet all universal self-care
requisites independently.
John will learn to manage treatment (e.g., medi-

cation) and rehabilitative measures (e.g., social skills training) that affect self-care behaviour.

Short-term goals address immediate needs and will be the basis for the nursing care plan which will identify what nurses and patients do to meet self-care demands and requisites. Goals should be stated in measurable outcomes and will serve as the criteria for evaluation of nursing care. John's impairment at this point is so great that he has difficulty accepting direction and supervision. Goals should reflect the minimum necessary to ensure basic health. Interventions should be set at a level that John can accept. When symptoms subside, nurses can gradually set higher goals.

John's short-term goals   To get out of this hospital so you will leave me alone.

Nurses' short-term goals Meet basic self-care demands

Nursing care plan   The following has been discussed with John, and he has agreed to accept nursing direction and supervision. Please do not change without discussion with the primary nurse. The plan will be reviewed in seven days.

Goal   Maintain intake of air/food/fluid
1. Patient will drink at least 3 litres of fluid per day and eat sufficient quantities of food to maintain his present weight of 160 pounds.

Interventions Nurse will:
1. Accompany John to the dining room, sit with him and encourage him to eat.
2. Provide supplemental food between meals as necessary and offer juice or water every 2 hours.
3. Document intake and output.
4. Weigh patient every other day.

Goal   Maintain care associated with elimination
1. John will have a bowel movement at least every 2 days. He will be able to report when asked.

Interventions Nurse will:
1. Document bowel movements.
2. Provide laxative if no bowel movement in 2 days and document results.

Goal   Maintain personal hygiene
1. John will:
   (a) Wash his hands and face and brush his teeth every day. The supplies are in his room. Check with him as per his schedule.
   (b) Shower every Monday, Wednesday, and Saturday.

Figure 16.1　Schedule 1

John and the nurse have discussed this schedule which the nurse designed and which John will try to follow. The nurse will remind him and encourage him but not force him to comply. John's primary care nurse will review the schedule every 7 days for changes.

7.00–7.30 a.m.	Wake up, wash hands and face and brush teeth
7.30–8.00	Nurse will meet you to go over your schedule
8.00–8.30	Breakfast, nurse will go with you to dining room
8.30–9.00	Go to medication room for medications. Try to stay out of your room for at least half an hour: walk in hall, sit in day room.
9.00–10.00	You can stay in your room; nurse will offer juice and/or water.
10.00–11.00	Monday, Wednesday and Saturday: shower with nurse's assistance. Tuesday: change bed linen with nurse's assistance. Thursday: get clothes ready for your mother.
11.00–12.00 noon	You may stay in your room, and the nurse will spend some time with you.
12.00–12.30 p.m.	Lunch; nurse will go with you to dining room.
12.30–1.00	Try to stay out of your room.
1.00–2.00	Go for a walk or to the patio with the group. Nurse will go with you.
2.00–3.00	Can be in your room
3.00–4.00	Visit with your mother
4.00–5.30	Can be in your room
5.30–6.00	Dinner, nurse will go with you
6.00–7.00	Try to join unit evening activity. Nurse will encourage you and stay with you.
7.00–8.00	You can get ready for bed, wash your face and hands and brush your teeth.
8.00	Go to the medication room for medication, and then go to bed for the night.

(Nurse should check water and be sure he has towel, soap, and clean clothes.)

(c) Change bed linen every Tuesday with nurse's help.

(d) Get his dirty clothes together for his mother to launder every Thursday with nurse's help.

Interventions 1. Nurse will:

(a) Ask John every morning and evening whether he has washed hands and face.

(b) Remind him before it is time to do (b;, (c), (d) above.

(c) Assist him as necessary.

Goal　　　　Maintain a balance of rest and activity

1. John will begin to develop a rest/activity pattern by following his schedule (see Fig. 16.1).

Interventions 1. Nurse will go over John's schedule with him each morning and remind him of the activities he can expect for the day.
2. At that time nurse should evaluate John's level of pathology to determine his ability to participate in activities.
3. Nursing staff will remind John to follow his schedule. Encourage but don't push at this time.

Goal   Maintain a balance of solitude and social interaction
1. John will begin to be able to tolerate minimal social interactions with support from the nursing staff.

Interventions 1. Attempt to establish an accepting relationship despite his obscene gestures and remarks. These are a result of his hallucinations and are not personal.
2. Orient to reality as needed. Reassure him that you know about the voices and are not angry with him.
3. Spend time with John in the morning and afternoon (see Fig. 16.1) talking about non-threatening topics.
4. Assist John to participate in low-stress socialization, such as walks.
5. Praise him for the time he is able to spend out of his room.

Outcome and evaluation

John's condition improved over the next three weeks and symptoms decreased in frequency and intensity but he continued to experience episodes of neck and head jerking and obscene gesturing. John also responded well to the low-demand initial care plan. At the end of two weeks he was independent in intake of air/food and fluid. He was no longer constipated but needed assistance to avoid the condition due to psychotropic medication (educative–supportive nursing system). He continued to need assistance with hygiene for another week, but after three weeks in the hospital he was independent.

Two weeks after admission the treatment team began to discuss discharge with John. The nursing staff reminded him that his goal was to get out of the hospital and that he could not do that if he stayed in his room all the time. His mother had agreed that he could come home if he could take care of himself and be of some help around the house. The treatment team suggested that he go to a halfway house to continue treatment and rehabilitation after discharge. John was ambivalent about what he wanted to do but knew that in either place he could not stay in bed all day. John and his primary nurse developed a new schedule

Figure 16.2   Schedule 2

John and the nurse have discussed how John could organize his day to be out of his room more. John wrote the following schedule after that discussion, saying: 'I will try to be out of my room as much as possible and will do this to be out. I want the nurse to remind me and help me do it'.

7.00–7.30 a.m.	Wake up, wash hands and face and brush teeth
7.30–8.00	Find the nurse and go over my schedule
8.00–8.30	Breakfast, go to my room when I am finished
8.30–9.00	Time for my first medication. Make up my bed and straighten up my room
9.00–10.00	Go to the scheduled activity
10.00–11.00	Monday, Wednesday, and Saturday: shower Tuesday: change bed linen Thursday: wash my clothes
11.00–12.00 noon	Walk in the hall or sit in the day room and the nurse will spend some time with me
12.00–12.30 p.m.	Lunch
12.30–1.00	Be in my room
1.00–2.00	Monday, Wednesday, and Friday: I will go to psycho-education group Tuesday and Thursday: I will try to go to relationship group, but I don't like it.
2.00–3.00	Be in my room
3.00–4.00	See my Mom
4.00–5.30	Be in my room
5.30–6.00	Dinner
6.00–7.00	Join unit evening activity
7.00–8.00	Watch TV or visit with other guys
8.00–9.00	Second medication time; watch TV
9.00	Get ready for bed

based on the agreement that John would be out of his room as much as he was in it (partly compensatory nursing system). He would need to be out of his room 12 out of every 24 hours. The nurses helped him plan how he would spend the time outside his room (maintain a balance of rest activity) and included opportunities to develop skill in maintaining a balance of solitude and social interaction (see Fig. 16.2). The nursing staff began psycho-education that included learning about his illness (schizophrenic disorder) and about his medication.

At the end of five weeks, with the support of his mother, John decided to go to a halfway house. He continued to hear voices but was no longer jerking his head and neck or making obscene gestures. He was occasionally frightened of the voices but was able to seek out staff for reassurance. He was still isolative and withdrawn. At this point he was independent in air, food and fluid. He had also learned to manage the constipation associated with medication, but he would need support to continue. He could also manage his personal hygiene including taking care of his own clothing and personal space with support. As would be expected, he continued to have deficits in both maintenances of rest/activity and solitude/social interaction. He could not consistently stay out of his room for 12 hours but he had established a regular bedtime and wake-up time. He attended most activities but his social skills were so limited that he had difficulty participating even when he was motivated.

Nursing care was judged to have been successful. John continued to show signs of impairment, but he was able to meet independently many self-care demands. The treatment team was not able to cure John's disorder, but we were able to treat and reduce his symptoms. Nursing staff began the rehabilitation process by helping John regain self-care skills in day-to-day living and begin to learn skills he did not have. John may never be able to enjoy mental health, but he can and did enhance his sense of well-being with the help of the nursing staff.

References

Farkas, M. and Anthony, W. (1988) An overview of psychiatric rehabilitation: the approach and its program, in *Psychiatric Rehabilitation Programs: Putting Theory into Practice* (eds M. Farkas and W. Anthony), Johns Hopkins University Press, Baltimore. (in press)

Freedman, D. X., Reginald, S. L., Meltzer, H. Y. *et al.* (eds) (1988) *The Year Book of Psychiatry and Applied Mental Health* (Chapter 1), Year Book Medical Publishers, Chicago.

Helzer, J. E. and Guze, S. B. (1986) *Psychiatry: Psychoses, Affective disorders, and Dementia*, Vol. II, Chapter 3, Basic Books, New York.

Underwood, P. R. (1983) Disintegrative life patterns, in *Psychiatric Nursing* (eds M. S. Wilson and C. R. Kneisl), 2nd edn, Chapter 13, Part 3, Addison-Wesley, Palo Alto.

Further reading

Clark, M. D. (1986) Application of Orem's theory of self-care: a case study. *J. Commun. Health Nurs.*, **3**, 127–35.

Fernsler, J. (1984) *A Comparison of Patient and Nurse Perceptions of Patients' Self-care Deficits Associated with Cancer Chemotherapy*. Proceedings of the Oncology Nursing Society's 9th Annual Congress, May 2–5, Toronto, Canada, p. 82.

Field, P. A. (1987) The impact of nursing theory on the clinical decision making process. *J. Adv. Nurs.*, **12**, 563–71.

Harper, D. C. (1984) Application of Orem's theoretical constructs to self-care medication behaviors in the elderly. *Adv. Nurs. Sci.*, **6**, 29–46.

McFarlane, E. A. (1980) Nursing theory: the comparison of four theoretical proposals. *J. Adv. Nurs.*, **5**, 3–19.

Moscovitz, A. O. (1984) Orem's theory as applied to psychiatric nursing. *Perspect. Psych. Care*, **22**, 36–8.

Munley, M. and Sayers, P. (1984) *Self-care Deficit Theory of Nursing*, Personal and Family Health Associates, New Jersey.

Nursing Development Conference Group. (1979) *Concept Formalization in Nursing*, 2nd edn, Little, Brown, and Co., Boston.

Orem, D. E. (1985) A concept of self-care for the rehabilitation client. *Rehabil. Nurs.*, **10**, 33–6.

Orem, D. E. (1985) *Nursing: Concepts of Practice*, 3rd edn, McGraw-Hill, New York.

Orem, D. E. (1988) The form of nursing science. *Nurs. Sci. Quart.*, **1**, 75–9.

Orem, D. E. and Taylor, S. G. (1986) Orem's general theory of nursing. *Nat. League Nurs. Pub.*, **3**, 37–51.

Padilla, G. V. and Grant, N. M. (1982) Quality assurance program for nursing. *J. Adv. Nurs.*, **7**, 135–45.

Reutter, L. (1984) Family health assessment – an integrated approach. *J. Adv. Nurs.*, **9**, 391–9.

Sandman, P. O., Norberg, A., Adolfsson, R. *et al.* (1986) Morning care of patients with Alzheimer-type dementia: a theoretical model based on direct observations. *J. Adv. Nurs.*, **11**, 369–78.

Whelan, E. G. (1984) Analysis and application of Dorothea Orem's self-care practice model. *J. Nurs. Ed.*, **23**, 342–5.

Woolery, L. F. (1983) Self-care for the obstetrical patient: a nursing framework. *J. Geriat. Nurs.*, **12**, 33–7.

Appendix A

SELF-CARE ASSESSMENT

LEVEL I – WHOLLY COMPENSATORY
LEVEL II – PARTLY COMPENSATORY
LEVEL III – EDUCATIVE SUPPORTIVE
LEVEL IV – INDEPENDENT

ASSESSMENT (*Yes Answer Requires Further Description)	YES	NO	I	II	III	IV	FURTHER DESCRIPTION
#1 AIR/FOOD/FLUIDS							
A. Breathing:							
*Problematic		×				■	
Difficulty breathing		×			■	■	
Danger of aspiration		×			■	■	
Danger of suffocation					■	■	
B. Smoking:							
Smoker	×			■	■	■	Must be reminded not to smoke in his room.
*Needs supervision of smoking	×				■	■	
Needs supply of cigarettes				■	■	■	
Needs funds to buy cigarettes							
C. *Fire Setting Potential Present		×				■	

D. Fluid intake:

*Problematic	X			X
Inadequate	X			X
Excessive				
Needs I & O	X			X

Does not take fluids unless reminded and offered

E. Food intake:

*Problematic	X			X
Inadequate				
Excessive				
Unable to eat in dining room				
Unusual mealtime/eating behavior				
*Needs nutritional teaching				
Recent weight changes	X			

Can't sit in dining room. Will not eat without reminders.

If so, _____ Lbs. _____ Loss _____ Gain _____ Over Last _____ Months

F. *History of ETOH abuse   ☒   Reports abuse.

G. *History of drug abuse   ☒   Reports marijuana and crack cocaine use.

H. Other (Describe)

GENERAL ASSESSMENT – AIR/FOOD/FLUIDS:

Overall Level of Self-Care Functioning: ☒   I ——— II ——— III ——— IV

Additional Comments: needs assistance and reminders in intake.

#2 ELIMINATION
A. Bowels:

ASSESSMENT (*Yes Answer Requires Further Description)	YES	NO	SELF-CARE LEVEL I	II	III	IV	FURTHER DESCRIPTION
*Problematic	X		X				Should improve with improved intake. Observe and document.
Unable to report problems independently							
Current problem – diarrhea							
constipation	X						
Uses corrective measures for problem							
diet							
medicine	X						
other							
Pattern Irregular	X						

B. Bladder:

*Problematic	X			
Unable to report problems independently				
Current problem – incontinence				
enuresis				
retention				
frequency				
discomfort				
Uses corrective measures for problem				
fluids				
medicine				
other				

C. Bathroom Behavior:

*Problematic				X	
Needs assistance finding					
Needs assistance using					
Notable elimination behavior					

D. Menstruation: N/A

*Problematic				.	
Patient has concerns					
Other					
Irregular Pattern					

E. Needs Teaching

F. Other (Describe)

GENERAL ASSESSMENT – ELIMINATION:

Overall Level of Self-Care Functioning: __X__ I _____ II _____ III _____ IV
Additional Comments

ASSESSMENT
(*Yes Answer Requires Further Description)

#3 BODY TEMPERATURE AND PERSONAL HYGIENE

A. Clothing:

ASSESSMENT	YES	NO	SELF-CARE LEVEL I	II	III	IV	FURTHER DESCRIPTION
*Problematic	×						Unable to attend to self.
Dressed inappropriately for weather	×						
Currently unkempt	×						
Unable to independently dress/ undress/change clothes	×						
Difficulty with laundering clothes	×						
*Unusual style of dress		×					
Needs additional clothes		×					
Needs resource for provision of additional clothing (identify)		×					

B. Hygiene:

						Unable to attend to self.
*Problematic	X					
Unable to independently: Bathe	X					
Shampoo	X					
Brush teeth	X					
Care for dentures						
Needs hygiene supplies (toothpaste, brush, etc.)		X				

C. Unable to maintain living area independently	X			

D. Needs teaching		

E. Other (Describe)		

GENERAL ASSESSMENT – BODY TEMPERATURE AND PERSONAL HYGIENE:

Overall Level of Self-Care Functioning: ____ X ____ I ____ II ____ III ____ IV

Additional Comments: needs constant direction and assistance to engage in any hygiene activities.

ASSESSMENT (*Yes Answer Requires Further Description)	YES	NO	SELF-CARE LEVEL				FURTHER DESCRIPTION
			I	II	III	IV	
#4 REST/ACTIVITY							
A. Sleep Pattern:							
*Problematic	×					■	In bed all day and night.
Irregular, inadequate							
Has current difficulty with Falling to sleep			■	■	■	■	
Frequent waking			■	■	■	■	
Early waking			■	■	■	■	
Excessive sleep	×		■	■	■	■	
Uses corrective measures for problems Medicine		×					
Other		×				■	
*Other sleep phenomena			■	■	■	■	

B. Work/School:

Employed

    Full time _____

    Part time _____

    Not at all ___X___

Student

    Full time _____

    Part time _____

    Not at all ___X___

*Problems

C. *Needs assistance with structuring activities of daily living

X		X		Defer for now.

D. *Needs assistance with structuring leisure time

X		X		Defer for now.

E. Leisure Activity:

   *Preference:

   *Resource for funds: defer

F. Exercise Patterns: Defer for now.

*Problematic	X				
Irregular physical exercise	X				
Physically inactive style	X				
Hyperactive					
Continually					
Periodically					
Responsive to corrective measures (identify)					
*Exercise preference defer					

GENERAL ASSESSMENT: REST/ACTIVITY

Overall Level of Self-Care Functioning: __X__ I _____ II _____ III _____ IV

Addition Comments: patient can't or won't structure day. Stays in room or bed at home and in hospital.

ASSESSMENT (*Yes Answer Requires Further Description)	YES	NO	SELF-CARE LEVEL				FURTHER DESCRIPTION
			I	II	III	IV	
#5 SOLITUDE/SOCIALIZATION							
A. *Special Precautions Needed							
Violence potential		×					
Suicide potential		×					
Elopement potential		×					
B. Mental Status:							Reports hearing voices. Observe for delusions.
*Problematic	×		×				
Confused							
Auditory/visual hallucinations	×		×				
Delusional thought content	?						
Needs reality testing	×		×				

C. Stimulus Barrier:

				Social interaction seems to increase head and neck jerking.
*Problematic	X		X	
Unable to tolerate external stimuli	X		X	
Able to tolerate only brief presence of others	X		X	
Unable to concentrate	X		X	

D. Interactional Style:

*Problematic	X		X	
Unclear verbal communication			X	
Tolerates only brief interactions	X		X	
Intrusive				
Withdrawn (stays in room)	X		X	

E. Sexuality Issues

						Notes
*Problematic	X					Patient reports voices tell him to make obscene gestures and speak obscene works. Actual relationship to sexual functioning unknown.
Hypersexual						
Uncomfortable with gender identity						
Identifies other problems of sexual functioning (identify)	X					
Birth control measures						

F. *Cultural Factors Affecting Hospitalization/Treatment

Language (non-English)					
Food preferences					
Religious beliefs					
Non-acceptance of need for hospitalization/treatment					
Other cultural factors					

G. Other

GENERAL ASSESSMENT – SOLITUDE/SOCIALIZATION
   Overall Level of Self-Care Functioning: ___ X ___ I _____ II _____ III _____ IV

Oriented to Unit: Yes ___ X ___ No _____ If No, State Reason _____

Informed of Patient Rights: Yes ___ X ___ No _____ If No, State Reason _____

_____
Mary Smith, R.N.
Signature/Title/Date

Developed by Langley Porter Psychiatric Institute, University of California, San Francisco.

Chapter 17

Roy's adaptation model: clinical applications

S. PURCELL and K. DORSEY

Introduction

Roy's adaptation model has been used internationally both in research and in clinical applications. The settings and studies suggest the flexibility of the model.

At the Alverno College Nursing Center for Wellness in Milwaukee, Wisconsin, the model has been used as a basis for a wellness programme on an outpatient service. Self-assessments of clients at the centre provide a useful tool to resolve health issues. The centre focuses on a healthier life style and presents information on health-oriented issues.

Hugh Chadderton, Director of the George Thomas Centre for Hospice Care, Cardiff, Wales, pioneered the use of the model in client interviews (Chadderton, 1988). Chadderton used the four modes of adaptation as the basis for his assessment tool. The format has provided a valuable format for more complex assessments of needs for the client and family.

Five graduate nursing students used the Roy adaptation model as a basis for practice in settings including obstetrics, paediatrics, outpatient clinics, intensive care units and medical/surgical, psychiatric and industrial health care offices. The researchers found that the model provided a vehicle for comprehensive nursing assessments. However, they found it difficult to utilize components of the model dealing with evaluations of residual stimuli in settings with rapidly changing circumstances (see Wagner, 1976).

Giger, Bower and Miller (1987) found that the use of Roy's model in an intensive care unit enhanced team communication and fostered a cohesive nursing care plan. The authors noted that control of the environment was facilitated by use of the model.

Leuze and McKenzie (1987) described the outcome of preoperative assessment based on the model tested at St Thomas Hospital, Nashville, Tennessee. Results revealed that nurses familiar with the model used the assessment tool more effectively, while organizing bio-psycho-social data.

At the National Hospital, Arlington, Virginia, a comprehensive administrative plan was implemented by Mastal, Hammond and Roberts (1982). In staff education and development, a tool utilizing the health–illness continuum proved to be time-consuming but essential. The model was still in use a year after implementation. The writers emphasized the importance of administrative support for implementation of a theory-based nursing practice model.

At the Roseburg Veterans' Administration Hospital, Roseburg, Oregon, the model was adapted for use in a nursing-home-setting nursing system as described by Dorsey and Purcell (1987). The four modes of adaptation provide structure for nursing assessments and intervention. Behaviour and related stimuli are assessed on admission, with monthly follow-up of goals and interventions which provide a holistic approach for long-term care.

A model for occupational health nursing was developed by Baughn (1977) to provide a systematic evaluation for the industrial settings. That author found that a more thorough assessment of bio-psycho-social needs was possible through the use of the model.

A theory-based curriculum for graduate students was implemented in Florida at the University of Miami School of Nursing. It provided a systematic process for geriatric nurse practitioner assessments following implementation of Roy's model. Changes in practice described by Brower and Baker (1976) indicated that the practitioners had expanded their assessments beyond disease processes to include the concerns of the elderly.

Farkas (1981) described a study which used the adaptation model to identify problems of the elderly in Calgary, Canada, who applied for nursing home admission. Study results revealed that adaptation problems in the physiological mode seem to be the determining factor for initiating a request for nursing home placement. The model served as a useful method for identifying the dynamics of interactions that play a key role in nursing home adjustments.

In studying the use of the adaptation model in an intensive care setting, Aggleton and Chalmers (1984) identified the quality of the nurse–patient relationship as a determining factor in accurate data collection. The authors recommend evaluation of the model in a variety of settings as a necessary step towards building credibility in clinical application.

Sato (1986) described a study which compared the accuracy of nursing diagnosis based on first-level assessment, then on first- and second-level assessments. Investigations found that nurses using first-level assessments made as many accurate diagnoses as did those using both levels of assessment.

The Roy adaptation model provides a framework for the identification of bio-psycho-social problems in a variety of settings through the four

Figure 17.1 Nursing care plan for W.G., based on Roy's adaptation model

1. *Physiological mode*	*Behaviour*	*Stimuli*
Nutrition	Refuses breakfast other than coffee; eats one-quarter to one-half of the remaining two meals; weight loss of 2 kg since admission.	Focal: nursing home dining room environment Contextual: depressed by nursing home patients in the dining room Residual: misses old friends from senior residence
Elimination	Bowel and bladder function intact	Focal: potential for altered function 2° to decreased food intake Contextual: no physical exercise Residual: no history of bowel/bladder problems
Skin integrity	Intact, dry normal ageing appearance; wrinkled gnarled fingers; nails clipped and clean.	Focal: normal ageing process Contextual: some grooming evident Residual: absence of pressure sores
Oxygenation	Blood pressure 110/70 Respiration 20 Pulse 80 and regular	Focal: intact circulatory and respiratory systems
Neurological function	Temperature 37.0°C Wears glasses Hearing aid in drawer, used on request	Focal: intact hypo-thalamus Focal: ageing changes Residual: rejects use
Activity/rest	Sleeps 10 hours at night, awakens fatigued; dozes in bed between meals Role mode within normal limits for age	Focal: rejects scheduled time for rest; no participation in activity and exercise programmes. Contextual: shares room with patient who has a multiple stroke history, cannot talk; lack of privacy. Residual: had self-directed activities; preferred life-style and had private room in prior residence.

Figure 17.1 (cont.)

Nursing process for physiological mode

Diagnosis: Actual/potential social isolation manifested by refusal to participate in nursing home programme, including nutritional maintenance.
Goal: The client will participate in team planning of his care within two weeks.
Interventions: 1. The nurse will assess client's functional level of activity, explore prior self-care and sleep practices. After assessment the nurse assists the client to write a specific activity/rest schedule and post it in his room.
2. The nurse will encourage client to make choices which will be adapted within the limits of the nursing home.
3. The nurse will set up a meeting time each morning during which progress and problems can be explored. The key to successful information exchange is the daily meeting and establishing a trust level.
Evaluations: The client makes his list of goals and meets daily with the nurse but continues to eat poorly.
Modification: Take client to kitchen to see how food is prepared and to meet cook and dietician. Client selects preferred place for meals and they are served there. Client begins to plan making diet choices.

2. *Role mode*

Role mapping
    Primary role: 75-year-old male resident in nursing home
    Secondary roles: widower, carpenter, retired
    Tertiary roles: bridge player, worker of crossword puzzles, history of successful independent life-style
Role selected: retired carpenter with history of independence in problem-solving

Instrumental behaviours	*Stimuli*
Made all decisions about living arrangements, including nursing home placement	Focal: consumer-oriented Contextual: nursing home setting different from senior residence; is financially able to live elsewhere Residual: has demonstrated ability to make effective choices in past

Expressive behaviour	
'Living in this place makes me feel like I will die soon.'	Focal: nursing home setting Contextual: able to perform all activities of daily living but sees self in sick, hopeless role

Nursing process for role mode

Diagnosis: Actual altered/deficit in role function secondary to reaction to nursing home placement

Figure 17.1   (cont.)

Goal:	The client within three months will make the appropriate transition to living in a nursing home or will explore appropriate alternative living arrangements within his financial and physical limit capabilities, within three months.
Interventions:	1. The nurse will suggest participation with team in planning outcomes including short- and long-term goals.
	2. The nurse will give positive encouragement to client's suggestions.
Evaluation:	The client was not aware that it might be possible to leave.

3. *Self-concept mode*

Component	Behaviour	Stimuli
Physical self Body sensations Body image	'I am tired all the time.' 'Don't the nurses know what I need. My wife did not mind caring for my needs.'	Focal: how client sees self Contextual: nursing home setting, in bed most of day; has functional cognitive level Residual: during stress, more accurately aware of loss of wife
Self-ideal	'Nobody wants me. That is why I'm here.'	Focal: reaction to nursing home admission, sees self as useless and undesirable Contextual: sees self as rejected because of nursing home setting Residual: history of pride in self, appropriate social interactions; dealing with Erickson's integrity versus control

Nursing process for the self-concept mode

Diagnosis:	Actual/potential alteration in self-image secondary to reaction to nursing home admission. Erickson (1968) identifies as part of the maturational crisis for the elderly the development of ego integrity for resolving dependency–independency needs.
Goal:	The client will examine current crisis for opportunities to enhance self concept.
Interventions:	1. The nurse will explore anxieties and assist client find choices to relieve anxieties.

Figure 17.1   (cont.)

2. The nurse will encourage the client to verbalize positive aspects of himself utilizing prior success experiences.
3. The nurse will arrange daily meetings with the client to enhance his self-esteem through the interest and reaction of the nurse.

Evaluations: The client once again was independent in his activities of daily living, i.e., dressing, grooming. He made friends readily and organized a bridge club.

4. Interdependence mode

Support system	Contributive behaviours	Stimuli
Primary nurse	Daily conferences	Focal: daily conferences
Health care team	Advocate role	were held between
		client and nurse.
	Plan ways with client to meet goals	Weekly conferences were held with team.

Nursing process for the interdependence mode

Diagnosis: Actual/potential social isolation in nursing home setting.
Goal: Client will work with staff to plan alternative placement or adjustment to nursing home setting within three months.
Interventions: 1. The nurse will participate in daily planning sessions with the client.
2. The nurse will facilitate meetings with health care team members.
Evaluation: At the end of three months, the client selected an alternative living setting which met his needs and was discharged. On occasion he returns to visit to share his successes with others.

adaptation modes. The following case study illustrates the use of Roy's adaptation model in a specific setting. The format in Fig. 17.1 was adapted from that developed by Sato (1986).

Case study

Mr W. G., at age seventy-five, was admitted to a nursing home after closure of the senior residence where he had resided for five years. Arthritis was his initial diagnosis. On admission, Mr W. G. stated, 'This is the end of the road for me, I might as well give up. No one wants me.'

The client, a self-taught carpenter, had always taken pride in his independence and good health. Married late in life at sixty, Mr W. G. was widowed when his wife, a nurse, died in a car accident. On retirement at sixty-five he moved to a senior residence which provided housekeeping services, including meals. In his new environment, Mr W. G. enjoyed playing bridge and working crossword puzzles. He was stunned when the facility closed with only two weeks' notice. On his physician's advice, Mr W. G. was admitted to a nursing home. The client's behaviour changed after admission, suggesting lowered self-esteem. He refused to participate in activities, his appetite decreased, and he lost interest in his appearance. Mr W. G.'s interactions with staff alternated between being hostile and being inappropriately friendly. Two weeks following admission, Mr W. G. became totally dependent on staff. His mental health issues included anxiety, hostility and low self-esteem.

Discussion

Relocation may be stressful in anyone's life. However, Rosswarm (1983) states that the person's perception of relocation is the key to coping effectively. The nursing care plan (see Fig. 17.1) explores strategies to resolve depression by changing the client's perception of the relocation experience.

The challenge to self-esteem that can occur during relocation may result in feelings of loss and grief which immobilize the individual according to Hirst and Metcalf (1984). The authors also point out that feelings of powerlessness may develop when experiencing institutionalization.

Dunning (1976) says that one of the developmental tasks for those over 65 years is to accept the help of others while maintaining the value of self. Anxiety results when there is an inconsistency between self-beliefs and perception of a crisis. Behavioural changes include activity dysfunctions as well as alterations in eating patterns (Perley, 1976).

By altering Mr W. G.'s perception of his relocation to the nursing home, he begins to make decisions and regains mastery. As Mr W. G. utilizes his life-long problem-solving skills, his depression resolves, as evidenced in resolution of his maladaptive behaviours.

Nursing interventions suggested in Fig. 17.1 are adapted from concepts developed by Roy (1976).

Summary

The case study illustrates the ability of Roy's adaptation model to facilitate assessment on a variety of bio-psycho-social components. Appropriate interactions of each component can then be developed.

The client expressed hostility, anxiety and lowered self-esteem through essentially the same behaviours. By focusing on the underlying problem, adjustment of perception of relocation, the physiological problems of reduced appetite and rest/sleep problems were resolved as the client coped with the focal stimulus of nursing home placement.

Roy's adaptation model enabled the nurse in the case study to isolate behaviour and related stimuli, and to develop interventions that facilitated adaptative coping with the experience of nursing home placement. The client increased his self-esteem, and relieved anxiety and reduced hostility by implementing coping strategies made possible through implementation of Roy's adaptation model.

References

Aggleton, P. and Chalmers, H. (1984) The Roy adaptation model. *Nurs. Times*, **80**, 45–8.

Baughn, S. (1977) A nursing theory and model for occupational health nursing. *Occupat. Health Nurs.*, **2**, 7–12.

Brower, T. and Baker, B. J. (1976) Using the adaptation model in a practitioner curriculum. *Nurs. Outlook*, **24**, 686–9.

Chadderton, H. (1988) Personal communication to authors.

Dorsey, K. and Purcell, S. (1987) Translating a nursing theory into a nursing system. *Geriat. Nurs.*, **8**, 136–7.

Dunning, J. (1976) Development of interdependence, in *Introduction to Nursing: an Adaptation Model* (ed. C. Roy), Prentice Hall, New Jersey.

Erickson, E. (1968) *Childhood and Society*, W.W. Norton, New York.

Farkas, L. (1981) Adaptation problems with nursing home applications for elderly persons: an application of the Roy adaptation nursing model. *J. Adv. Nurs.*, **6**, 363–8.

Giger, J., Bower, C. and Miller, S. (1987) Roy adaptation model: ICU application. *Dimens. Crit. Care Nursing*, **6**, 215–24.

Hirst, S. and Metcalf, B. (1984) Promoting self esteem. *J. Geront. Nursing.*, **10**, 72–7.

Leuze, M. and McKenzie, J. (1987) Preoperative assessment *Association of Operating Room Nurses (AORN)*, **46**, 1122–3.

Mastal, M., Hammond, H. and Roberts, M. (1982) Theory into hospital practice: a pilot implementation. *J. Nurs. Admin.*, **12**, 9–15.

Perley, N. (1976) Problem in self consistency: anxiety, in *Introduction to Nursing: an adaptation model* (ed. C. Roy), Prentice-Hall, N.J.

Rosswarm, M. (1983) Relocation and the elderly. *J. Geront. Nurs.*, **9**, 632–7.

Roy, C. (1976) Nursing Intervention Based on Roy Adaptation Model, in *Introduction to Nursing: an adaptation model* (ed. C. Roy) Prentice-Hall, N.J.

Sato, M. (1986) The Roy adaptation model. *Case Histories in Nursing Theory*, National League for Nursing, New York, Pub. No. 1, 5–2152.

Wagner, D. (1976) Testing the adaptation model in practice. *Nurs. Outlook*, **6**, 682–5.

Chapter 18

The eclectic approach: clinical applications

B. BENFER and P. SCHRODER

Case study

Susan Smith, a 23-year-old single female, was admitted to the psychiatric unit following a suicidal gesture. She had taken an overdose of Haldol, a medication that had been prescribed for her because of increasing psychiatric symptoms. Susan had been in outpatient treatment for a year, since she had begun experiencing auditory hallucinations with the voice of a priest telling her that she was bad. A precipitating event to her overdose had been a sexual encounter with a male student from the same university that Susan attended. Susan had lived at home and attended a local vocational college before starting at the University a year and a half before. During her time at the university, her ability to concentrate on her studies and to carry out activities of daily living had gradually deteriorated, although she continued to be able to function well in some structured classes. At times she was easily agitated, and her language became fragmented when there was an increase in stress for her.

Susan's parents accompanied her to the hospital. They described her as an only child, admitting that she might have been overprotected. In her childhood years she was fearful of school, clung to her mother, and had very few friends. As a young child Susan had been very ill with rheumatic heart disease and was left with some residual weakness. Following the illness, she had been unable to participate fully in usual childhood activities, but there was no restriction on her activities at the present time. Initially in her early years in school Susan had achieved high grades, but when she was 12 her grades dropped to near failing. The drop in grades coincided with a sexual assault by an uncle that was not known to the parents until a year later. At the same time, it was noticed that Susan had become more fearful and withdrawn. At the age of 15, Susan did socialize a few times with peers that did not meet with parental approval, and the parents discovered that she had begun to use street drugs with them. The parents threatened to send Susan to live with her grandmother, and Susan promised to no longer use drugs or socialize with the group. Her grades in school improved, but she did not develop new friends, and was seen by peers and teachers as a loner.

While Susan stayed close to her mother, looking to her for affirmation of what she should say and do, she did not appear to have a close relationship with her father. Susan's father is described as a strict disciplinarian, who was away from the home a great deal, since he works the evening shift at a nearby factory. Susan saw little of him in her formative years.

Nursing assessment

Upon admission to the unit, Susan denied being depressed. When questioned about her overdose, she minimized the seriousness of it, saying that dying was her destiny, and that the voice of a priest told her to overdose and that everything would be OK. She giggled frequently throughout the interview, but would not share with the nurse what was humorous. She became enraged when told that she could not leave the hospital with her mother, then repeatedly demanded that she be allowed to call her mother immediately even though her mother had not yet had time to arrive home. Susan calmed down temporarily when her therapist arrived on the unit to meet her. Susan's attire was dishevelled, and she wore extensive make-up. She was immediately attracted to young male patients on the unit, and made inappropriate remarks to them. She had to be reminded of unit guidelines about not wearing her nightgown without a robe into the lounge at night.

Planning the nursing care and treatment of Susan requires that the nurse be skilled in obtaining data for a thorough assessment, as well as having a sound conceptual framework and philosophical approach upon which to base interventions once data have been obtained. Building upon the framework set forth in Chapter 10, the authors of this chapter will formulate an approach to Susan's care, using psychodynamic concepts based upon a knowledge of Susan's growth and development as well as her present strengths and weaknesses, and will postulate how the nurse can make maximum use of the milieu for this particular patient.

One of the first priorities for the nurse is to collect the necessary data in order to make nursing diagnoses and develop the plan of care. With Susan, it would be essential to collect data relative to her lethality as well as her depression, both current and past, to ascertain any threat that the patient poses to herself at the present time. The nurse will want to further assess whether any suicidal gestures are a result of depression and hopelessness, or whether she is acting on input from voices. If she is engaging in impulsive acts in response to voices, the nurse would have more awareness that a problem exists in terms of Susan's ability to differentiate between internal stimuli and reality. Whether the patient is genuinely depressed or acting impulsively in response to internal stimuli, the nurse should at least initially assume that an immediate suicide threat exists, and take steps to ensure Susan's safety from her own impulses. This will take priority over other psychological needs if both cannot be met simultaneously.

Obtaining information about the voices Susan hears will be one focus for the nurse, who will want to find out when the voices started, the frequency with which they occur, and the content. If hallucinations began after Susan's experimentation with street drugs, there could exist a linkage to the ingestion of unknown substances. In such a case, part of Susan's problem could be a drug-induced psychosis. The nurse would want to keep in mind that Susan could have continued to take drugs without the knowledge of her family. Additionally, the nurse will elicit information whether Susan experiences the auditory voices at times of stress, and if the voices are accusatory or offer relief from a threatening external world for her. Family history is also useful. The history of the family can be used to determine whether close family members suffer from similar problems, thus suggesting a hereditary factor, or to give treaters a clue as to environmental factors that could have had an impact on Susan. The history from the mother reveals little evidence to suggest that heredity is of any importance in Susan's case.

In addition to objective data, information about attitudes and feelings should be a part of the psychosexual history. It would be overly simplistic to assume that problems Susan experiences in heterosexual relationships stem entirely from the sexual assault that took place when she was 12 years old. The rape would indeed be a significant event that would impact on the child's developing sexual identity as well as personal identity, but the nurse should also obtain information relative to what it means to Susan now. Clues exist that the rape was traumatic for her, that she had been unable to talk about it at the time, and that she is presently confused in terms of relationships with males whether the relationship is sexual or not. In addition to what Susan says verbally, the nurse would note whether non-verbal clues, such as body language of fidgeting, increase when the topic is on sexuality.

Not only would the nurse seek information relative to problems in Susan's life, but attention would be given to areas of strength and those things which Susan has done well in the past or presently.

Diagnostic and dynamic conceptualization

In conjunction with the psychiatrist, social worker, activity therapist, and psychologist, the nurse would be part of the treatment team that would form a diagnostic and dynamic picture of the patient. Each discipline would contribute data which had been collected from the patient or the family, or from interaction with the patient during the initial hospitalization. The therapist could also contribute to the understanding of the patient. In planning Susan's treatment, several events from Susan's developmental years would be deemed as significant. Specifically this would include her physical illness when she was two years old, her difficulties in separating from her mother, her difficulties in school, the sexual assault when she was 12 years of age, her use of street drugs to try to fit in with peers, and the distant relationship which she had with her father. Based on research of Mahler, Pine and Bergman (1967) and Mahler and Furer (1968) it can be assumed that while there was initially normal healthy symbiosis between Susan as an infant and her mother, her childhood was not problem-free. The process of separation and thus formation of a differentiated view of self was thwarted by Susan's bout with a life-threatening illness that required protection for physical reasons, and that interfered with her psychological development. Susan would have, by empathic communication, picked up her mother's anxiety. That anxiety would have threatened the child's security and her efforts to move away from mother to try new behaviours that a child needs to learn in order to have a separate sense of self apart from mother. The insecurity and need to have mother's presence at all times carried over to when Susan began school, still frightened and anxious if her mother was not there. The fusion between mother and child likely served a need for both of them, with the mother's sense of well-being also dependent upon the presence of the child. This is not to say that the mother was bad; anxiety related to a child's welfare would have been a natural sequela to the severe illness, leading to overprotectiveness. With Susan's security so closely tied to mother, Susan would have been ill-prepared to be involved in the tasks of learning to relate to peers, learning to compete, to compromise and eventually to co-operate with peers, all activities important to a child in order to learn competence and cooperation.

From the therapist, the team learned that Susan had suffered a severe stress trauma as a result of being raped. Susan had been at an age when she was just beginning to enter puberty, which in itself is a time of anxiety and stress regarding the process of physical maturation as well as psychological development. It is noteworthy that problems during this process can readily cause an adolescent to remain fixated within childhood behaviour patterns, and continue to use childhood defences. Susan had been attracted to her uncle in her search for a caring father figure, and not having male siblings or having her father around the house often left Susan ill-prepared and unknowledgeable about dealing with males in general as well as not knowing how to deal with emerging sexual feelings. Susan had responded to hugs of affection, and the uncle took advantage of her naivety, and forced her to have intercourse, then threatened her if she told anyone. In order to handle the physical and psychological assault that created overwhelming anxiety and confusion, Susan blocked it out of conscious memory, by the use of the defence mechanism of repression, with no recall of the incident. However, when Susan became sexually involved with a fellow student, the defence of repression no longer was effective. The subsequent anxiety was a factor in the disintegration of her coping skills. Susan's more detailed recall surfaced in the therapy process.

Living within the protected environment of the family, Susan managed to function marginally through her formative years, and did develop some adaptive ability, so that when she was not under undue stress or was not in new or unfamiliar situations, she could cope with life. While living at home, she was able to complete successfully a course of general study at a local vocational college. However, when she left home for the environment of the larger university, and without the dependent relationship everyday with her mother, the fact that there was decompensation was not surprising. At the time of admission to the hospital, she had regressed to using coping mechanisms that were more appropriate to a child and less adaptive as an adult, such as giggling when anxious, waiting for all decisions to be made for her, and labelling herself or others as good or bad.

Ego strengths and weakness assessment

Using the ego functioning scale of Bellak, Hurrich and Gediman (1973) as described in Chapter 10 of this text, the nurse would find it helpful to assess where Susan would fit on the scale of ego weakness or ego strength. As seen in Fig. 18.1, Susan would receive a rating of four on most items, or slightly below midpoint. Such a rating reflects impairment, but also potential for growth in each area. The deficits in judgement and regulation of drives, impulses and affect are three areas which can easily

Figure 18.1 Rating of Susan on ego functioning scale

	Ego weakness							Ego strength		
	1	2	3	4	5	6	7	8	9	10
Reality testing				×						
Judgement			×							
Impulse control			×							
Object relations			×							
Thought processes				×						
Autonomous functions				×						
Synthetic–integrative functioning				×						
Mastery-competence				×						

be addressed in a nursing plan of care. Similarly, problems in relationships that are identified with a low score on object relations are generally responsive to psychiatric intervention, such as consistent daily one-to-one contact. Areas of greater strength for Susan are in terms of her thought process, with Susan being able to think clearly when not under stress. Equally, Susan has a higher score in autonomous functioning, an area that has been less impacted by her illness.

Nursing care

Utilizing the data available, the nurse would need to further define areas to address in Susan's care. Several areas will need the nurse's attention including the patient's potential lethality, her poor judgement, the lack of ability to relate well to others within the milieu, her poorly defined self-image, issues of sexuality, resolution of Susan's fear of males, her need to learn more adaptive coping skills, and her dependency, particularly on female authority figures. However, within this chapter we have selected to focus on only three of the issues. It is expected that the patient's problems will be phrased in terms of nursing diagnoses, with defined interventions and patient goals. For this chapter we will be dealing with impaired interpersonal relationships, disturbance in self-concept, and impaired impulse control.

Impaired interpersonal relationships

A nursing diagnosis of impaired interpersonal relationships can be used to encompass a wide range of interactional patterns. These can range from withdrawl from interactions with others to inappropriate intrusion into other's lives and conversations, to extremes in intensity within a relationship. The nurse identified that this nursing diagnosis was appropriate for Susan, based upon several factors. These included the patient's inappropriate seductive behaviour toward male patients and staff and her lack of knowledge of how to relate to males, her inability to engage in casual conversation, her history of confusing sexual closeness with other forms of relating, her over-dependency upon her mother and therapist with severe separation anxiety when they were not physically present, her history of withdrawal and isolation from peers and lack of friends, presently as well as during her school years, and a history of being unable to form and maintain sustained relationships outside of the immediate family. The nurse made the assessment that Susan's primary form of relating has been to become immediately overattached and fused with others, or to distance herself completely from others. Since the patient's ability to relate satisfactorily with others will be essential to her functioning outside of the hospital, the nurse deemed this to be a major nursing care issue that would require attention throughout the patient's hospital stay.

The origin of difficulties in impaired interpersonal relationships lies with earlier developmental tasks which were not completed. Specifically, as a child, the patient has often had beginning difficulties in the separation–individuation from the parenting figure. During latency (6–12 years) and puberty (ages 12 to 17 years) a child typically makes much progress toward a basic sense of identity, and then learns intimacy instead of isolation. Even when there have been earlier problems, corrective learning experiences during these phases allow the child to develop in spite of the earlier inadequacies. For patients such as Susan, major traumatic events (such as rape) prevent the child from being able to use opportunities to grow. The child who already is inept with peers is thrust into still more experiences that he/she is expected to learn prior to an adult stage of development. While other children are learning how to compete, to compromise, and cooperate in mutual endeavours, all tools necessary in the developmental task of learning to form satisfactory relationships, the traumatized child has not learned the same skills. Instead, he/she may remain isolated, with the resultant loneliness often contributing to depression. Without play-mates, the child is more likely to engage in fantasy or private thought that is not validated with others, furthering the difference between themselves and others.

The nursing care of patients with impaired interpersonal relationships will focus a great deal on patient teaching. Through individual contacts as well as group participation, the nurse cannot only teach, but can provide the patient with opportunity to test out new patterns of relating to others that will increase the patient's sense of being understood and accepted, making him less fearful of contacts with others.

Disturbance in self-concept

A nursing diagnosis of disturbance in self-concept requires that the nurse make a distinction or differentiate between disturbances in self-concept, self-identity and low self-esteem as identified by Sundeen *et al.* (1989). In practice, the nurse will frequently find that the patient's difficulties in one of these areas is not isolated from the others, and will select the diagnosis that seems to fit best for each case. A justifiable argument could be made to select any one of these as a nursing diagnosis for Susan, but the authors chose to focus on the self-concept.

Self-concept involves the perceptions which an individual has of himself or herself as separate from others. Being based upon interpersonal and experiential situations throughout life, self-concept includes not only others' observations and feedback, but also one's own perception of self in relation to reality.

Sullivan (1953) formulated the concept of the self-system as developing in infancy to include the good me or positive picture of oneself that is a result of experiencing tenderness and approval from others. The bad me or negative self-view arises from experiences which increase the anxiety state of the individual, and the not me which are those aspects of the person which are rejected and disowned as being a personification in response to overwhelming anxiety that is either not understood or which create awe, dread or horror for the person. While later experiences can alter the self-views developed earlier, an individual tends to incorporate input which is ego syntonic, or that which matches the view held of oneself. Input that is ego dystonic, or different from our own self-concept is more likely to be discarded or rejected. An integrated self-concept is necessary for a stable ego identity, and determines the individual's later stability, integration, and flexibility (Kernberg, 1975). The mental mechanisms of projection and introjection are closely linked to the process of developing a stable self-concept.

The concept of self includes self-esteem, perception of body image, and an individual's sense of identity; of who we are in total. Self-concept strongly influences the degree to which an individual has a sense of mastery over his/her environment, and shapes the competence to take an active role to master one's own destiny.

In the case of Susan, the nurse based her decision to make a nursing diagnosis of disturbance in self-concept upon the patient's diffuse sense of identity, as Susan continued to rely heavily upon others to define who she was at any given time. Additionally, Susan's image of herself was that she was of little value and her life was not worth preserving. She lacked confidence in handling any aspect of her own life other than the most trivial detail, and there was not an acceptance of herself as a person with any worth. With the team, the nurse made the assessment that Susan's overdose was not a direct suicide attempt, but rather a reflection of her distorted self-concept and low self-esteem, as well as a lack of impulse control. (In practice, during the initial hospitalization, a tentative nursing diagnosis of potential for suicide or self-injury would be prudent, but the authors have deliberately elected other nursing problems in the assumption that discussion of suicidal behaviour may have been addressed elsewhere in this text.)

Susan's early illness left her in a position of relying heavily upon her mother for input beyond the time when a child usually has begun to look to others as well. Because of Susan's isolation from others, there was inadequate input from peers, teachers, and others that could have broadened her self-concept in her formative years. The absence of her father, and thus his emotional unavailability to her, did not provide opportunity for her to develop a self-concept in relation to males, and the rape would have made her even more fearful of any exploration in terms of defining herself in relation to male figures. Compounding her lack of interpersonal relating with other children, Susan would have failed to develop competencies and skills that would have helped solidify a positive self-concept. Without external validation, she would have relied upon possible distorted impressions of her capabilities and who she was. Her ideal self, or the person she thought she should be, was a vague image of a good girl, loosely associated with a definition of good or bad coming from her religion. When her defences failed to work for her, that image became a projection as onto the voice of a priest in her fantasy.

When Susan moved from the secure, predictable environment of home to college, her familiar stable figure of mother was no longer available to mirror an identity for her, and Susan's self-concept would have become more tenuous. In her therapist, Susan found another person to serve this role, developing a transference to that therapist. The nurse would anticipate that if Susan perceives her as caring and nurturing, a transference will also take place with Susan putting the nurse in that role of mirroring an identity for her.

The experience of hospitalization will open the door so that Susan will be accessible to new input in regard to her self-concept, through new experiences and the potential for new relationships. Through aiding Susan to identify and express her thoughts and feelings, Susan can develop a greater sense of self. This in turn will lead to increased self-esteem and self-acceptance, the essence of personality integration (Stuart and Sundeen, 1987). The earlier identification of ego strengths will be helpful in that the nurse will attempt to enhance areas of strength for an improved self-concept.

Impaired impulse control

Technically speaking, impaired impulse control would at the current time be more appropriately deemed a nursing care problem rather than a nursing diagnosis, in that the North American Nursing Diagnosis Association (NANDA) has not accepted it as an official nursing diagnosis. However, there is little doubt that impaired impulse control is a major issue for many patients that calls for skilled nursing assessment and intervention.

Impaired impulse control is closely related to the ego function of regulation and control of drives, affect and impulses (Bellak *et al.*, 1973), as well as being related to the ego function of judgement. Many professionals view impulsiveness negatively; however, acting upon an impulse is neither good nor poor judgement. Rather, there is an absence of judgement. Impulsive behaviour is an unpremeditated, irrational action, usually in response to a basic need. That need may be pleasure-oriented, that is, to do spontaneously something without giving thought to consequences or results, such as impulsively purchasing an article of clothing because it's attractive rather than needed, and without concern to finances. Additionally, impulsive behaviour may be driven toward relief from an unpleasant strong emotion, such as striking another person when angry, or cutting upon oneself rather than face an unpleasant encounter. Impulsive behaviours that are maladaptive usually are in response to feelings about something that is threatening to the ego integrity of the person, in other words, something that threatens the individual's self-concept, their idealized image of self, or self-esteem. Impulsive behaviour that is in response to such a threat is more likely to be of an aggressive nature.

It should be noted that an individual can have impaired impulse control by over-control as well as when there is lack of control of impulses. With over-control, a person can come across to others as rigid, non-adaptive, with little tolerance for deviation from routine. With under-control, an individual may be able to keep impulses in check most of the time, but then engage in impulsive behaviour at times of stress. The impulses may be directed toward self, such as alcohol or food binges, or may be directed toward others, such as hitting, shouting, or other forms of assault. The nurse made the assessment that Susan suffered from impaired impulse control based upon the history of the patient's overdose with her medication, her sexual liaison with a male that she knew only slightly, and her yelling and weeping when her mother left the hospital. Additionally, some of her behaviours following admission, for example, wearing a scanty nightgown to the lounge and her seductive behaviour, were seen as having some elements of poor impulse control as well as impaired judgement. Susan also found it difficult to tolerate any frustration, another indication of poor impulse control. At times Susan exercised over-control of impulses, while at other times, there was undercontrol.

Initially the nurse will find it helpful to use structure and unit routine to help Susan appropriately deal with impulses and to provide safety for both Susan and other patients. Later, patient teaching in regard to alternate ways of handling feelings as well as ways to relate to others will become the primary focus in helping with the impairment in impulse control.

Establishing goals

Having identified three major nursing care problems currently interfering with Susan's adjustment, the nurse will set forth long-range goals in relation to those problems. Hopefully Susan will have made much progress toward those goals during her hospitalization, although continued work will remain to be done outside of the hospital as well. The long-range goals will include the aim that Susan will be able to form and maintain meaningful relationships outside of her immediate family; that Susan will be able to identify and implement adaptive coping behaviours in response to her impulsive thoughts and drives, and that Susan will formulate a concept of herself as an individual with improved self-esteem based upon achievement of realistic goals and tasks. While these goals do not encompass all that must take place in order for Susan to have improved mental health, they do give the nurse a sense of direction for interventions with the patient. Additionally, short-term goals and measurable objectives can be developed by which the nurse can measure Susan's progress toward the longer-term goals.

Since Susan's life is not in a vacuum, but rather takes place within the unit environment, the various aspects of that milieu must be considered in helping Susan to develop new coping skills.

Milieu

As identified by Colson *et al.* (1986), the task of the hospital milieu is to contain and process affects of the patients, and it is a place where team members strive to identify and understand the broad array of personal reactions that accompany their work and use this information as an aid to understanding patients and planning their treatment. The use of milieu therapy requires a high degree of team effort among all disciplines, but the role of the psychiatric nurse is of paramount importance. Knowledge and expertise is required, due to the close relationship that the nurse must have with the patients throughout the entire twenty-four-hour day. This means that nurses must not only assess the individual needs, the ego strengths and weaknesses of each patient, know the problems and goals of each patient, but must also provide an environment for the group of patients that is safe, yet one that stimulates learning and growth.

Determination of those facets of the milieu that will be helpful to a particular patient incorporates a consideration of not only that patient, but other patients, staff, the environment itself, and the interplay between these various components. Stuart and Sundeen (1987) point out that there are several basic assumptions regarding milieu approaches in in-patient psychiatric treatment. These include: (1) patients have strengths and conflict-free areas of their personalities; (2) they can influence their own treatment constructively as well as the treatment of others and to a degree, the organized structure of the hospital; (3) successful treatment is dependent on pervasive, therapeutic staff involvement; and (4) all levels of staff have potential for exercising a therapeutic influence.

Benfer and Schroder (1985) have articulated the specific actions that must go on within a milieu in order for it to be therapeutic. These include: (1) providing for basic needs of the patient; (2) offering organization and structure to the patient's life; (3) giving support and aiding intrapsychic growth; (4) assisting the patient with interpersonal and interactional skills; and (5) promoting coping skills in a teaching and learning environment. To determine the kind of activity in each of these five areas that fit the needs of the patient, the assessment of the patient's ego strengths or weaknesses can be one parameter for that judgement. In the case of Susan, it is useful to focus on strengths and weaknesses both in terms of present functioning as well as past functioning. An example of strength would be her intellectual capabilities, demonstrated by her college work except for most recent times. Susan's talent of playing the piano would be another strength which would be particularly useful as the nurse searches for non-threatening ways to help Susan begin to relate to others.

Using the framework set forth by Benfer and Schroder (1985), the nurse can look at the more specific milieu needs experienced by Susan.

Providing for basic needs

In terms of the degree of assistance needed by Susan in handling activities of daily living, a need for a safe environment, and assuring Susan that her needs for shelter, food, space and safety are met, there will be variation from that which is needed initially and that which will be needed later. Upon admission, Susan will need a safe, controlled environment. Not only must the nurse protect Susan from physical danger, but Susan is at risk for potential acts which could be embarrassing to her or interfere with others' acceptance of her. Except in situations where there is a strong emotional reaction or increase in anxiety, Susan has relative strength in the area of autonomous functioning, being able to focus her attention, perceive what is said to her, ability to recall, and carry out routine activities with minimal difficulty. If Susan has a sense that the nurse is looking after basic needs, she will feel more secure and receptive to interventions.

Organization and structure

Structure offered by the unit's routine and boundaries will give Susan guidelines for appropriate behaviour, as will the supervision provided by nursing staff. Since Susan tends to become more disorganized and fragmented with stress, the external structure offered and the continuity will help her reorganize her thoughts and retain better contact with reality. Susan's reality testing was impaired at the time of admission, but this was more likely a projection of her internal world onto reality rather than a true hallucination. Part of the poor reality testing can be attributed to her limited validation with others. Later, when Susan's reality testing has improved, there will be less need for structure, especially when the nurse sets up situations where Susan can try new behaviours and as she becomes more sure of herself.

Giving support and aiding intrapsychic growth

Susan has perhaps her greatest ego weakness in the area of object relationships, with extreme dependence on parenting figures, and anxiety when there is separation. She has minimal internalization of relationships, being unable to recall, remember or experience a relationship when the other person is not present. Her relationships with males is chaotic, with Susan making primitive efforts to establish closeness, but being unable to handle the emotions when others do try to get close to her. Correction of these weaknesses requires improvement in relationships and an enhanced self-concept, as was identified earlier in the nursing care problems. Additionally, Susan has relative weakness in the ego functioning area of synthetic–integrative functioning, with her life being experienced more as bits and pieces, non-related and without continuity since she has used repression as a major defence much of her life. The nurse's role in helping Susan recognize feelings, tie thoughts, feelings and actions together, and communicate directly are all activities that fall into the realm of giving support and aiding intrapsychic growth. While some actions by the nurse in the other areas of the milieu will be generally viewed by the patient as being cared for, the patient may or may not be aware of the part the nurse plays in helping her with intrapsychic growth. Ideally, the patient will instead be aware of how she has grown; the work she has done, and take credit herself for the change and incorporate it into her own self-concept.

Early support will be given by offering Susan continuity, consistency in contacts, and acceptance. As Susan improves, the support will become more acknowledgement and approval of things that Susan does for herself and her accomplishments.

Assisting the patient with interpersonal and interactional skills
Earlier in this chapter, it was mentioned that one of the nursing care problems was Susan's impairment in interpersonal relationships. Thus, work within this area of the milieu will be of prime importance. Helping patients with interpersonal relationships involves supporting the patient as he/she learns socialization skills and learns to be more at ease with others, and giving immediate feedback and validation. Not only can the nurse assist the patient, but other patients can play an important therapeutic role in offering the needed support and validation. The milieu becomes an arena where the patient can learn about his/her own interactions, apply what has been learned, and then adopt the improved or new ways of interaction instead of continuing to use the former non-productive methods of relating. The patient is given opportunity to practise new skills first on a one-to-one basis, then she can be introduced gradually to groups when new skills can be further developed and refined. Groups within the milieu can also give the patient opportunity to develop skills in addition to interpersonal ones. For example, a patient can learn to play a sport such as volleyball, or learn to cook or sew, or learn ways to express artistic skills not developed previously.

Susan could be expected to be more comfortable with one-to-one relationships initially, and would need the nurse to be sensitive to the timing for advancing her to group activities. With the identified strength of being a good learner, one could expect Susan to do well in this area.

Promoting coping skills within a teaching environment

Successful experiences with the nurse and other patients will be paramount in the development of Susan's strengths and will directly impact upon her self-esteem. Through being able to do activities well, and then to receive affirmation from others that they also see her as doing well, will help Susan to feel positive about herself. Susan's sheltered early life has hindered her learning many skills others in her age range would have mastered. Individual work with Susan prior to group participation could prevent her from continuing to feel different, and thus isolated, from age mates. The focus of teaching, however, would not fall solely on activities. Part of the teaching includes how to express feelings, how to initiate a conversation, how to control undesired thoughts, how to appropriately express sexual feelings, as well as other topics individualized for the patient.

A key component of the promotion of coping skills includes allowing the patient to assume responsibility for those areas of his/her life that can be managed, and takes into consideration the readiness to assume responsibility, as well as capability. Susan would probably be hesitant about making decisions for herself, lacking confidence in herself to do so. However, with encouragement and support, it can be assumed that she could do well. Later in her treatment, she would be encouraged to participate in patient government, committees, or similar activities that involve responsibility. This would help her to gain confidence in decision making as well as help her to develop skill in working with others.

Summary of nursing care

After reviewing what the milieu can offer, and assessing Susan's particular ego strengths and weaknesses, the nurse is in a position to implement Susan's plan of care. Several activities and interventions will serve to promote growth in all three problem areas identified. The nurse would begin by establishing a working relationship with Susan on a one-to-one basis, provide reality orientation as needed, and offer continuity through meeting with her on a regular, consistent basis. The milieu would be used to provide the necessary check for Susan's impulsive behaviour as it arises, so that there will be neither danger nor embarrassment due to loss of control. Susan would be encouraged to talk about topics where she felt secure, with the nurse taking care not to force Susan to talk about events or experiences she was not ready to discuss. Attempts would be made to help her begin to clarify distortions of reality, separating thoughts and feelings from actions.

Initially, external stimuli would be kept to a minimum, with Susan participating in unit activities only to the degree that she could tolerate without a sharp increase in anxiety. From the beginning, Susan would be encouraged to make decisions for herself in regard to choice of activities, to take care of herself and her activities of daily living, and to have the opportunity to withdraw if things became too stressful for her. Gradually the nurse would provide less direct nurturance, as that would run the risk of making Susan too comfortable and not encouraging her to reach out to others. Feedback to Susan would be a constant process, as would encouragement for her to look at her feelings and behaviour, identifying what does not work well for her and what she would like to be different in her life. Using the learning process, the nurse can aid the patient in the exploration of alternatives which she can try, and then provide opportunity within the milieu for the new behaviours to be integrated. Throughout, use will be made of Susan's strengths, such as being good at sports once she learns them, sewing well, doing attractive art work with another patient in making unit posters, or helping another patient style her hair.

As Susan becomes more comfortable with groups, she would be supported in taking an active role with the group; to share her observations, and feedback to and from other patients would be encouraged. Structured groups, such as self-awareness groups, values clarification groups, medication groups, etc. would also be used to work toward the goal of improved self-concept. Anticipating the likelihood of a strong transference reaction from the patient, the nurse could expect the patient to use the primitive defence of splitting, whereby authority figures would be seen as all good or all bad, depending upon the patient's internal state and the degree to which there had been gratification of needs. An attitude which would convey acceptance of both positive and negative feelings toward the nurse by the patient, without rejection or disapproval, would give Susan additional security to express her ideas or thoughts without fear. Being able to talk to the nurse individually, and later within a group, about feelings about self and others would be important for Susan in working toward resolution of all three nursing problems identified. Ownership of one's own emotions is a key component of self-concept; it's essential in being able to form and maintain relationships, and feelings that are talked about are far less likely to be acted upon, thus providing the necessary control of impulses and drives previously operational for Susan on an unconscious basis.

Summary

Throughout the chapter, the authors have followed the case example of Susan, focusing upon three nursing care problems of impaired interpersonal relationships, poorly defined self-concept, and impaired impulse control. By using concepts drawn from the nursing process, ego strengths and weaknesses, and concepts related to the therapeutic milieu, the reader can identify methods by which successfully to make nursing interventions with the identified patient or similar patients.

References

Bellak, K., Hurich, M. and Gediman, H. K. (1973) *Ego-Functions in Schizophrenics, Neurotics and Normals: a Systematic Study of Conceptual, Diagnostic, and Therapeutic Aspects*, John Wiley, New York.

Benfer, B. and Schroder, P. (1985) Nursing in the therapeutic milieu. *Bull. Menninger Clin.*, **49**, 451–65.

Colson, D., Allen, J., Coyne, L. *et al.* (1986) An anatomy of countertransference: staff reactions to difficult psychiatric hospital patients. *Hosp. Commun. Psych.*, **37**, 923–8.

Kernberg, O. (1975) *Borderline Conditions and Pathological Narcissism*, J. Aronson, New York.

Mahler, M. and Furer, M. (1968) On human symbiosis and vicissitudes of individuation. *Infant. Psychosis*, **1**, 740–63.

Mahler, M., Pine, F. and Bergman, A. (1967) *The Psychological Birth of the Human Infant*. Basic Books, New York.

Stuart, G. and Sundeen, S. (1987) *Principles and Practice of Psychiatric Nursing*, C. V. Mosby, St Louis, MO.

Sullivan, H. S. (1953) *The Interpersonal Theory of Psychiatry*, Norton, New York.

Sundeen, S., Stuart, G., Rankin, E. *et al.* (1989) *Nurse–Client Interaction – Implementing the Nursing Process*, 4th edn, C. V. Mosby, St Louis, MO.

Part Four

ISSUES RELATED TO TEACHING, LEARNING, PSYCHIATRIC AND MENTAL HEALTH NURSING, AND THE SCOPE OF PSYCHIATRIC NURSING RESEARCH

This section, Chapters 19–21, has two major objectives. First, it examines the dynamics of supervision (particularly within the clinical area) from the viewpoints of the teacher and learner. The teaching–learning models described in the first two chapters originated from the authors' accumulated teaching, clinical and research experience over the past decade. Essentially, these chapters examine the conditions and processes which are considered necessary to move the learner towards clinical excellence.

Secondly, the existing contribution of nursing research towards the state of the art in psychiatric and mental health nursing is considered. (Banister and Kagan, 1985.) This final chapter provides an overview of existing research, its limitation, its contribution to the existing knowledge base, and suggests areas for future research.

Reference

Banister, P. and Kagan, C. (1986) The need for research into interpersonal skills in nursing, in *Interpersonal Skills in Nursing: Research and Applications* (ed. C. Kagan) Croom Helm, London.

Chapter 19

Teaching psychiatric and mental health nursing: a teaching perspective

W. REYNOLDS

Introduction

In this chapter a conceptual model (the psychodynamic learning model) for teaching and learning is described. This model originated from the writer's accumulated teaching, clinical and research work, over the past decade. It is proposed that the conditions and processes within this model are necessary, and have the capacity, to move the nurse learner (basic and post-basic) from novice, or basic competence, toward clinical excellence, in a variety of clinical settings (community and hospital) and with all psychiatric clients (children, adolescents and adults).

I will focus on the teaching and learning of psychotherapeutic nursing activity. In Chapter 1, psychotherapeutic activity was defined as the manner in which the nurse personally (as a professional with certain learned competencies) influenced the mental health status of the client, and it was suggested that psychotherapeutic work was the primary function of the psychiatric nurse. Thus, my rationale for concentrating on one aspect of the nurse's role is based upon the view that psychotherapeutic skills, utilized in many forms, are the major therapeutic tools available to psychiatric nurses, and my view that these skills are amongst the most difficult ones to teach, learn and evaluate (see Reynolds, 1985; Reynolds and Cormack, 1987; Reynolds, 1988a).

An operational definition of intensive clinical supervision will be discussed, and an argument will be advanced in favour of nursing theory and clinical practice being taught/supervised by the same individual, who is both college- (academically-) based and clinically-based (as a nurse practitioner). Essentially, I am proposing an expansion of dual classroom/clinical teaching roles. This proposal will be illustrated and supported by: anecdotes borrowed from my personal experience of clinical supervision with students, a critique of some of the existing learning theories, and reference to some of the available (educational) outcome studies. An essential part of my theme includes: the need for a theory-based approach towards teaching and learning, and the teacher's responsibility and potential contribution towards the building of a theoretical basis for psychiatric nursing. It is my contention that unless psychiatric nurse teachers are closely involved with the clinical data that arise from clinical practice, and possess analytical competencies, progress towards defining the goals, strategies and boundaries of our practice will be slower than it need be. Unless psychiatric nursing evolves as a field of scientific enquiry it will continue to be dependent upon the medical paradigm to define it's role and function. As was proposed in Chapter 1, that role (medically-defined) may sometimes damage the mental health of those we purport to help.

The need for psychiatric nurse teachers to practise clinical nursing

Numerous contributors to the literature have advanced arguments to support the view that those who purport to teach psychiatric nursing should also practise nursing. Possibly the most compelling rationale is that advanced by Hildegard Peplau. That writer (see Peplau, 1987) proposed that nurse educators have a major part to play in the development of a theory-based approach towards psychiatric nursing. During a major review of Peplau's work, Reynolds (1988b) suggested that unless nurse educators were closely associated with the clinical data (verbal and non-verbal aspects) arising from nurse–client interactions, then it would be difficult for nursing to evolve as a field of scientific enquiry.

In Chapter 1, Reynolds and Cormack discuss Peplau's (1988) suggestion that psychiatric nurses face a major decision: whether assisting psychiatrists is their primary function, or whether they will make that function secondary and instead develop their own primary function by taking the option of elaborating a different viewpoint and treatment approach. They quote extensively from Peplau's literature and conference work during the 1980s. For example, Peplau (1986) argues that psychiatric nurses have a responsibility to identify the focus of psychiatric nursing. By focus, she meant the phenomena to which the skills of the psychiatric nurse are addressed so as to achieve favourable outcomes for clients. In her paper to the Canadian psychiatric nurses, Peplau (1988) emphasized that: 'This issue is important, it is the named focus of the work that determines what theories the practices require, the most relevant foci for nursing research, and the major information which the public needs and wants from nurses for purposes of self-maintenance of health.' Peplau (see Chapter 5) goes on to suggest that the phenomena commonly observed by nurses during their relationships with psychiatric clients should be the focus for nursing intervention, and the clinical supervision of learners. Phenomena may be defined as: behavioural human responses to traumatic life events.

Examples of phenomena include human responses such as anxiety, lone-liness, hallucinations and negative self-concept. It is proposed here that if nurse are to make themselves experts in a humanistic alternative ap-proach to such problems (that differs from the medical viewpoint of treat-ment), then it is necessary for students of psychiatric nursing to study the clinical data associated with their nurse–client interactions within a non-threatening relationship with their teachers. Peplau (1986) proposes that it is during educative clinical experience, followed by supervised review of interaction data, that skill in theory application and in the use of theory-derived interventions are learned, refined and validated.

In my view, Peplau's conceptualizations are amongst the most important nursing statements made during the 1980s. These statements provide clear and positive suggestions for the development of the psychiatric nurse–teacher's role. Unfortunately, this role has not been accepted through-out the worldwide community of nursing. Peplau (1988) states that close supervisory review of interaction data is the costly part of nurse education; it requires an intensive one-to-one relationship, and it takes time for well qualified and highly skilled teachers to review clinical data. She points out that not all societies are willing to provide the resources for in-depth skill training. It is my suggestion here that unless nurse educators are willing to closely supervise their students during clinical practice (a process that includes role-modelling and analysis of the clinical data from nurse–client interactions), their contribution towards the development of the psychia-tric nurse's role will be negligible. Isolation from practice will not so much result in them (the educators) not knowing the answers to the questions, so that they will not even know what the questions are.

Reynolds and Cormack (1985) alluded to that final point when they stated that students shared a common problem during clinical practice. The problem relates to their struggle to formulate operational nursing activity from a multiplicity of theories. For example, students frequently ask questions such as: 'What do I do when a client does not keep a sched-uled appointment?' or 'What do I do or say when a client says he feels hopeless or lonely?' Thus clinical supervision seeks not only to help stu-dents to understand psychotherapeutic theory, but how to implement it. When teachers demonstrate an ability and a willingness to share the risks of clinical practice with their students, they will become aware of the questions being generated by clinical work, and the focus for teaching will switch from cognitive (inside the head) achievements towards clinical excellence. After all, teachers should be concerned with what learner nurses are able to do, not just with what they know.

Barriers to progress

There is evidence in the literature of an increasing awareness on the part of nurse educators in the UK of a need to educate and train nurses more effectively in interpersonal techniques. Examples include: Nicol and Withington (1981), Millar (1981), Briggs (1982), Marsen (1982), Reynolds (1982, 1985) and Burnard (1985). There has also been an increased interest in non-traditional learning methods. This approach has become almost trendy (see Robinson, 1986; Sweeney, 1986; Richardson, 1988), and has been described variously as self-directed learning, experiential learning, student-centred, and adult learning (androgogy). Often such terms have been used as a synonym, i.e., as if one meant the other. It is not my intention here to become involved with semantic discussions. My major point in this: with the exception of Nicol and Withington (1981) and Reynolds (1982) all of the literature referred to here reflects a trend: the tendency to focus exclusively on classroom-based teaching environments. In my view this represents a major barrier to progress in the UK, because college-based work should be regarded as preparatory for clinical work. It is a primer, a simulation of the real work that will follow. It is not a substitute for supervised clinical practice; it is merely part of a sequence.

Currently, there is a poverty of UK literature about the clinical supervision of psychiatric nurses. However, in recent years a small trickle of papers describing structured clinical supervision programmes for psychiatric nursing students, and arguments for a greater concentration of teaching resources in clinical areas have appeared in the UK journals. These teaching methods closely follow the approach used in the American system of nurse education (see Reynolds, 1984), where teachers often have a dual classroom–clinical teaching role. These teaching programmes are both student-centred and patient-centred.

Reynolds (1982) defined patient-centred teaching as being clinically focused, and described an activity which examined and became involved with the students' working day and client contacts. This view was later repeated by Ellis and Watson (1985) who referred to patient-centred teaching as learning with the patient. Central to the patient-centred idea is the view that the teacher should provide a therapeutic role model. In addition, various methods of collecting raw clinical data from student–client interactions are employed, such as taped segments of one-to-one counselling interviews, and a sociometric analysis of interaction during therapeutic groups. These data are utilized during supervisory sessions with teachers, and are intended to facilitate the students personal and professional development.

In spite of the fact that Maukish (1980) seriously questioned the ability of American nurse teachers to practise nursing, my personal experience of the American system suggests that teachers in the USA have made greater progress towards the development of a dual educational–clinical role than UK-based teachers (see Reynolds and Smoyak, 1983; Reynolds, 1984). In the USA, nurse teachers have made attempts to remain in contact with clinical practice, either through accepting responsibility for the supervision of their students' clinical work, or through private practice, for example, working part-time as a family therapist. This contrasts with the general tendency of most UK teachers not to practise clinical nursing, and reflects the cultural differences towards the arrangements for nurses' clinical supervision alluded to by Peplau (1986).

In the UK, different solutions have emerged towards providing learner nurses with clinical supervision. The common tendency (with some exceptions) has been to divide the responsibility for teaching nursing theory, and the supervision of nursing practice between different people (tutors and clinical teachers). In many instances the responsibility for clinical supervision and assessment of students' competence is delegated to clinically based nursing staff who are not usually trained teachers. In many cases (through no fault of their own) they may not even be skilled clinicians because many registered nurses have not been provided with continuing professional development for many years. This is serious because there are widely held views in the literature on the education of nurses that the current basic (UK) training programmes are failing to provide learners with the knowledge and skills they require to become competent practitioners in the health care programmes. This criticism has been particularly strong in respect of the interpersonal skill area, the extent to which nurses have failed to implement the nursing process and (in most instances), the lack of a theoretical basis for practice. Chapman (1983, p. 270), in support of that view, suggests that:

> In some situations any move by the nurse to get involved with the patient is frowned upon. While talking to the patient is given a degree of credibility, it is considered unprofessional to get emotionally involved or to demonstrate empathy. Instead the nurse is told to spend less time talking to the patient and to hide any feelings of sympathy she may have for his predicament. So talk becomes superficial and the patient is jollied along rather than allowed to express fears, anxieties and sadness.

In recognition of this problem, the Scottish National Board for Nursing, Midwifery and Health Visiting has decided that one of the mandatory post-basic experiences for registered nurses should be a module that focuses on learning, teaching and counselling. The hope that this strategy will resolve (in the long term) the existing supervision problem, may prove to be a false one. The probability is that the complex relationship between theory and practice (which will be discussed in some depth at a later point) will defeat the best efforts of the Scottish system to mass-produce clinical supervisors. I would suggest that the mass utilization of clinicians as part-time educators is likely to fail because most clinicians may be unable to meet all of the minimal conditions that I consider to be necessary for adequate supervision to exist, namely that:

1. Clinical supervisors should possess and practise the skill that is to be taught and learned.
2. They should also understand the dynamics which operate within the supervisor–supervisee relationship (e.g., anxiety, low self-efficacy, avoidance, etc.), knowing how to treat such problems.
3. They should be familiar with and competent in the theory of nursing that has been taught to the student.
4. They should be highly visible, approachable, and readily available to the learner nurse (when needed).

Because it is unlikely that many UK clinicians would be able to meet all of the minimal criteria for adequate supervision, alternative solutions may be necessary. One alternative would be to hire more teachers and to invest post-basic educational money on re-skilling teachers. In that way, full-time, professional supervision could be provided. I would also suggest that this route provides exciting prospects for nurse consultancy roles, primary nursing and theory development and testing. However, at the present time it would not appear that sufficient interest exists in the UK (by those who allocate budgets) to make that degree of financial commitment to nurses' education.

While cost may be an important factor that inhibits the development of the teacher's clinical role, other variables may be of equal importance. Following a series of semi-structured interviews with Scottish nurse educators, Reynolds (1986) identified several factors that influence their roles. These included:

1. *Traditional role stereotyping*
   This may be defined as the perceived expectations of the educational institution. Administration and classroom (college-based) work takes priority over clinical work. It is mandatory and non-negotiable.
2. *The low status of clinical teaching*
   Those who teach clinically are generally lowly placed on a hierarchical grading structure. The clinical teaching grade is similar to but not exactly analogous to the most junior faculty grade in the American system. It reflects the British bias towards having two levels of educators by splitting the responsibility of teaching theory and practice between two individuals. It would appear that Cormack's (1976) view that clinical practice is valued less than administrative ability, is as true of nurse education as it is for clinically based nurses. Generally speaking, those who are provided with status and financial reward are teachers who have moved further away from ward-based teaching. By contrast, those attempting to teach and practise complex psychotherapeutic skills (usually clinical teachers) receive the lowest amount of status and financial reward. I would propose here that there is a need to reconsider this paradoxical reward system, and even to reverse it.

3. *The high student:teacher ratio in clinical areas*

Understandably, for the previously stated reasons, many nurse tutors feel that they are unable to become involved with the clinical supervision of students and restrict their teaching input to college learning environments. Unfortunately, it follows that those teachers who do teach in clinical areas (mainly clinical teachers), will have to accept (as a consequence) responsibility for larger numbers of students. Because successful outcome during clinical supervision may be dependent upon the supervisor's ability to create a non-threatening one-to-one relationship, a student overload often results in ineffectual teaching because it dilutes the amount (and often quality) of the teacher–student relationship. It may also be a perception, on the teacher's part, that teacher presence in clinical areas makes little difference to learning. This discovery also acts as an incentive to avoid or leave clinical areas. Some support for these views emerged from Reynolds' (1986) data who concluded that student overload in clinical areas reduces and minimizes the effect of empathy training for student nurses.

Conceptual models for learning

A theory-based approach towards teaching provides consistency and direction to the teacher's approach. Essentially, the teacher who does not have a theory of learning is in a similar position to a nurse who does not have a theory of nursing. As Fox (1983, p.7) states:

> She might try the first idea to come to mind and see if that worked. If it did not work, then she might try the second idea she thought of, and the third until one worked sufficiently well. Or, she might seek to determine what others have done before her in similar situations. Or, she might rely on directives from those in authority, or more senior to her.

The difficulty with that approach, which clearly lacks any theoretical or scientific basis, is that solutions are often accepted without question or rationale. Even if a solution is found (to a nursing or educational problem), it may not be the best one, or one that will enable another person to achieve an optimal amount of learning.

While several theories of learning exist, this section will mainly concentrate on three conceptual models of learning: Rogers' student-centred approach, Bandura's social learning theory, and Festinger's theory of cognitive dissonance. While these conceptual models will comprise the main focus for the discussion that follows about teaching and learning, the debate will be supplemented by reference to theorists and authors who support and complement the theoretical perspectives of Rogers, Bandura and Festinger. I should emphasize that I use the term model as a synonym for theory (i.e., one means the other). While some writers (see Pearson and Vaughan, 1988) suggest that the terms are not interchangeable – for example, a model is a representation of what something looks like, and a theory is a set of proposals which give a reasonable explanation to an event – I find this semantic debate unconvincing.

Rogers' student-centred approach

General principles   As was stated in Chapter 7, Rogers' approach to education grew out of his earlier theoretical formulations about the nature of counselling and personality development. Essentially, human beings are said to be creative, trustworthy, forward moving and realistic, when they are free of defensiveness. These capacities will be achieved or released in a relationship that has the characteristics of a helping (open, two-way critical approach) relationship. This holds true, in Rogers' view (see Rogers 1969 and 1977), irrespective of whether we are talking about a nurse–client relationship or a teacher–student relationship. Reynolds (1985, p. 245) alluded to that point when he stated that: 'A permissive democratic supervisory structure will promote learning more effectively than an authoritarian structure in which students are given directives. After all, teachers help students just as nurses help clients.'

Rogers (1969, p. 18) suggests that teaching is more difficult than learning because: '. . . what teaching calls for is this: to let students learn.' What Rogers meant is that learning does not mean the lifeless, sterile, futile, quickly-forgotten stuff that might be crammed into the mind of the helpless student. He was talking about the insatiable curiosity that drives an adolescent boy to absorb everything he can read or hear about engines in order to improve the speed of his motorbike. He was also talking about the student nurse who on finding her client's verbalizations difficult to understand, sought permission to record it on audiotape in order to study the meaning of her client's communication.

Two kinds of learning   Rogers (1969) divides learning into two general types. One type is the learning of meaningless information by a student whose background provides no context for the material being studied. Rogers calls that learning which involves the mind only. He further states (Rogers, 1969, p. 19) that: 'It is learning from the neck up. It does not involve feelings or personal meanings; it has no relevance to the whole person'. In support of that view, several studies conducted in the USA have suggested that traditional classroom teaching alone will not enable helping professionals to understand or help other people. Following a review of 81 studies, Taft (1955) reported a lack of correlation between the amount of theory taught and the ability to understand other people. This point was demonstrated by Chance and Meaders (1960), who explored the relationship between increased psychological-mindedness (knowledge of psychology and personality theories) and empathy. The results showed that empathy significantly decreased as psychological-mindedness increased. Studies by Arnhoff *et al.* (1954) and Weiss (1963) offer additional support for this view. Smith (1966) concluded that the development of psychological-mindedness appears to be a dubious way of increasing empathic ability.

By contrast, Rogers proposes that there is such a thing as meaningful, experiential learning. In congruence with that view, Reynolds and Cormack (1982) suggested that it was necessary for the student to be provided with evidence that her theory of nursing could work, i.e., make a difference. They provided descriptions of student nurses' experiences during clinical practice. As one learner explained: 'I appreciated the enthusiasm of the charge nurse and his interest in me, but I would have preferred it if he had demonstrated his nursing skills rather than talked about them.' (Reynolds and Cormack [1982], p. 233).

One might wonder why the charge nurse didn't demonstrate his skills and then allow the student to imitate or practise them. Rogers' conceptualization of the learning process suggests that it may well be the observation and practice of nursing, followed by analysis of its effect which renders it meaningful. That point is entirely congruent with Peplau's (1986) view that supervised review of nurse–client interaction data results in skilled application of theory. Rogers' view that there should be some point to learning is a core concept for nurse educators to consider. After all, we can teach a child about the meaning of hot, but it is a difficult concept to grasp unless you personally experience it. When heat is experienced, knowing about it becomes meaningful (avoidance of pain, or a method of cooking, etc). Similarly, there is little point in telling a student nurse that you shouldn't argue with an angry person, unless she is allowed to observe and practise that approach. When that happens learning is likely to be meaningful and remembered out of sheer necessity, i.e., it may mean that physical violence is avoided. That is the value of demonstration and imitation. After all, we would not expect a child to learn how to tie up her shoelaces by providing her with a lecture or a tutorial, so why should we expect talking alone, about issues that have little immediate relevance, to facilitate clinical excellence?

Some of the central themes which underpin Rogerian theory were expressed by Heidegger's (1968) thoughts. That writer stated that the primary task of teachers is to permit the student to learn, to feed his or her curiosity. Merely to absorb facts is only of slight value in the present, and usually of even less value in the future. Learning how to learn is the element that is always of value, now and in the future. He goes on to say that, in true teaching, there is no place for the authoritarian nor for the person who is on an ego trip.

The student–teacher relationship Rogers' conceptualization of learning suggests that the teacher's capacity to experientially know his learner is critical. Like the nurse–client relationship, the student–teacher relationship is important to outcome. Numerous barriers to learning exist, in much the same way that barriers to problem solving exist within the nurse–client relationship. Like the nurse–client relationship, the student–teacher relationship is a psychodynamic process; it is specific, goal-orientated, and requires relationship building skills on the part of the teacher. Reynolds (1985) proposed that the ability of teachers to help students learn would be enabled by understanding their learners needs. Empathic awareness of the learner is essential to all phases of the teaching/learning process. That process is similar to the nursing process in the sense that teachers and learners ought to: assess learners needs, plan teaching goals and strategies, implement teaching–learning strategies, and evaluate learning outcomes.

Reynolds (1985, p. 244) emphasized the specific, goal-orientated and psychodynamic nature of the supervisory relationship, in the following manner:

> ...the student–teacher relationship will progress through the same phases as the nurse–client relationship, namely (a) orientation, (b) testing out, (c) working together, and (d) termination. During the working phase of the relationship, students should feel free to express themselves, be confident enough to interpret what is going on in their nurse–client relationships, and as a consequence grow in their ability to experiment with new ideas and skills. If the relationship fails to develop beyond orientation or testing-out phases, the teacher's ability to help the student will be very limited.

When a teacher meets a new learner, who is a stranger, the learner will often attempt to avoid the teacher. Avoidance may occur in many forms. For example, the student might remain silent, verbally criticise the teacher, or busy himself with tasks that frustrate the teaching–learning process by minimizing the amount of interaction between student and teacher. These problems can be overcome, or at least reduced, when teachers make themselves acceptable to the learner. Essentially, student-growth is like client-growth, it is dependent upon a non-threatening relationship between teacher and student. In that sense, the supervisory (teaching) relationship can be said to be a treatment modality, or a method of facilitating learning. As with the nurse–client relationship, it is the teacher's responsibility to study the dynamics that operate within that relationship (the origins, nature and variations of the relationship) and from that, to formulate solutions that will resolve any difficulties that exist.

Support for that view comes from numerous contributors to the literature. Bregg (1958) claimed that the interaction between teacher and student is an important influence, not only on the learning experience, but also on the student's growth into professional stature and maturity. Gregg, Bregg and Spring (1979) defined individual supervision as a working relationship developed between a student and teacher for the purpose of guiding the student's learning of therapeutic nursing interventions and clinical excellence. It is argued by those writers that a democratic supervisory structure promotes a compassionate, flexible and thinking person. The development of a thinking person is an important contribution to nursing because, as Barker (1988) suggests, there is a need to cultivate the questioning tradition which is the mainspring of real professionals. These points have been emphasized by several other writers. Thus, von Bergen and Cline (1956, p. 152) suggested that: 'In order to learn how to give help, the student needs to experience receiving help. This experience is made available to her through her relationship with the instructor.' Smith (1957, p. 8) suggested that: 'The kind of understanding and help given to students during clinical practice may be more significantly related to the kind of nursing care she is able to give, than the content of some of our nursing courses.'

The importance of the trust relationship has been addressed by writers who have been concerned with the emotional impact of nursing work particularly in respect of psychosocial issues. Benfer (1979) suggested that the experiencing of trust within the supervisory relationship can act as a support system for the care giver. Peplau (1957) pointed out that what nurses actually experience when clients are anxious, express feelings of worthlessness, resentment or hatefulness influences these situations. Peplau stated that understanding by the nurse of her own participation when clients express various behaviours, can only be learned by examining what is felt, thought and done by the nurse. Zetzel (1953) suggested that the emotional impact of clinical work is a potentially maturing one for the student, provided that she experienced a kind of supervision that provides security and freeom.

The research evidence The available research evidence in support of the statements made in the preceding text tend to be very encouraging indeed. An interesting study by Schmuck (1966) showed that when teachers listen to their students, and are empathically understanding, their students tend to like each other better. A correlation was shown to exist between student liking and a more positive attitude towards education.

The previous study is a sample of many small studies that began to accumulate. However, it could still be asked, does the student actually learn more when those attitudes (an open two-way critical approach and empathy) are present? Aspey (1965) did a careful study of six classes of young school children. He found that in three classes where the teachers' facilitative attitudes were highest, the pupils showed a significantly greater gain in their reading achievement than in those classes with a lesser degree of those qualities. Aspey and Roebuck (1975) later enlarged this research into a programme that extended for more than a decade. The overwhelming evidence that they accumulated makes it very clear that the attitudinal climate of the learning environment, as created by the teacher, is a major factor in promoting or inhibiting learning.

Rogers' theory suggests that empathy (the ability to place yourself in the student's world) is a core facilitator of learning outcomes. Support from that view comes from a study conducted by Hughes and Huckill (1982). That study sought to investigate the relationship between a teacher's characteristics and teaching outcome. It was found that empathy, as measured by the empathy construct rating scale, was the primary predictor of teacher success.

At the present time very little research is being conducted in respect of clinical environments in nursing, and education outcomes. The impact of structured clinical supervision is a fertile area for nurse scientists to investigate. However, Reynolds (1986) found that where structured, intensive clinical supervision (based on Rogerian principles) was provided, there was a greater tendency for students' scores on an empathy instrument to increase among ratings than in clinical situations where students were provided with minimal supervision from nurse educators. These data are not conclusive, but they are encouraging, and warrant further investigation.

Bandura's social learning theory

Central to Bandura's theory is the view that antecedent factors, in other words, the previous experiences in a person's life, are potent influences on whether a behaviour can be learnt, mislearnt, avoided, or forgotten. An important factor, though one that is sometimes not considered by supervisors, is that in order to behave in a skilled way it is necessary to have some degree of confidence in our ability to do so. Many writers have referred to the complex relationship between cognitive self-assessment and behavioural outcomes (see Bandura, 1977a; Davidson, 1985).

The concept of self-efficacy   Bandura (1977b) elaborated on the concept of self-efficacy. He argued that possessing a skill or competence does not necessarily lead to its use. Whether it is used or not depends to some extent on a cognitive factor, a belief in our capacity to perform well. This is what Bandura calls the person's sense of self-efficacy.

Anxiety and defensive behaviour   A great deal of human behaviour is activated by events which become threatening through association with painful experiences. A prime function of most anticipatory behaviour is to provide protection against potential hazards. Some of this arises from what Bandura (1977a) calls vicarious expectancy learning. He states that '. . . although emotional responses often are learned from direct experiences, they are also frequently acquired observationally.' By this, he meant that many intractable fears arise not from personally injurious experiences, but from seeing others respond fearfully toward, or be hurt by, threatening experiences. Similarly, evaluation of places, persons, or things often originates from exposure to modelled attitudes. Much of this can be observed in students' avoidance techniques in clinical areas, or students' methods of coping with the student–teacher relationship. Reynolds (1985), when commenting upon the tendency of a few students to resist the teaching process, provided the following example from a student's diary:

> Immediately after this interaction (a shopping trip), the teacher asked me if it was beneficial. I said no: however, at the bus stop (while returning to the ward) I felt awful for saying so, when in fact it was not true. I just felt tired and hungry, and I did not give his question any consideration. In fact I had learned a lot about my client, as I had never seen her in that situation before. (Reynolds, 1985, p. 244).

In fact this student was also concerned about her prolonged absence from the ward. In spite of the fact that this form of nursing care had been negotiated (and ostensibly approved), the need to be liked by clinical associates can often engender feelings of threat in an apprentice type training programme, such as the UK ones. Reynolds (1982, 1986) and Reynolds and Cormack (1982, 1985, 1987) also reported that students delayed or avoided interactions with clients until their self-efficacy problems had been addressed. Commenting on that point, Reynolds (1986, p. 43) stated that: 'It would appear that the teacher–student relationship can resemble a psychotherapeutic interaction between a therapist and a client.'

Treating self-efficacy problems Self-efficacy is a theoretical framework, postulated by Bandura, to explain and predict psychological changes achieved by different modes of treatment. As previously stated, it was hypothesized that expectations of personal performance determine whether coping behaviour will be initiated, how much effort will be expended, and how long it will be sustained in the face of obstacles and aversive experiences (Bandura, 1977b). In many situations people who possess skills also hold negative beliefs about their abilities which prevent them from using the skills. They may not lack appropriate responses, and they may also hold the expectation that the response will be well received; what they may lack, however, is a sense of their own capacity to act in a desired way. This view appears to bear some resemblance to the notion of internal locus of control put forward by Rotter (1966). It would appear that behaviour and cognitive self-assessment are often locked together in a negative self-fulfilling prophecy. The role of the teacher/supervisor is to break this self-fulfilling prophecy.

Breaking the self-fulfilling prophecy Bandura's model for promoting change does not involve approaching the person's beliefs directly. Rather, he suggests an indirect approach via behaviour. Bandura argues that it is possible to give the individual experience of successful outcomes by prolonged exposure to graded modelling. Support for that view comes from Ellis and Watson (1987) who described how they introduced student nurses to group psychotherapy, first in a classroom, and then in a series of structured, and then unstructured, clinical groups. This teaching programme was similar in many aspects to that described earlier by Reynolds and Cormack (1985), where a core feature was the role modelling function of the supervisor. Ellis and Watson (1987, p. 220) state that: 'At first, learners viewed their performance more negatively than the supervisor's assessment, perhaps due to strong feelings of anxiety and low self-efficacy. However, as their experience and self-confidence improved, they tended to view their behaviour more positively and perceived an improvement in their performance.'

Bandura argues that it is possible to give the individual experience of successful outcomes using guided and reinforced imitation, in a situation where anxiety is kept within tolerable limits. This may be achieved if the teacher demonstrates the skill, or the learning situation is organized so that outcomes can be experienced over an increasingly wider range of tasks. In this way, a sense of self-efficacy is developed. Self-efficacy, according to Bandura, has the useful function of inoculating people against occasional setbacks. Thus, in order, to become skilled, and develop self-efficacy, there is a need to observe and practise a skill. Reynolds and Cormack (1982) proposed that while talking, role play, and simulation exercises may be a useful graded introduction to a skill, on the job competence will be acquired only when the learner practises in the real world. Bandura's (1977 (a) and (b)) work has suggested that a great deal of skilled behaviour is learned vicariously, in other words, established at a distance through observation of others. In recognition of that view, Reynolds (1987, p. 267) stated that: 'It is possible, therefore, that without an initial role model to learn from, the individual might well not acquire behaviours, or the idea that certain behaviours can effectively bring rewards.'

The role-modelling of the teacher

During a personal communication to this writer, Peplau (1983) emphasized the logic of role modelling. She stated that 'If you wanted to learn to play the violin, presumably, you would not only seek out a teacher who played the violin, but someone who could play it better than you could. In order to have that confidence you would expect your teacher to demonstrate competence in violin playing.' It is likely that most, or many, nurse teachers would agree with the logic of this position. However, the organizational structure of nurse education, and the multidimensional demands of a teacher's role (administration, interviewing, curriculum development, reading reports and attending meetings, etc) has resulted (at least in the UK) in many teachers adopting a pragmatic approach, attempting to meet the perceived demands of the institution as quickly and easily as possible. This has resulted in a somewhat paradoxical situation in the UK. Reynolds (1988a) emphasized that paradox in the following manner:

> Let us suppose that garage mechanics were trained like this. The tutor mechanic (who hadn't fixed cars for several years) taught the apprentices about the theory of car mechanics, in isolation from practice. Next, the apprentices are sent to the garage (workplace) where they largely work with other apprentices, unskilled labourers, or on their own. The trained mechanics work mainly on their own (in the office doing administrative work). The tutor mechanic sometimes visits the apprentices, but only talks to them about what they are doing. In that case it would not be surprising if our cars left the garage in a worse state than when they entered for diagnosis and repair. Perhaps that is why (on some occasions) clients are damaged by the health care systems, because this anecdote replicates the personal experience of many student nurses.

This rather amusing anecdote emphasizes the interface between theory and practice. Interaction between the learner, client and supervisor not only provides the learner with a role model, it provides the learner with the opportunity to experience reinforcement. Reinforcement or reward, comes from the experience of observing your theory working and the discovery that some clinical behaviours can be personally rewarding. However, some learner nurses will avoid interaction with clients. That problem is best overcome within a competent, safe and democratic supervisory relationship that is initially established in less threatening circumstances (in the classroom laboratory). Reward comes from helping the client and receiving positive feedback from the client and supervisor. It also results from the avoidance of a common student experience, namely, what Festinger (1964) terms cognitive dissonance. Cognitive dissonance is a major contributor towards much of the stress and anxiety experienced by learners during clinical learning, and occurs when their behaviour (nursing practice) is incompatible with their beliefs (theory of nursing).

Festinger's theory of cognitive dissonance

Festinger's (1964) theory of cognitive dissonance, complements and supports Bandura's (1977a) concept of self-efficacy. Festinger argues that anxiety occurs when a person's values are not consistent with his behaviour. This experience is what Festinger (1957) termed cognitive dissonance.

That phenomenon was graphically described by Rickard (1981, p. 6) who stated that:

> The position of learner nurses is one of having to spend two or three years formulating their own ideas and standards without alienating themselves from the hospital community. The learners exist in a no-man's-land between the values promulgated by the Nursing School, and the practices of ward staff. If learners accept the School's values, they may reject some of the ward practices. If they accept all that happens on the wards, then their own values are likely to be incompatible with those of the School.

Rickard was largely referring to the situation in the UK where there is a tendency to separate theory and practice. In the USA, where theory and practice are generally controlled by teachers, the impact of cognitive dissonance (see Reynolds, 1984) would appear to be less severe. Rickard goes on to say that:

> The ward staff may describe the educationalists as having 'their heads in the clouds', while the School may regard the ward staff as victims of an institutionalizing culture. This puts great pressure on learner nurses to reduce their anxiety by totally accepting one set of values and rejecting the other. To pick out the trust in each and thus accept neither side completely involves an even greater psychological discomfort (Rickard, 1981, p. 6).

Festinger's view is that the anxiety associated with cognitive dissonance arises when a learner's behaviour and vicarious learning (observations) are incompatible with the theory of nursing that has been taught. For example, they may have been introduced to the idea that suicide potentiality can be assessed and predicted. Confusion and anxiety may arise if clinical associates appear to have no criterion for assessing those at risk of self-harm. Additionally, the principles of communication taught to learners may have been based on Rogers' theory of non-directive counselling. They might have been led to believe that empathy, the ability to understand another person's world from his point of view, is considered to be the core characteristic of an effective interpersonal relationship (see Reynolds and Presley, 1988). Imagine their confusion if their role model (who is in a position of authority) demonstrated a more directive counselling approach, or even told the client how he ought to be feeling?

Reynolds (1985) suggested that it was essential that the supervision of nursing practice and the teaching of nursing theory were taught by the same person. The rationale for that view stemmed from the belief that in order to teach clinical nursing, the teacher must practise those skills using a theoretical model that is familiar to the learner. Reynolds further suggested that it was unfortunate that nurse teachers (in the UK) had delegated responsibility for the clinical supervision of student nurses to practising nurses, because: '. . . these nurses may not have teaching skills, or the time or motivation to teach. Furthermore, clinicians may not share the teacher's perception of the nurse's role. For example, if clinicians do not view counselling skills as being a primary function of the psychiatric nurse, it is unlikely that students will observe or practise counselling, unless their teacher is actually present'. (Reynolds, 1985, pp. 144–5).

Treating cognitive dissonance

While Reynolds was making a case for teachers to practise on the grounds that their classroom work would be more realistic and credible, he was also commenting upon the relationship between theory and practice. Essentially, he was stating that theory and practice have to be linked. This means the learner thinks about it in the classroom, practises it in the classroom and the clinical area, and evaluates the outcome of nursing interventions with his supervisor. In this way: (1) critical thinking is encouraged; (2) learning becomes meaningful; (3) self-efficacy is raised when learners achieve; (4) learners acquire new behaviours; and (5) cognitive dissonance is minimized. This process is likely to become disjointed if several people become involved, in much the same way that inconsistencies may occur in the delivery of nursing care if the nurse–client relationship becomes fragmented among several care-givers. In my view success is dependent upon a prolonged and intensive relationship, over time, between learner and teacher/supervisor. That view is supported by Hughes (1985) who suggested that working with the student during various phases of the supervisory relationship (testing out, problem solving and termination), was potentially exhausting, and required total concentration and commitment on the part of the teacher. It is for these reasons that I express concern about the attempts in Scotland to train clinicians as teachers (supervisors).

If clinical nurses (in the UK) are unable to meet the previously mentioned criterion for adequate clinical supervision to exist, it follows that someone else needs to accept responsibility for that role. In my view that resource should (like the American system) be provided by the nurse education department. I predict that if the educational institutions enabled teachers to practise nursing with their students, that this experience would facilitate the personal growth of both teachers and learners. For example: clinical practice would enable teachers to help their learners (during supervisory review of clinical data) to adapt to ongoing clinical developments, and to validate and refine the nursing approach. A recent example from my own supervisory work emphasizes the need for the teacher to be closely associated with the clinical data. A student (staff nurse grade) who was counselling a male client, diagnosed the following problems: negative self-concept, loneliness, anxiety, and a tendency to harm himself by cutting his wrists. The counselling method used was a client-centred

(Rogerian) approach. Following a review of the clinical data from several counselling interviews, it appeared that the amount of gratification received from self-harm attempts, the strength of the negative thoughts, and the emptiness in the client's life merited the use of an alternative theory approach. A modified cognitive-therapy approach was introduced and combined with some of the Rogerian principles. The essential point being made here is that the kind of help and understanding given to students during clinical practice has a potent effect upon the kind of nursing care that a learner is able to provide for a client.

Conclusion

This chapter has reviewed the learning outcome from the writer's personal experiences, and theoretical constructs borrowed from several theories of learning. I would suggest that now is the time to combine these various concepts into a new model or theory of learning. I propose that the concepts to be described in the final part of this chapter describe a new model of learning which may be utilized by nurse educators to design teaching and learning experiences that are intended to produce clinically excellent practitioners in psychiatric nursing. I believe that the model to be described here meets the criteria for a model which have been identified by Pearson and Vaughan (1988). It contains the three basic components of any practice model: (1) the beliefs and values on which the model is based; (2) the goals of practice or what the practitioner aims to achieve; (3) the knowledge, skills and attributes the practitioner needs to develop in order to gain these goals. The concepts (or constructs) within this model, the psychodynamic learning model, also provide nurse scientists with numerous fresh targets for research.

The psychodynamic learning model

This model has its antecedents in many old ideas and insights into the learning process. It did not spring forth, entirely brand new, inspirational from the brow of Zeus. However, I would propose that it is a fresh conceptualization of the teaching–learning process, from the perspective of nurse education. I call it the psychodynamic learning model because I believe that learning (or failure to learn) is largely about the mental and developmental process that occurs within the confines of a relationship with a significant other. It also recognizes that the supervisory relationship is a constantly changing and dynamic experience.

Concepts of practice

1. Nurse educators have a responsibility for contributing toward the development of a theoretical basis for practice.
2. It is during educative clinical experience followed by supervised re-

view of the verbal and non-verbal aspects of nurse–client interaction data that skill in theory application and in the use of theory-derived interventions are learned, refined and validated. When teachers are willing to share the risks of clinical practice with their students, they become aware of the questions being generated by the clinical data.

3. There is a need for teachers and learners to develop tools/methods of capturing raw clinical data (recording them) so that they can be studied and reviewed. Clinical data help to explain clinical phenomena and tell us whether the language of the nurse is constructive or destructive. Physicians are guided by clinical data in the form of laboratory reports and other measurements. The problem in nurse–client verbal and non-verbal interactions is the ambiguity of the data. You have to make it more concrete, in the sense that you hold it still while you look at it.

4. The term supervision describes an intensive one-to-one relationship between teacher and learner, the antecedents of which begin in the classroom and continue throughout simulated practice in the classroom laboratory into the clinical areas. In this manner, time is made available to develop a permissive, democratic supervisory structure, necessary to cultivate a thinking, flexible and compassionate person.

5. The clinical phase of the supervisory process needs an identifiable structure which consists of three specific and purposeful phases. These phases are:

Phase	Purpose
(a) The pre-clinical conference	To discuss nursing strategies and purpose
(b) Interaction with the client	To assess needs or operationalize nursing theory
(c) The post-clinical conference	To review the clinical data and evaluate the effect of nursing care

6. The student–teacher (supervisory) relationship will progress through the same phases as the nurse–client relationship, namely (a) orientation, (b) testing out, (c) working together, and (d) termination. During the working phase of the supervisory relationship, students should feel free to express themselves, be confident enough to interpret what is going on in their nurse–client relationships, and as a consequence, grow in their ability to experiment with new ideas and skills. If the relationship fails to develop beyond orientation or testing-out phases, the teacher's ability to help the student to learn will be very limited.

7. Critical supervisory behaviours include: empathy, warmth and genuineness and the ability of the supervisor to develop an open, two-way critical approach. The supervisory relationship is a psychodynamic process. As with the nurse–client relationship, it is the teacher's responsibility to study the dynamics that operate within that relation-

ship (the origins, nature and variations of the relationship) and from that, to formulate solutions to resolve any difficulties that exist. There is no place within supervision for the omnipotent expert, the authoritarian, or the person on an ego trip. Supervision is a support network that is designed to help our students grow.

8. Supervisors should demonstrate nursing skills to learners in recognition of the fact that learning is partly vicarious. This should be done during simulated nurse–patient interactions and during clinical practice. Student-centred, or adult learning methods in the classroom environment are preparatory for the clinical work that will follow. It is a primer, a simulation for real clinical work with clients. It is not a substitute for supervised clinical practice; it is merely part of a sequence.

9. Unless nurse teachers practise nursing, they will become de-skilled, and their teaching becomes irrelevant to the development of nursing theory, or the manner in which care is delivered.

10. The minimal conditions of adequate supervision are that:
    (a) Supervisors should possess and practise the skill that is to be taught and learned.
    (b) They should understand the dynamics which operate within the learner–teacher relationship (e.g., low self-efficacy, cognitive dissonance, self-fulfilling prophecy, avoidance, etc.) and be capable of treating these conditions.
    (c) They should be familiar with, and competent with, theories of nursing that guide the student's actions and thoughts.
    (d) They should be highly visible, approachable, and readily available to the learner (when needed).

11. Learning is most easily retained when it is experiential and meaningful. In other words there has to be a reason for knowing something. In order to discover reasons, learners need to be provided with an opportunity to operationalize (practise) their theory. That enables them to learn that specific behaviour can result in rewards. Feedback comes from the client, self-awareness, and interaction with the supervisor, in a climate that is safe and frees the learner from defensiveness.

12. The conditions mentioned in 11 are more likely to occur when theory and practice are controlled/supervised by the same person; it should never be divided between two or more persons. This is due to the time needed for teacher and learner to experientially learn about each other, the need for structured and graded exposure to a skill, and the need for consistency between the nursing theory and clinical practice. This will minimize the effects of cognitive dissonance, and reduce self-efficacy problems by exposing learners to success. Success (and adequate self-efficacy) inoculates learners against occasional setbacks.

13. The teaching/learning process is similar to the nursing process in the sense that teachers and learners ought to: assess learners' needs, plan

teaching goals and strategies, implement teaching and learning strategies, and evaluate learning outcomes.

14. Knowing the student is central to successful learning outcomes. This involves the previously stated need for non-directive counselling skills. It also suggests that there is a need for student–teacher contracts and students' and/or teachers' diaries as part of this process of learning about another. Data arising from such tools may form the basis for the development of performance indicators, which may be used to study the quality and nature of the teaching–learning environment.

It is suggested here that the conditions and processes described within this model are necessary, and have the capacity, to move the nurse learner from novice to basic competence, and ultimately, toward clinical excellence. The model has application to all groups of nurses, irrespective of the level of education (i.e., diploma, masters or doctoral level). The concepts which comprise this model, also provide a focus for educational outcome studies. Clearly much remains to be done.

References

Arnhoff, F. *et al.* (1954) Some factors influencing the reliability of clinical judgements. *J. Clin. Psych.*, 272–5.

Aspey, D. N. (1965) *A Study of Three Facilitative Conditions and Their Relationship to the Achievement of Third Grade Students*. Unpublished PhD thesis, University of Kentucky.

Aspey, D. and Roebuck, F. (1975) A discussion of the relationship between selected student behaviour and the teacher's use of interchangeable responses. *Human. Ed.* **1**, 3–10.

Bandura, A. (1977a) *Social Learning Theory*, Prentice Hall, New Jersey.

Bandura, A. (1977b) Self-efficacy: towards a unifying theory of behaviour change. *Psychol. Rev.* **84.**, 191–215.

Barker, P. (1988) The Lundbeck Leading Article. Reasoning about madness: the long search for the vanishing horizon; Part 1. *Commun. Psych. Nurses J.*, **8**, 7–13.

Benfer, B. (1979) Clinical supervision as a support system for the care giver. *Perspect. Psych. Care*, **17**, 13–17.

Bregg, E. (1958) How can we help students learn? *Am. J. Nurs.*, **58**, no. 8, 1120–2.

Briggs, K. (1982) Interpersonal skills: training for nurses during introductory course. *Nurs. Ed. Today*, **2**, 22–4.

Burnard, P. (1985) *Learning Human Skills: a Guide for Nurses*, Heinemann, London.

Burnard, P. and Morrison, P. (1988) Nurses' perceptions of their interpersonal skills: a descriptive study using six category intervention analysis. *Nurs. Ed. Today*, **8**, 266–72.

Chance, J. and Meaders, W. (1960) Needs and interpersonal perceptions. *J. Perspect. Psych. Care*, **28**, 200–10.

Chapman, C. (1983) The paradox of nursing. *J. Adv. Nurs.*, **8**, 269–72.

Cormack, D. (1976) *Psychiatric Nursing Observed*, RCN Research Series, London.

Davidson, C. (1985) The theoretical antecedents of interpersonal skills training, in *Interpersonal Skills in Nursing: Research and Applications* (ed. C. Kagan), Croom

Helm, London.
Ellis, R. and Watson, C. (1985) Learning through the patient. *Nurs. Times*, **81**, 52–4.
Ellis, R. and Watson, C. (1987) Experiential learning: the development of communication skills in a group therapy setting. *Nurs. Ed. Today*, **7**, 215–21.
Festinger, L. (1957) *A Theory of Cognitive Dissonance*, Row Patterson, Evanston, IL.
Festinger, L. (1964) *Conflict Decision and Dissonance*, Tavistock Publications, London.
Fox, D. (1983) *Fundamentals of Research in Nursing*, 4th edn, Appleton-Century-Crofts, Norwalk, CT.
Gregg, D., Bregg, E. and Spring, F. (1979) Individual supervision: a method of teaching psychiatric concepts in nursing education. *Perspect. Psych. Care*, **14**, 115–29.
Heidegger, M. (1968) *What is Called Thinking?* Harper Torchbooks, New York.
Hughes, C. (1985) Supervising clinical practice in psychosocial nursing. *J. Psychosoc. Nurs.*, **23**, 27–32.
Hughes, R. and Huckill, H. (1982) Participant Characteristic, Change and Outcome, in Clinical Teacher Education. Report No. 9020, University of Texas, Austin, TX.
Marsen, S. (1982) Developing skills in communication – 1. An interaction approach. *Nurs. Ed. Today*, **2**, 12–14.
Maukish, I. (1980) Faculty practice: a professional imperative. *Nurs. Educator*, **5**, 21–4.
Millar, E. (1981) Learning to Communicate. *Nursing: First Series*, 1197–9.
Nicol, E. and Withington, D. (1981) Recorded patient–nurse interaction: an advance in psychiatric nursing. *Nurs. Times*, 1351–2.
Pearson, A. and Vaughan, B. (1988) *Nursing Models for Practice*, Heinemann Nursing, Oxford.
Peplau, H. (1957) What is experiential teaching? *Am. J. Nurs.*, **57**, 884–6.
Peplau, H. (1983) Personal communication to W. Reynolds.
Peplau, H. (1986) Psychiatric Nursing Skills: Today and Tomorrow – a World Overview. Paper presented at *A Celebration of Skills*, Third International Congress of Psychiatric Nursing, Imperial College, London, September.
Peplau, H. (1987) Interpersonal constructs for nursing practice. *Nurs. Ed. Today*, **7**, 201–8.
Peplau, H. (1988) Substance and Scope of Psychiatric Nursing. Paper presented at the 3rd Conference on Psychiatric Nursing, Montreal, Canada.
Reynolds, W. (1982) Patient-centred teaching: a future role for the psychiatric nurse teacher? *J. Adv. Nurs.*, **7**, 469–75.
Reynolds, W. (1984) Psychiatric nursing in the USA. *Nurs. Mirror*, **158**, 25–7.
Reynolds, W. (1985) Issues arising from teaching interpersonal skills in psychiatric nurse training, in *Interpersonal Skills in Nursing: Research and Applications* (ed. C. Kagan), Croom Helm, London.
Reynolds, W. (1986) A Study of Empathy in Student Nurses. MPhil thesis, Dundee College of Technology.
Reynolds, W. (1987) Empathy: we know what we mean but what do we teach? *Nurs. Ed. Today*, **7**, 265–9.
Reynolds, W. (1988a) Nurse teachers should practise nursing? Debate (chaired by A. Altschul), PNA Conference, University of Stirling, 21st June 1988.
Reynolds, W. (1988b) The primary and secondary role of the psychiatric nurse. Keynote speech delivered to psychiatric nurses, 88: Our Value, Vision, Variety and Vitality (Te Ao Maramatanga) Wellington, New Zealand, 6th October, 1988.
Reynolds, W. and Cormack, D. (1982) Clinical teaching: an evaluation of a problem

orientated approach to psychiatric nurse education. *J. Adv. Nurs*, **7**, 231–7.

Reynolds, W. and Cormack, D. (1985) Clinical teaching of group dynamics: an evaluation of a trial clinical teaching programme. *Nurs. Ed. Today*, **5**, 101–8.

Reynolds, W. and Cormack, D. (1987) Teaching psychiatric nursing: interpersonal skills, in *Nursing Education: Research and Developments* (ed. B. Davis), 122–150.

Reynolds, W. and Presley, A. (1988) A study of empathy in student nurses. *Nurs. Ed. Today*, **8**, 123–30.

Reynolds, W. and Smoyak, S. (1983) Interview – Bill Reynolds. *J. Psychosoc. Nurs.*, **21**, 38–46.

Richardson, M. (1988) Innovating androgogy in a basic nursing course: an evaluation of the self-directed independent study contracts with basic nursing students. *Nurs. Ed. Today*, **8**, 315–24.

Rickard, T. (1981) Cognitive dissonance: the learner's experience. *Brit. J. Psych. Nurs.*, **I**, 6–7.

Robinson, K. (1986) Learners in the driving seat. *Senior Nurse*, **4**, 9–10.

Rogers, C. (1969) *Freedom to Learn*, Merrill Publishing, Columbus, OH.

Rogers, C. (1977) *Carl Rogers on Personal Power*, Delacorte, New York.

Rotter, J. (1966) Generalised expectancies for internal versus external control of reinforcements. *Psychol. Monog.: Gen. Appl.*, **80**, 1–27.

Schmuck, R. (1966) Some aspects of classroom social climate, and some aspects of peer liking patterns. *School Rev.*, **71**, 59–65 and 337–59.

Smith, D. (1957) Lets help our students learn and grow. *Nurs. Outlook*, **5**, 16–19.

Smith, H. (1966) *Sensitivity to People*, McGraw-Hill, New York.

Sweeney, J. (1986) Nurse education: learner-centred or teacher-centred? *Nurs. Ed. Today*, **6**, 257–62.

Taft, E. (1955) The ability to judge people. *Psychol. Bull.*, **52**, 23.

von-Bergen, R. and Cline, A. (1956) Some aspects of learning how to supervise. *Nurs. Outlook*, **4**, 152–4.

Weiss, J. (1963) Effects of professional training and amount of accuracy of information on behaviour. *J. Consult. Psychol.*, **27**, 257–62.

Zetzel, E. (1953) The dynamic basis of supervision. *Social Casework*, **34**, 143–9.

Chapter 20

Psychiatric and mental health nursing: learning in the clinical environment

M. CHAMBERS

Introduction

The aim of this chapter is to look at learning in the clinical environment mainly from the perspective of the learner nurse. However, as the relationship between learner and teacher is more or less inseparable there will be areas of overlap between what is written here and that in Chapter 19.

An initial examination of some of the essential concepts surrounding the process of psychiatric nursing will generate ideas which will form the foundation for the exploration and discussion of learning in the clinical environment. The main areas for further discussion will be: (a) conditions for learning, and (b) a model for practice. Whilst the major emphasis will be on the learner nurse it is anticipated that many of the issues raised will be relevant to any nurse who is actively engaged in the care of psychiatric patients.

It is recognized that learning is a life-long process and nowhere is this more true than in the area of psychiatric nursing. Here, each patient and each interaction presents new challenges, new opportunities for growth, both for nurse and patient alike. What both must learn is how best to use the opportunity to fulfil their own potential. The nurse has an additional responsibility in that she must facilitate and guide the patient whilst simultaneously learning about herself.

Setting the scene

Psychiatric nursing

Let's begin by having a brief look at psychiatric nursing and what it means to me. The beliefs I hold clearly influence how I see the skills of psychiatric nursing being developed and the crucial importance of learning in the clinical environment. The question of what is psychiatric nursing has occupied the thoughts of many nurse theorists for some considerable time, but especially in the last 40 years.

Travelbee (1979) pointed out that there was almost a complete lack of definition of psychiatric nursing. This remark would seem to ignore the seminal work of Peplau (1952) when she began to analyse the nature of psychiatric nursing. She considered it to be an interpersonal process and emphasized that within that process the nurse takes on a number of roles. However, her work at that time did not seem to fully recognize the personal position and potential for growth of the nurse herself.

Stuart and Sundeen (1988) point out that most psychiatric nursing texts focus on the functions and role of the psychiatric nurse. The particular definition which they offer is that psychiatric nursing is an interpersonal process that strives to promote and maintain behaviour that contributes to intergrated functioning. The patient or client system may be an individual, family, group, organization or community. This particular definition picks up on the important aspect raised by Peplau, that of the interpersonal process.

The American Nurses Association's Division of Psychiatric Nursing and Mental Heath Nursing, as cited in Stuart and Sundeen (1988), defines psychiatric nursing and mental health nursing as 'a specialized area of nursing practice employing theories of human behaviour as its science and purposeful use of self as its art. It is directed toward both preventive and corrective impacts upon mental disorders and their sequelae and is concerned with the promotion of optimal mental health for society, the community, and those individuals who live within it.' This definition does consider the use of self, and the science of human behaviour, and emphasizes the optimal mental health for society, the community, and those individuals who live within it. However, it does not make explicit the self-learning and development of the psychiatric nurse as a person and practitioner.

This chapter is developed around the belief that . . . psychiatric nursing is a process of relationship building between nurse and patient where the nurse seeks through that relationship to facilitate the growth of the individual patient to the maximum point of his or her capability, and to do so in a manner which will enable him/her to resume or take on a new role or function in everyday living as a member of a family or chosen society. Fundamental to this relationship is a learning process whereby the nurse, as a member of a caring team, can assess her therapeutic contribution and seek actively to promote her personal and professional growth and development.

This definition recognizes the importance of the nurse–patient relationship as the major element of the therapeutic process. It also gives cognizance to the fact that the nurse is learning and developing – therefore reinforcing the dynamic nature of psychiatric nursing. In addition, by bringing into focus the importance of developing the patient to the maximum point of his capability, it is incorporating one of the principles of Peplau's (1952; 1969) interpersonal model for psychiatric nursing, namely, helping clients to gain intellectual and interpersonal competencies beyond those they had at the point of illness. Implicit in this also is the rehabilitative aspect of psychiatric nursing. By highlighting the importance of personal growth for both parties it makes explicit the caring element embodied in psychiatric nursing. According to Mayeroff (1971):

> . . . to help another person grow is at least to help him to care for something or someone apart from himself, and it involves encouraging and assisting him to find and create areas of his own in which he is able to care. Also, it is to help that other person to come to care for himself, and, by becoming responsive to his own need to care, to become responsible for his own life. Growing includes learning to the degree that one is able, where learning is to be thought of primarily as the re-creation of one's own person through the integration of new experiences and ideas, rather than as the mere addition of information and technique.

What Mayeroff is saying here is, in essence, what the psychiatric nurse is trying to achieve.

The crucial element of psychiatric nursing is, therefore, the nurse–patient relationship, and this holds true and constant irrespective of what model of care is being practised, whether it be behavioural, psychotherapeutic, or sociotherapeutic. This reinforces the view held by Cormack (1985) who stated that the nurse–patient relationship is neither borrowed from nor imposed by other professional groups. This suggests that it is indeed non-productive to engage in argument about the origins of nurse–patient relationships. Instead, more energy should be directed at analysing examples of where such relationships have shown evidence of success. In this way much more progress will be made in establishing a sound theoretical basis for the practice of psychiatric nursing and enhance the quality of nursing knowledge.

Strang (1982), for example, described what happened when nurses on a drug dependency unit took on more responsibility for therapeutic intervention as part of a move toward individualized patient care. Here, the nurse was conducting work which had previously been considered the domain of the doctor or psychiatric social worker. It soon became evident that the use of the nurse as a psychotherapist was a powerful force in the sessions, especially as the nurse also had extensive contact with the patient outside these sessions in ward activities – for example, occupational therapy and ward group therapy.

It is unfortunate, however, that many still see psychiatric nursing as consisting of a series of different roles and functions. This is primarily because the value of the central tenent – the nurse–patient relationship –

is neither properly recognized nor valued. It could be suggested that this is why many psychiatric nurses, even today, cannot adequately describe what it is that they do, and if they cannot, then how can anyone else? Indeed the aforementioned article illustrates this in that there was almost an element of surprise when the force of the nurses' interventions was recognized. Surely this is the role of the psychiatric nurse and therefore does not require special conditions or treatment before it becomes evident!

However, psychiatric nurses have a responsibility to demonstrate that they have the necessary skills to function in this manner. Altschul (1972) indicated that psychiatric nurses tend not to have any identifiable perspective to guide them in their dealings with patients. The initial findings from a study, albeit small (Chambers, 1989), would support this statement even today. Time has moved on by nearly two decades since then, and in the interim some very sophisticated post-basic nursing courses have been developed, but without any thorough examination of basic preparation. This is like building a house with a magnificent facade, but without sound foundations – eventually it will collapse.

The process of psychiatric nursing

It is evident therefore, that the essential component of psychiatric nursing is the nurse–patient relationship. This relationship, being therapeutic in nature, has to reflect, and be developed around the three essential qualities of a therapeutic relationship as identified by Rogers (1957) namely, empathy, warmth and genuineness. For psychiatric nurses to be effective practitioners they must have the ability to utilize these elements in their work, that is, in their relationships with patients. In addition they must know how to think and possess the necessary principles, concepts and facts with which to be able to use the self as a therapeutic agent. The latter element is most important as the ability to use self in this way will promote the process of growth for both nurse and patient. Kreigh and Perko (1979) suggest empathy as the essential core of psychiatric nursing. Empathy of itself is not enough; the nurse must have other skills, as already outlined, in order to take the patient beyond the present into the future. The process of psychiatric nursing is therefore made up of: the need for clear recognition and understanding of the essential elements of a relationship; appropriate thinking and problem-solving ability incorporating facts, principles and concepts; a theoretical framework to guide interventions; and the skills to use self therapeutically.

Conditions for learning

Having outlined the major facets of psychiatric nursing we must now address the issue of how best to learn the necessary skills. The only way that this can be achieved is by working with real people in their home

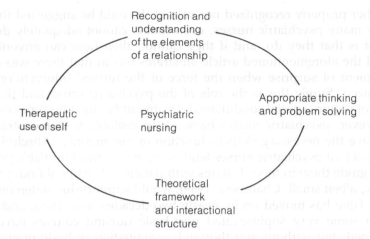

Figure 20.1 The process of psychiatric nursing

environment, wherever and whatever home means for that individual person.

Irrespective of the clinical environment in which the learner nurse should find herself there are certain conditions which must be present for learning to take place. These can be divided into: (a) those extrinsic to the person, and (b) those intrinsic to the person. However, this differentiation is somewhat artificial as both groups are interrelated and cannot therefore be separated. In this instance, for the purpose of clarity of presentation, they will, where possible, be discussed separately.

External factors

Learning environment

Much has now been written about the ward as a learning environment, for example Fretwell (1978), Orton (1979), Ogier (1982), Lewin and Jacka (1987); however, few published studies have concentrated exclusively on the psychiatric ward. It must be emphasized that there are many learning situations outside the ward environment and as more and more patients are cared for in the community these situations will increase. However, of the points raised here, the majority are of relevance irrespective of setting. Some of the characteristics which make up a good ward learning environment as identified by researchers include:

1. The ward sister/charge-nurse takes an active role in teaching; is democratic and patient-orientated.
2. Anti-hierarchical with regard to ward organization and management.

3. Good ward communication systems.
4. Strong emphasis on team work.
5. The availability of trained staff.

With the exception of the role of the ward charge person, all the above concentrate on organizational aspects or ward management and the availability of teachers.

(a) **Learners' perceptions** Pearson (1979) focused on the effectiveness of ward teaching as perceived by learners and found that the major issue was the teaching orientation of the charge nurse or ward sister. In a more recent study, Hyland, Millard and Parker (1988) found that 50% of the nurses whom they sampled felt that ward sisters or charge nurses were rude to them and did not make them feel at home. It was the behaviour of the charge person that determined student ward preferences. Firth *et al.* (1986) found that if students perceived the availability of support from the charge person then there was a reduction in emotional distress. These studies raise many issues about the ward as a learning environment, for example, the work of Hyland *et al.* and the issue of the charge persons' rudeness to learners. Why are they rude? Is it because of factors related to themselves as individuals, e.g., their interaction skills or anxieties about their role as ward charge person? Are there factors related to the students, to the organizational system in which the individuals are placed, or perhaps a combination of the above? Are there other areas not yet identified? Unfortunately, at present, there is no simple answer, and research into this vital area must continue.

(b) **Initial encounter** Meanwhile, what about the learners who daily enter hospital wards – many for the first time. For some it will be their first encounter with psychiatric patients as well as their first encounter with the hospital as a complex organization. Some students will be keen to embrace the challenge and may experience little or no anxiety, whilst for others it may be the opposite. If the ward climate is not perceived as safe they may be unable to express their emotions lest it jeopardizes their opportunity to become a nurse.

Through the period of theoretical preparation and orientation to the hospital, the learner will have become partially familiar with the hospital. However, it is only on entering the ward for a particular period of allocation that she really appreciates her vulnerability. She will fear making mistakes resulting in being told off by the charge person or other senior personnel. This distress will be magnified if at some time in the past she has had a bad experience with authority figures.

It is well known that some wards have particular reputations either as good or bad which quickly pass around the learner group. If the learner doubts her capabilities, which is inevitable at this early stage, she may be tempted to focus on incidents which reinforce the beliefs she currently holds of herself. Consequently she will be ignoring those which convey a more appropriate evaluation of her performance. This may be detrimental if there is no one around with whom she can communicate her anxieties.

(c) **Breaking the ice** Before commencing clinical placements, learners should be taken on a visit accompanied by the teacher and introduced to both staff and patients. For community placements this may be more problematic; none the less, it should be possible to meet the community nurse responsible for the learner and to be introduced to other community staff in the health clinic or wherever the community service is based.

In terms of psychological preparation, the learner must be encouraged to believe in herself, not to be too self-doubting, not always to interpret situations that go wrong as her fault, and to question practice, despite the risks.

It is the responsibility of the teacher to instil confidence, provide assertiveness training, support and reassurance. This can be greatly enhanced by the teacher establishing strong links with ward personnel and paying regular visits to the ward or community setting to work alongside the learner.

Preparation for practice

(a) **Relationship between theory and practice** It is not possible to consider preparation for practice without referring to the theory-versus-practice debate; however, it is the intention here to keep it short, but simultaneously raise levels of awareness.

Considerable research effort has gone into looking at the relationship between theory and practice. The study most pertinent in this instance is that of Clinton (1981) who looked at the classroom teaching and ward experience of students during a psychogeriatric placement. Clinton raised a number of very interesting points regarding ward-based teaching in relation to perpetuating the split between theory and practice, which can be summarized as follows.

1. Factors which render nursing care invisible to the nurse teacher:
   (a) They visit wards infrequently.
   (b) Much of the care is given at times when they are not available – early in the morning and late in the evening.
   (c) Insufficient time is available on the ward due to pressure of teaching in the school of nursing.
   (d) Clinical teachers avoid contact with patients by taking students away from direct patient care to give tutorials.
2. Division of labour:

(a) This ensures that the least qualified provide most of the direct patient care.
(b) Reinforces the belief that discrepancies are inevitable as long as there are shortages of both staff and resources.

A considerable reduction in the problems of relating theory to practice could be achieved if nurse teachers were free, or indeed prepared to work in the ward environment in the manner as described by Alexander (1985).

Working in the ward environment does not mean simply visiting the ward at regular intervals – although this, too, is necessary. It means working on the wards for prolonged periods of time with learners. Here the learner will have the opportunity to see the expert in action. However, this does put certain demands on the teacher, and for many it is now such a long time since their last meaningful patient contact that their skills are somewhat rusty. Teachers in this position cannot be expected to take on this role without proper up-dating.

Preparation for practice is greatly enhanced when liaison and relationships between the school of nursing and ward staff are congenial and where both are perceived by the student to be compatible in both aim and purpose. In essence they form a partnership – a marriage. If not the marriage, at least the period of courtship should begin as early as possible, preferably at the curriculum planning stage. Here, all staff come together to decide on which curriculum and nursing model best reflects their philosophy of care. This coming together will enable all to work for common goals, which should include high-quality nursing care coupled with high-quality learning experiences and opportunities for learners and trained staff alike.

As a learning milieu it should not be possible to separate clinical areas from the school of nursing – the whole of the hospital is the learning environment – the training school. Too often there is a tendency to separate one from the other; hopefully it is a thing of the past. However, nursing is still steeped in tradition and unfortunately in many instances it is very difficult to implement change without meeting lots of resistance generally because change is perceived as a threat.

There is one other factor worthy of note and that is the assumption that what is taught in the classroom is correct, or the ideal. Could it be that it is no more ideal than what is taught on the ward? As already stated, many nurse teachers are very out of touch in terms of working with patients. It is much easier to talk about what should be done and how to do it when, by and large, the situation is under one's control (as it is in a classroom) and not influenced by a patient going through a major life crisis.

(b) The classroom experience What has been outlined above in relation to promoting ward-based learning, for example, a democratic, anti-hierarchical environment, should also be true of the classroom. The educational process should be student-centred, leading to autonomous, self-thinking, sensitive individuals who can further enhance their skills though clinical practice and supervision.

There is still too much emphasis on teacher-directed learning. Students of nursing are young adults and as such should be given greater responsibility for their own learning. Jones (1981) outlined how attempts were being made to accomplish this independence in one school of nursing in England. This does not mean that learners should have total autonomy, but rather that their contribution to the planning and organization of learning experiences should be recognized and respected. After all, they are the consumers of the system, and as the emphasis is now on consumer satisfaction and quality assurance then it is imperative that they are given the opportunity to become more actively involved. However, this is dependent on a number of factors including the teachers' style of leadership.

(c) Style of leadership   Weinholtz and Ostmoe (1987) cite the work of Hersey and Blanchard (1977) who suggested that individual leadership styles tend to fall into one of four major categories depending on the amount of emphasis the teacher puts on task or relationship behaviour (see Fig. 20.2). They also propose that each of these leadership styles may

Figure 20.2   Four leadership styles available to clinical instructors

Style	Instructor behaviour
Telling (high task, low relationship)	Instructor dominates communication, providing learners with information and/or directions concerning responsibilities expected of them in the future.
Selling (high task, high relationship)	Instructor closely controls the flow of communication but fosters two-way communication with learners and re-inforces them for their contributions.
Participating (low task, high relationship)	Instructor stimulates free communication among learners, offering occasional information and reinforcement as needed.
Delegating (low task, low relationship)	Instructor allows the learners to control the learning situation and serves primarily as an observer or low-profile participant.

Printed with permission of Appleton-century crofts, Norwalk, CT, USA.

be more appropriate in certain situations. The leader should be able to move between styles as and when appropriate. However, if in the main a democratic style of leadership is adopted within the educational encounter then there is more likelihood of a positive outcome where the student will be able to use the educational experience as a medium for growth, in both educational and personal terms.

Whether or not teaching/learning is taking place in the ward or classroom environment, one of the major determinants likely to influence positive outcome is that of the teacher–learner relationship.

Teacher–learner relationships

Because this is such a crucial element, in the teaching/learning process, it presents difficulties as to where exactly it should be discussed; it requires a mention at all levels. However, it does seem to fit here as we have just considered the ward climate, the classroom climate and leadership styles and are about to move forward to look at the process of andragogy (adult learning) a central tenet of which is the teacher–learner relationship. This relationship is analogous to that occurring between nurse and patient. Many of the same issues enter into it and have the same potential to either enhance or hinder. Because of the hierarchical nature of nursing, which unfortunately still does exist despite the rhetoric to the contrary, there is a tendency for the teacher to be seen as an authority, in authority, if not authoritarian.

The concept of the teacher–learner relationship and what it means to individual teachers and learners will be influenced by a number of factors, including their self-image and self-concept, and the overall educational philosophy of the institution, including the curriculum model. The personal beliefs and attitudes of teachers will also be of importance. However, if both teacher and learner are to gain from the experience then the teacher must be prepared to shed some professional veneer and relate to the learner as one human being to another. This will allow for a much more open, honest relationship with the learner more likely to question and experiment, consequently gaining as a person. As already stated for some teachers, this may present a little difficulty but if entered into in the right spirit and with colleague support the advantages will outweigh the initial discomfort.

(a) Adult learning There is now considerable literature available on the process of teaching adults (andragogy), the best known of which is that by Knowles (1980). According to Knowles there are four assumptions in the andragogical process all of which are directly relevant to learning psychiatric nursing skills. They are as follows:

1. The learner moves from dependence to independence.
2. The learner's experience becomes an increasingly rich source of learning.

3. In the context of orientation to learning, adults wish to apply what they learn, so that education should be organized around comprehensive categories.
4. Adults are ready to learn material relevant to their life situation.

We will now consider the above in relation to learning psychiatric nursing skills.

It is hoped that, as the learner becomes more competent, she can move on to taking more responsibility for patient care as well as being capable of entering into relationships of a more complex nature and in greater depth. Indeed learners long for the opportunity to explore their own potential and skill. Sometimes they are held back because of reluctance on the part of trained staff, lest the learner or the patient gets hurt.

The idea of moving in a graded way may seem very idealistic and far removed from the practicalities of life; however, this is no reason for not at least trying. It is a sound educational principle, as outlined by Ausubel, Novak and Hanesian (1978), to move from the known to the unknown. Given the nature of the work carried out by psychiatric nurses there is, arguably, a moral responsibility to achieve this form of progression!

The issue of the learner's range of experiences becoming an increasingly rich source of learning is also fundamental to learning psychiatric nursing. It is both from and through experience that learners acquire sensitivity, perception, thinking, and problem-solving skills. Of course this cannot be achieved alone, and it is here that the teacher plays a vital role. Through utilizing a variety of approaches, the teacher can help the learner to acquire the necessary insights into practice. This particular point will be examined in more detail in a later section. It is only through practice based on theoretical principles with sound constructive feedback that high levels of skills will be acquired.

With regard to readiness to learn, one must assume that most students come into psychiatric nursing because they want to. (It is also acknowledged that some will enter for other reasons.) As such, it might be presumed that they possess an element of self-motivation and therefore a readiness to learn.

In addition to learning skills specific to psychiatric nursing, the learner will also acquire a range of skills relevant to everyday living. Interaction skills and a grounding in the understanding of 'human-ness' are important irrespective of setting. Overall, the learner will gain a greater understanding of herself and others which will be of benefit wherever she should go.

Internal factors

Individual differences

Learning is a multifaceted activity in which an individual uses a variety of stimuli to organize thoughts, feelings and behaviour. Much will be in-

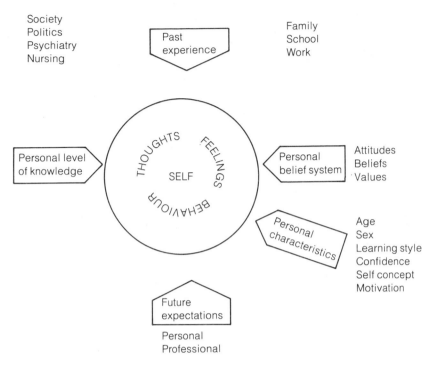

Figure 20.3 Learning set

fluenced by past experience and future expectations as well as what is happening in the here and now.

From Fig. 20.3 it is clear that a number of factors operate in the learning arena. It is impossible to discuss all of them in detail here, so only those of particular significance will be looked at, and then only briefly, as each in itself is worthy of a book, let alone a brief section in a chapter.

(a) Self-concept The concept of self is one of the most important aspects of one's being. What a person believes about herself is a function of her interpretation of how others see her, which she infers from their behaviour towards her. Her concept of self, therefore, rests in part on what she thinks others think of her. It is recognized that the family is most influential in the development of the self-concept. As the individual gradually moves away from the family others take over the role of significant others, and in the case of the learner nurse the teachers, in all areas, will become an important force. What the learner perceives and how she interprets what she perceives are conditioned by her concept of self. If she has a positive self-concept, then she will be able to explore the work openly and honestly because she has sufficient positive experiences and successes to lead her to believe 'I am OK'. On the other hand, if she has a negative self-concept she will be unsure, timid, with high anxiety and therefore more likely to make mistakes. This then becomes the cycle of the self-fulfilling prophecy.

Rogers (1961) developed his theory of the fully functioning person, whilst Maslow (1954) described the concept of self-actualization. Here we will concentrate on Rogers' view as it fits more closely with some of the ideas expressed earlier.

Central to Rogers' view of the fully functioning person is that the individual moves away from facades that are not true to the self and also emphasizes the need to move away from pleasing others who impose artificial goals, and gravitate towards becoming autonomous, self-directing and self-responsible. In additions he is open to change and exploring her potential, is open to her own self and the lives of others, trusts and values herself; and attempts to express herself in new ways. An understanding of this concept is extremely important for the learner nurse and her teachers in order to prevent unnecessary distress and enhance potential for learning. This reinforces the ideas expressed in the section concerned with breaking the ice and teacher–learner relationships – for example, the need to encourage the learner to take risks and the importance of openness and honesty in relationships.

It is also clear that there is a need for the teacher to get to know the learner in order to establish how she sees herself and encourage a more positive approach if necessary. It further reinforces the view that nurse teachers must shed their facades and face the truth about themselves as individuals, and all that that encompasses. The study by Hyland and co-workers, referred to earlier, is an example of where the potential to reinforce learners' positive self-concept was being missed – as, clearly, learners did not feel at ease or at home in certain wards.

(b) Self-ideal   Self-ideal is another very important and related concept. It is to do with the individual's perception of how he/she should behave, based on certain personal standards (Stuart and Sundeen, 1979).

There are a number of factors which influence one's self-ideal, for example, setting goals that are within one's capabilities. Self-ideals are also influenced by culture, so that the individual will be checking out her behaviour in relation to that of her peers to establish its consistency with the culture. Other influential factors include ambition, the need to achieve, and prevention of failure and anxiety. These factors form the basis for a realistic self-ideal, thus facilitating personal growth and development. Alternatively, the self-ideal may be negative and unrealistic.

For the fully functioning individual there will be a congruence between the perceptions of self and the self-ideal. In other words she sees herself more or less as she would like to be. From the perspective of the learner nurse this would include both the personal and the professional self. Working in the ward situation the learner will be checking her behaviour and responses in relation to other members of her peer group and that of trained staff. She will be seeking confirmation that her performance is congruent with that of a professional psychiatric nurse – she will be developing her professional self-ideal. Consequently, there is a need for appropriate ward-based role models otherwise the learner will suffer from incongruity. She may not be able to work out what her self-ideal should be in the absence of role models. Such incongruity could create a situation whereby the learner may decide to terminate her training.

(c) **Self-esteem** This is the individual's personal judgement of her own worth obtained by analysing how well her behaviour conforms to her self-ideal (Stuart and Sundeen, 1979). High self-esteem tends to come from success and is rooted in unconditional acceptance of self even when things go wrong. It is also correlated with low anxiety, effective functioning in groups, and a willingness to accept others. Low self-esteem is associated with the reverse situation.

It is recognized that self-esteem increases with age and that it is at its most vulnerable during adolescence and early adulthood (Stuart and Sundeen, 1979). Nurse teachers should be familiar with this concept in order to better understand both themselves and the learners for which they are responsible. Considering that the majority of learners begin training in their teens and early twenties, when they are at their most vulnerable with regard to establishing self-esteem, the teachers both in the ward and the classroom are clearly influential. According to Maslow, self-esteem is a prerequisite of self actualization and that once self-esteem has been achieved the individual can then concentrate on fully achieving his potential.

(d) **Motivation** Another important and related issue is that of motivation. Considerable research has taken place in this area with the best known work being that of McClelland (1959) who looked at achievement motivation. Through the use of projective tests, subjects were asked to write short stories in response to pictures. Those individuals scoring high on achievement motivation showed a preference for more difficult tasks, were more self-confident, and were prepared to wait longer for gratification. McClelland also pointed out that those with high need to achieve scores generally came from a family where emphasis was placed on independence.

Research by Birney, Burdick and Teevan (1969) highlights another important and related facet, that of fear of failure. In our society there is support for those who succeed, and in our present (UK) political climate, which focuses largely on individual achievement, this is magnified. Birney believes that fear of failure may have many causes but he points out three: lessening of self-esteem, lowering of public image, and loss of reward accompanying poor attainment. It is important therefore that clinical supervisors are aware of the above research and structure their clinical supervision in such a manner as to reduce the likelihood of the above happening. Inherent in this is the all-important element of reinforcement.

(e) Reinforcement Reinforcement is anything which, when it follows a behaviour, increases the possibility of that behaviour happening again. This reinforcement can be either positive or negative, and can take a number of forms. Here we will be talking about direct and vicarious reinforcement.

Direct reinforcement Direct reinforcement is as described above – anything which, when it follows a behaviour, increases the likelihood of that piece of behaviour occurring again. As the concern here is with learning psychiatric nursing skills, the emphasis will be on positive reinforcement as that is what is most commonly used. This will normally take the form of feedback on work completed and will be either written or verbal. As we are concerned with learning in the ward environment the majority of this feedback will be verbal. To be of maximum benefit it should be given as soon as possible following the behaviour and in a manner that will convey to the learner that her behaviour was of such a standard as to warrant praise. There will be occasions when the learner will have to receive feedback which is negative (not to be confused with negative reinforcement), but if this is delivered in a caring manner the learner, whilst not liking it, will be able to appreciate that it is necessary.

Teacher feedback is a very important part of the learning process and can be enhanced if the relationship between teacher and learner is good and the teacher has respect, a respect that is achieved not ascribed.

Vicarious reinforcement Learners also learn through the observational process of seeing others being praised for a particular aspect of behaviour. Kanfer (1965) indicated that behaviour learned in this manner is of the same magnitude as that acquired through direct reinforcement. Work by Berger (1961) and Marlett (1968) seems to indicate that under certain circumstances changes in behaviour acquired through this process may exceed those achieved by direct reinforcement. 'A vicarious reinforcement event not only provides information concerning probable reinforcing contingencies, knowledge about the types of situations in which the behaviour is appropriate, and displays of incentives possessing activating properties, but it also includes affective expressions of models undergoing rewarding and punishing experiences' (Bandura, 1969).

Considering that the majority of learning opportunities (at least in the

UK) are available in the ward environment then, clearly, the importance of vicarious reinforcement cannot be overlooked by teachers. To date, it would appear that no one has really considered this as a serious issue.

The study by Reid (1985), in which she looked at the teaching/learning on medical wards, found, by direct observation and learner reports, that they were unsupervised most of the time. Learners tended to work either alone or with another learner. If this is examined within the framework of vicarious learning, which emphasizes the importance of role modelling, it gives major cause for concern.

(a) **Role model** 'One of the fundamental means by which new modes of behaviour are acquired and existing patterns are modified entails modelling and vicarious processes' (Bandura, 1969). When learning by this vicarious process it is not only psychomotor components of the model's behaviour that the observer experiences, but also the concomitant emotions. This will entail appropriate emotional coping skills which psychiatric learners need to see in operation. This is both in terms of how the role model directs and facilitates patients' coping skills and also how she handles her own emotions. It can be deduced, therefore, that the role model within the ward situation is crucial to learning nursing skills. As previously mentioned, the study by Reid and others has indicated that learners spend considerable periods of time in the company of other learners. These learners may be senior, but where and how did they acquire their skills – was it solely from other learners? In psychiatric nursing this poses particular problems – considering that the main therapeutic tool the psychiatric nurse has is herself. If learners cannot see this process in action, and if models are not available within the clinical environment, then where and how are the appropriate therapeutic skills going to be learned? How are psychiatric nurses going to fulfil their therapeutic role? How are they even going to realize that they have one? Where does this leave the psychiatric nurse of the future?

This section has looked at the conditions for learning, including external and internal factors. It must be emphasized, however, that only a small sample of the factors involved have been examined. It will be left to the reader to pursue the others, as indicated in Fig. 20.3, and also to investigate other areas which they consider important and which have not been included in any part of this text.

In summary then, to maximize the potential for learning in the clinical area, the conditions must be right in that: the environment must be safe; relationships between teacher and learner must be centred around honesty, trust and respect; learners fears must be recognized and catered for; learning must be structured; opportunity must be available for the learner to be active in the learning process; and appropriate role models must be available.

A model for practice

Having said something about the conditions for learning we will now move on to look at a possible model for practice. This will consist of an exploration of the various theoretical ideas around which the model is developed before considering its operationalization.

Theoretical underpinnings

It has already been stated that the best way to learn psychiatric nursing skills is to work with real people in their usual living environment, thus leading to a meaningful experience. This enables the learner to make sense of what is happening and what it is she is learning, and it also enables her to relate it to previous learning. In addition she will be able to explore and experience the appropriate emotional states, and experiment with her own coping strategies. The theoretical framework which best accommodates this approach is that of experiential learning.

Experiential learning

Burnard (1989) has pointed out that experiential learning means different things to different people. This comment was based on the findings of a survey of nurse educationalists in England and Wales. The definition of experiential learning which will be used here is that of Kolb (1971): '...experiential learning is a process in which a particular experience is, on reflection, translated into concepts which become in turn guidelines for new experiences.'

Experiential learning dates back to the first writings of John Dewey (1916) an American philosopher of science and education. Since then a number of others have contributed to the growing body of literature. Perhaps the best known work is that of the late Carl Rogers, who pioneered the philosophy of student-centred learning. More recent work is that of Kolb (1971) in the USA and of Heron (1975) in the UK.

With regard to the epistemology underpinning experiential learning, little was available until the work of Heron (1981). He believes that there are three domains of knowledge within the epistemology: propositional knowledge, practical knowledge, and experiential knowledge. It is suggested that whilst each of these domains is free-standing they are also interrelated. Simply put, propositional knowledge can be thought of as textbook knowledge; practical knowledge is self-explanatory – knowledge which is acquired through the development of skills; and experiential knowledge is that acquired through personal encounter, let it be with a person or object, it is personal knowledge. An important point about experiential knowledge is that it is relative, constantly changing, as personal experiences and memories change. It is not possible to record this type of knowledge, as doing so would automatically transform it into proposi-

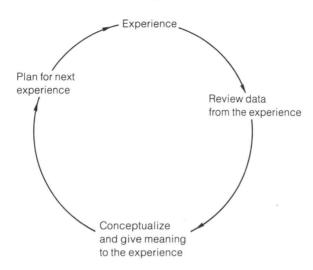

Figure 20.4 Experiential learning cycle (adapted from Kolb and Fry, 1975).

tional knowledge; however, there are occasions when it is necessary. A central component of experiential knowledge is reflection, which will be discussed later.

(a) Learning cycle The most frequently cited learning cycle is that of Kolb and Fry (1975), a modified version of which is outlined in Fig. 20.4. Burnard (1987) adopted this learning cycle for nurse education to enable teachers to use clinical nursing practice as the foundation for planning theoretical input.

Burnard's model (see Fig. 20.5) is useful in terms of providing a framework for reflection and examination of an overall clinical experience. It does, however, seem to imply that reflection should take place in a group and secondly that it should happen in the school of nursing. This presents certain difficulties in that some considerable time may have elapsed from the actual experience and the subsequent reflection; thus, the degree and intensity of the situation is lost as may some pertinent material. It is difficult to generate the same atmospheric conditions in the classroom, although approximations can be achieved through the use of games and exercises. It can be restricting and prohibitive for some individuals to engage in this type of work in a group, at least initially.

The model suggested here (see Fig. 20.6) is where the learner reflects on her interaction immediately it happens on the ward, reviews the data collected, conceptualizes, and gives meaning to the experience, using her theoretical framework, and then discusses the outcome with her mentor before setting new goals for the next interaction.

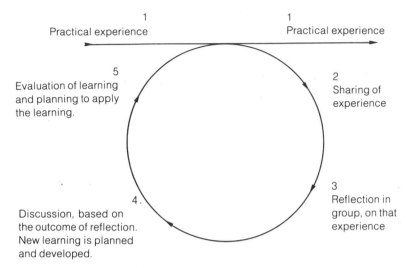

Figure 20.5 Experiential learning cycle for nurse education (from Burnard (1987), with permission from Blackwell Publications).

This particular approach allows for immediate feedback within the ward setting. The establishment of new goals and strategies for the next encounter is made easier, hence the situation is much more alive and meaningful. The learner is then free to enter into another interaction quickly, if appropriate, and feel confident that she can handle it.

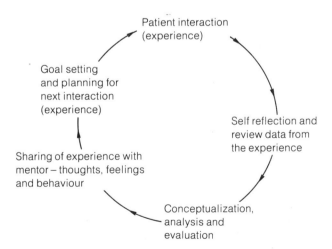

Figure 20.6 An experiential learning cycle for psychiatric nursing in clinical practice

The process suggested by Burnard (1987) would then enable learners to reflect on the clinical experience as a whole, and would be complementary to, and not instead of, that which took place within the clinical setting. Indeed, there could be a particular interaction which the learner may wish to share and examine with colleagues in the classroom.

Of course, it could be argued that in order to make the reflection meaningful, time should elapse to allow the associated emotions the opportunity to settle, thus enabling a more balanced and productive self-examination of the situation.

(b) Reflection Reflection is a significant element in adult learning, and not something which happens automatically or at one level. According to Mezirow (1981) it involves seven levels ranging from reflectivity – that is, awareness of seeing, thinking or acting – through to theoretical reflectivity – an awareness that taken-for-granted assumptions may be less than sufficient to explain perceived reality.

The importance of reflectivity with regard to learning psychiatric nursing skills is that the learner must be given space to engage in this process and must be allowed to work at her own pace and not be pressurized by her teacher mentor to reach conclusions. Indeed, part of her growing as a person and as a psychiatric nurse will be achieved through reflection – setting new personal goals which she can critically analyse and test, setting the whole process in motion again. This then develops within the learner a willingness to engage in self-assessment and analysis and develop a keenness to experiment – as well as an openness in the sharing of experiences. Reflection must therefore become an integral part of the learning process. In 1952 Peplau wrote that the kind of person the nurse becomes influences the quality of the learning that takes place in the patient she nurses. Consequently the nurse needs to be open and as free from defences as possible if she is going to be able to use herself as a therapeutic agent.

(c) Therapeutic use of self Therapeutic use of self as operationally defined by Uys (1980) refers to the ability of the nurse scientifically and purposefully to employ her/his entire person, or a combination of elements that constitute her/his unique individuality, and identity as a tool for promoting health and limiting disease.

If the nurse is unfamiliar with herself she will be of less value therapeutically. This does not mean, however, that she must be the epitome of psychological adjustment. Rather, it means that she needs to have sufficient insight into her own strengths and weaknesses and recognize that, whatever her shortcomings, these will not interfere with her relationships. A detailed account of this process is given by Uys (1980) but briefly it consists of a series of antecedent steps:

1. Self-knowledge: becomes aware of/pays attention to own behaviour/ thoughts/feelings, for example, 'What am I doing? What am I feeling?' Studies the antecedents and consequences of behaviour as well as the interpersonal situations, for example, 'Why did I do that? Why do I feel this? What feelings do those thoughts cause? Has this or something similar happened before?'
2. Self-growth: takes ownership and responsibility for behaviour/thoughts/ feelings, for example, 'Did I do that? Then it is my responsibility. If I feel angry, no one made me angry; it is my reaction; it is my responsi- bility.' Modifies behaviour/thoughts/feelings towards responsibility, assertiveness and health, for example, 'Since that is a destructive way of expressing my feelings, I will express them differently.' Develops feeling of self-acceptance and appreciation of own worth, for example, 'What do I like about myself? Why do people love me? I am OK.' Devel- ops skill of disclosing self appropriately, for example, discloses appro- priate amounts of information. Picks the right time for self-disclosure.
3. Acquires scientific knowledge; acquires in-depth knowledge about the spectrum of human behaviour in health and disease and the science of changing/influencing it, for example, studies psychology, sociology, etc.

One of the highlights from this framework is that the psychiatric nurse needs to combine an understanding of self with scientific knowledge. Consequently, interventions need to be scientifically based, used purpose- fully and flexibly, adapting to individual patient needs. This demonstrates the coming together of the art and the science of nursing.

Clark (1988) commented that the absence of an identifiable theoretical underpinning leaves the nurse open to undue influences from other quarters and they appear unwilling or unable to accept a therapeutic role for themselves in relation to other disciplines. Where psychiatric nurses have identified a major role and have become a powerful force is in the field of behaviour therapy nursing. Here, nurses have demonstrated their efficacy in using a range of behavioural approaches across all spectra of psychiatric illness; however, the number of nurses adequately trained in this area is small.

(d) Six category intervention analysis The work of John Heron from 1975 onwards has been most influential in helping psychiatric nurses develop a framework for patient interactions. A whole range of other disciplines including medicine, social work, business and management and the police force now use this approach. It would seem a little ambit- ious to classify Heron's work under the heading of scientific; however, its potency as a framework must be recognized. Some of the major attrac- tions of this approach include: the focus on intention and practitioner creativity; the balance between the authoritative and facilitative forms of interaction; and the emphasis on self-awareness and self-understanding, and the resultant personal development.

The six-category system deals with six basic kinds of intentions the practitioner can have in serving the patient/client. It is a practical working hypothesis and not a dogma. It is easy to understand and put into practice because it focuses on the intention and purpose of the interventions, which meet the needs of human beings.

What this approach has to offer the nurse is that it gives intention and purpose to interactions. By drawing attention to the importance of centredness – being self-aware – it therefore increases awareness of the persons with whom the interaction is taking place. If the nurse is here now, meaning aware of herself, then she will also be there now, meaning that she will also be aware of her patient. In other words she will be awake and therefore more likely to be therapeutically on target. This will be a result of the nurse knowing what intervention she is using and why she is using it. Whilst many psychiatric nurses do adopt this approach many do not possess the necessary skills; consequently, many avoid entering into any form of lengthy conversation with a patient which may have the potential to progress into a therapeutic encounter. This fear to enter into such conversations with patients was highlighted by Davis (1981). As the six categories of intervention are easy to learn, the nurse can see results quickly. These results will include an increase in her own personal self-confidence and a confidence in using the interventions as well as changes in the patient's ability to handle his emotions.

For the reasons already outlined it is recommended that training in the six categories become an integral part of psychiatric nurse education, as the interventions can be used irrespective of the overall therapeutic approach.

(e) Self-awareness A continuous theme throughout this section has been self-awareness. For example, it was referred to at the beginning when we were discussing experiential learning, and again just now when considering Heron's six-category intervention analysis. Here we will look at it in a little more detail so as to make explicit what is being considered, and its importance with regard to learning psychiatric nursing skills.

Self-awareness is about increasing/gaining a greater knowledge of self and others. The Johari window (Luft, 1970) is a helpful means by which to analyse the concept (see Fig. 20.7).

If we use this above window as a reference point, we can see that quadrant 1, the open area, includes those parts which are known to the self and others and includes thoughts, feelings and behaviour. Quadrant 2, the blind area, includes those things which others know about us but of which we are unaware. Quadrant 3, the hidden area, includes those things which only the individual knows about: hidden agendas and personal feelings.

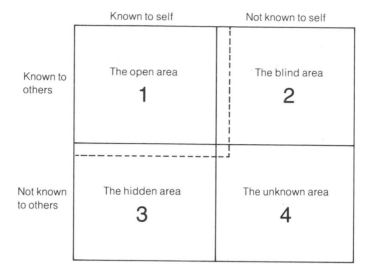

Figure 20.7   The Johari window

Quadrant 4, the unknown area, includes all those things which are unknown to self or others, but which may at some point be revealed. When attempting to increase self-awareness, the goal is to increase quadrant 1 – therefore decreasing the size of the other three quadrants (see Fig. 20.8).

The first step is to listen to oneself; this means experiencing genuine emotion, exploring one's thoughts, feelings and memories.

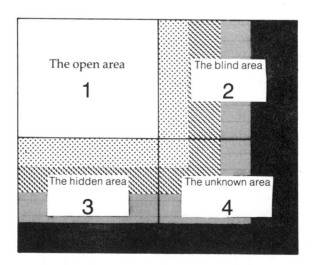

Figure 20.8   Increasing self-awareness

The second step is to reduce the size of quadrant 2 through the use of feedback from others but this requires active listening and the feedback from others must be received with openness.

The third step is to reduce the size of quadrant 3 through self-disclosure or sharing with others important aspects of oneself. Therefore increasing one's self-awareness consists of a process of listening to one's self and experiencing real emotions, being receptive to feedback from others, and being prepared to self-disclose. As we shall see later, this is what takes place during the post-interaction discussions between learner and mentor. It also resembles closely that which was discussed in the section concerned with the therapeutic use of self, reinforcing the belief that if one is to be at ease in the therapeutic setting, then one needs to understand one's self and feel comfortable with it.

An important feature in the process of increasing self-awareness is responding to feedback. In order to increase the effectiveness of the feedback it is best given in a sensitive caring manner. It is always better to be descriptive and specific rather than evaluative and general. If possible it should be directed towards behaviour that the individual can control. All mentors and teachers should be aware of the importance of delivering feedback in this way.

The learning experience

'Whatever theory or research evidence makes sense, its translation into practice is a complicated and tentative process. Our good intentions are often difficult to put into effect even where we know what is necessary to achieve them' (Jaques, 1984). The particular approach to learning in the clinical environment advocated here is based on a number of preconditions, and as such, may be problematic for some. However, most problems are surmountable if the end product is deemed to be of sufficient importance or value. The preconditions are that:

1. The ward environment is conducive to learning as outlined at the beginning of this chapter.
2. The learner will have a mentor on the ward, that is, someone with whom she can speak freely about any aspect of her work on the ward – including personal feelings – and who also acts as an appropriate role model. (It must be recognized that all qualified nurses have a responsibility to facilitate learning in the ward environment.) The mentor, however, has direct responsibility for one or two learners, preferably only one.
The personal qualities required of a mentor are similar to those identified by Rogers (1983) when considering the needs for the part of a facilitator. They are an ability to:

be aware of oneself
respond to the feelings of the learner
recognize one's own feelings
accept the trust of the learner
empathize with the learner

Some see the role of facilitator as synonymous with that of mentor. Here it is not considered in that way, but is perceived to extend beyond that. The mentor, therefore, is considered to have at least five functions including pastoral, facilitative, role model, assessor and supervisor.

3. The learner will have a tutor who will see her through her period of training, thus giving continuity and facilitating the building of a learner profile. Ward mentors will change from ward to ward; it is therefore necessary for the learner not to be the only constant variable in the triad.

4. This tutor will visit the ward to work with the learner and mentor as part of the triad system in the practice of psychiatric nursing. She will give support to both learner and mentor and help with the problems of transference and counter-transference, should they occur.

   The tutor will be in an excellent position to make judgements about the learner's progress as she has the opportunity to observe her in a number of different settings and involved in a variety of activities. This gives the learner a degree of security, hence increasing the opportunity for learner autonomy in terms of setting her own goals both personal and professional (some of which she may not wish to disclose). It will also provide the climate to enable the learner to assess her own performance and begin to look critically at her work within a supportive environment.

5. Primary nursing is the approach to care. Here the learner and the mentor have responsibility for a small number of patients. (This also reflects nursing in the community. However, the mentor would have responsibility for larger numbers of patients.) The learner, mentor and tutor will formulate individual patient goals and short-term nursing objectives. This facilitates the learning process further in that patients get to know both the learner and the mentor very well. During interactions, both can be present without either patient or learner feeling alarm or increased distress – it is part of the normal sequence of events. Obviously the patient does not get to know the tutor to the same extent, but as most of the direct supervision is conducted by the mentor this is not a major problem.

6. Preparation and additional training will be provided for the mentor in terms of how to facilitate learning – for example, how to set objectives, assess and evaluate the degree of learning, assess the ward as a learning situation, as well as assessing the degree of learning accomplished by the learner.

Setting objectives does not mean purely behavioural objectives but rather how to encourage the learner to set her own personal and professional objectives. The mentor, too, will set her own objectives for the learner, thus providing material for negotiation and encouraging student autonomy in the learning process. This is why training for mentors is so important, as many will be unaccustomed to the idea of student-centred learning and student autonomy.

7. The student will have periods of time during the day for reflection and to write up process recordings on her work. These periods will be followed by consultation with her mentor.
8. Multidisciplinary team work will be evident where the mentor, as primary nurse, can function as an equal member of the team, thus providing a good role model.
9. If possible, a staff support group will be in operation on the ward and it will be multidisciplinary in nature.

(a) Pre-placement visit Before beginning a particular placement the learner should be taken to the ward by the tutor. This will enable her to get a feel for the ward as well as giving her the opportunity to meet her mentor, if known. If not, this would be an appropriate time to identify her/him and to get acquainted. It is preferable for the learner to identify her own mentor; however, this may not always be possible.

During this visit the mentor can become familiar with the learning objectives for the placement and, together with tutor and learner, outline a learning map. For example, from the objectives it can be negotiated what aspects to focus on first, bearing in mind individual learning styles and previous learning. This acts as an advanced organizer (Ausubel, Novak and Hanesian, 1978) for the learner, as she will know what to expect when she comes to the ward. Whilst this might seem rather laborious and time consuming it is very worthwhile. After the initial introductions and sketching of the learning map, the tutor can leave the learner with her mentor. This will allow the learner freedom and autonomy to pursue issues important to herself with her mentor should she desire so to do.

It is advisable that the tutor, learner and mentor meet at regular weekly intervals to assess progress and set new goals. The tutor may have worked with the learner at other points in the week, but there should be a regular scheduled time irrespective of this.

The teaching/learning method

At the beginning of the chapter it was stated that the most potent therapeutic tool the psychiatric nurse possesses is herself. Therefore, it is this that must be developed during clinical placements. It is manifested in the relationship that the learner has with individual patients, irrespective of therapeutic approach, and needs to be the focus for learning. Travelbee (1979) identified one of the characteristics of a relationship as being one where both patient and nurse change and modify their behaviour; if changes do not occur in either or both participants, then it is assumed that a relationship has not been established:

> As a result of the relationship the ill person grows in his ability to face reality, to discover practical solutions to problems, to become less estranged from the community, and to derive pleasure from communicating and socialising with a fellow human being. The nurse grows as a human being as a result of the encounter with the emotionally ill person. The practitioner learns new ways of assisting the ill person to move towards meaningful participation in the human community. She learns more about self and, over a period of time, develops the ability to audit and change her behaviour.

Using the primary nurse system as described by Fairbanks (1980) the learner can act as associate nurse. Here she will be involved with a small group of patients, thus increasing the potential for getting to know them as individuals and of establishing a therapeutic relationship.

The learner will of course interact with a number of patients at different levels, at different times in different situations, ranging from small-talk, to a more in-depth therapeutic interaction. It must be emphasized that the patient's permission should always be obtained before beginning any interaction. For example: 'Is it alright with you, Mrs Smith, if I sit and talk with you for a while?'

There will of course be times when spontaneous learning situations arise within the ward – for example, when a patient cries or gets angry. The learner may not have been prepared for this. In most times of crisis individuals cope to the best of their ability, and learner nurses are no exception. However, it is hoped that a trained member of staff would be available quickly if required. In any event learner nurses should, ideally, not be left alone with very disturbed or potentially disturbed patients, however, reality must be acknowledged and it does happen.

Whatever the incident, time should be set aside as soon as possible afterwards to discuss what happened, how the learner coped, and what her feelings were. If it was a particularly difficult experience and something which had importance for the whole ward, then it may be necessary to raise it at the next staff support group.

Before discussion of the teaching/learning cycle in action, it is important to look at the medium whereby the cycle will become operationalized and translated into a learning experience.

Considerable discussion takes place within nursing literature about the importance of experiential learning and reflection, but very little has been said as to how nurse teachers can develop and use it in a meaningful way.

It is insufficient to think of it simply in terms of learners gaining from an experience. The learning must be planned for and developed in a systematic manner. One way in which this can be achieved in clinical practice is through the use of process recording.

Process recording

Travelbee (1979) defined process recording as a systematic method of collecting data prior to interpreting, analysing and synthesizing the data obtained. A process record is a written account of what transpired before, during, and following a nurse–patient interaction (mostly the verbal aspects).

The purpose of process recording is to improve the quality of patient care and simultaneously that of the learning experience, as it encourages the learner or practitioner to attend to what is happening. In other words they become conscious of their interactions and bring into focus those elements as outlined in Fig. 20.1 at the beginning of this chapter, and also the points raised when referring to Heron's six-category intervention analysis. This is in contrast to the more intuitive approach which is still prevalent today. In addition, process recording facilitates: the integration of theory and practice; increased self-awareness through the identification of thoughts and feelings, verbal and non-verbal communication, and how others are affected as a result; development of learner's observational skills; competence in the collection, analysis and synthesis of data (in the case of the learner nurse this will be done initially under the supervision of her mentor); development of the learner's ability to identify nursing problems and the competencies necessary to solve them.

In this instance we are considering process recording as a means of helping the learner nurse to develop the skills necessary to become competent psychiatric nurses. However, all nurses in the clinical setting should be encouraged to utilize some form of process recording as part of their ongoing personal development. It can help private reflection or alternatively it can be the basis for discussion with peer(s) individually or in groups.

(a) Ground rules for process recording The nurse has a responsibility to inform the patient during her first interaction with him that what is discussed during their interactions will be shared with others, for example, her mentor. As this is confidential information then it must be treated accordingly. As a precaution, the learner can use a fictitious name within the body of the text. The learner and mentor need to decide on the following: (1) the nature of the recording – will it be a descriptive narrative or a column format? (The narrative helps the learner to organize and synthesize information.) (2) The type of information to be included. It must be such as to help the nurse plan, analyse and evaluate nursing interventions. She must know what aspects to focus on during the interaction. (3) What

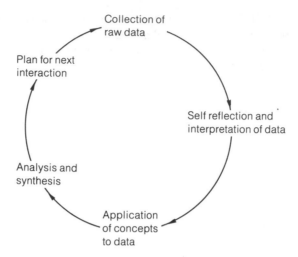

Figure 20.9 Process recording cycle

background information is required before commencing the interaction – for example, patient's age and previous admissions. (4) What information and knowledge of specific treatment modalities is required, including effects and side effects. (5) What knowledge of the dynamics of psychiatric illness is necessary.

(b) Stages of process recording As can be seen from Fig. 20.9, the stages of process recording mirror very closely those of the experiential learning cycle for clinical practice. A brief description of each of the stages will be given here; a more detailed account can be found in Travelbee (1979).

Collection of raw data: stage 1. This includes the verbal and non-verbal communication of both the learner and the patient during the interaction. It includes all data received via the sense organs prior to interpretation of the meaning of the data. It does not include assumptions, suppositions or feelings; however, it is useless without interpretation.

Interpretation: stage 2. This is one of the most difficult phases for the learner. Here she must be able to explain that which is not explicit, to comprehend the probable meaning of data and recognize the relevance to nursing. This takes place after the interaction has been completed and can be at different levels ranging from assumption to hypothesis. A competent nurse operates mainly at the hypothesis level. This presupposes a knowledge of the concepts and principles underlying psychiatric nursing practice; this is necessary in order to be able to explain and predict patient behaviour, as well as allowing for some degree of validation.

Application of concepts: stage 3. In order to be able to apply concepts, the nurse must possess an understanding of the body of knowledge underlying nursing practice, that is, the principles and concepts used to explain and predict behaviour in nursing situations. However, it must be recognized that it is not possible to know everything and every possible concept. What is important is a willingness on the part of the learner (or qualified nurse) to recognize this and to engage in the process of continuing education.

Analysis: stage 4. After collection of raw data, their interpretation and the application of concepts to the data, the next stage is to analyse it. This involves separating the data into component parts in order to critically assess its nature and significance. It is important to look at each part and its relationship to the whole.

Synthesis: stage 5. This is concerned with the process of putting the analysed parts of the data together to form a complete whole. On completion of the analysis the learner puts the parts of the data back together again and examines the results of the analysis. It is as a result of the analysis and synthesis that the learner is able to plan future interactions.

(c) Items to be included in the process recording This may vary depending on individual circumstances but should include:

1. Date, time, place and duration of the interaction.
2. The learner's thoughts and feelings prior to the interaction. It can be difficult for learners and trained nurses alike to focus on feelings, and many prefer to examine their thoughts in relation to the feelings. However, it is an essential part of self-awareness training and the therapeutic use of self to be able to focus on personal feelings and be able to examine their effect on performance. Learners need to be directed to focus on their feelings.

   There is a variety of reasons why learners and others avoid examination of personal feelings; some of these feelings have already been discussed – for example, fear of failure or criticism. Another very important factor is the socialization process, both in terms of the family and society at large. Children often have to deny feelings, and males in particular may be told not to cry.
3. Objectives for the interaction – these are the statements of the goals for the interaction. The learner will have worked these out in advance with her mentor; they are designed to give structure to the interaction and to identify the desired changes in the patient's behaviour as well as acting as a means of evaluation. In addition, the learner may specify her own personal objectives.
4. The interaction. This will include as much as possible of the communication, both verbal and non-verbal, as well as any periods of silence,

and will be recorded using the previously agreed format. It will also include the learner's thoughts and feelings about the patient and his behaviour. Major and recurring themes in the patient's conversation will be recorded, as well as those areas about which he is reluctant to speak. Anxiety levels will be noted together with any circumstances which appear influential in either their increase or decrease.

Some feel that it is not advisable to keep verbatim notes during patient interactions as it is too distracting for both patient and learner. Unfortunately it is very easy to forget exactly what happened during an interaction, especially if feeling a little anxious. Reynolds (1982), using a similar approach, outlined the importance of this type of recording. An alternative would be to video-record the interaction, but this, too, has its problems – not least of which would be getting both verbal and written permission from the patient.

The learner must be made aware of the consequences of falsifying data. Whilst not a common problem, it can arise, especially if the learner is afraid of making a mistake.

5. Learners' thoughts and feelings following the interaction. This is concerned with the learner's examination of her own thoughts and feelings immediately following the interaction. For example, was she relieved that it is over, does she feel sad, happy or indifferent? What is the significance of these thoughts and feelings and to what does she attribute them?

    The learner needs to ask herself to what extent her feelings about the patient prior to the interaction interfered with the interaction and its outcome. What did she learn about the patient that she did not know prior to the interaction? What did she learn about herself as a result of the interaction?

6. Evaluation of the interaction. This will be assessed in terms of how well the objectives for the intervention were achieved. If the learner can give examples of responses, or identify changes in the patient's behaviour – for example, he was able to wash his hands without checking the wash basin (something he could not do before the interaction) – it can be assumed that the objectives have been achieved.

    If the learner has not achieved her objectives, then this needs to be recognized and decisions reached as to how they can best be realized next time. Were the objectives realistic? Was it the intervention that was inappropriate? Did the opportunity not present itself?

    The learner must begin to analyse why particular interventions succeeded or failed and be able to consider alternatives. This forms part of the problem-solving and conceptualization process of psychiatric nursing.

7. Planning for the next interaction. After the evaluation the learner makes plans for the next interaction and identifies the potential nursing

problems. These plans and objectives should be written immediately.
8. Identification of the customary pattern of reacting. Here the learner identifies and describes her customary pattern of behaving or responding in situations. For example, she may feel uncomfortable with a lengthy silence; therefore she interjects too quickly and the therapeutic nature of the silence is lost. It is important for the learner to examine her own behaviour and identify her strengths and weaknesses. It must be emphasized that she cannot do this alone so here her mentor is a most valuable asset and a crucial element in developing increased self-awareness.

The teaching/learning cycle

On joining the ward team it is important to give the learner the opportunity to see what happens on a daily basis before getting her involved in detailed process recordings of patient interactions. It is also important that she gets the feeling of belonging to the ward team and being capable of making a useful contribution. Over the first one to two days she can be gradually introduced to the learning process as outlined below.

Guided observation

The importance of a good ward-based role model has already been referred to. What is going to be emphasized now is that it is insufficient to observe only. The learner needs to be given guidance as to what to observe: for example, the mentor might say 'Watch how I introduce myself to Mrs Jones', or 'Observe my sitting posture and non-verbal behaviour'. On completion of the interaction, learner and mentor discuss what took place, and why, and plan for the next observation and interaction.

On second observation the learner could be told: 'Now observe the interactions I am using and identify them from Heron's six categories', or 'Note the form of words I am using and also my non-verbal behaviour'. Again, this would be followed by a discussion. By adopting this graded approach and making it clear to the learner what to observe, she will feel more at ease and know what to look for. As she is moving from the known to the unknown, and from the more simple to the complex, the learning map is following the laws of learning theory (Skinner, 1953; Ausubel *et al.*, 1978).

Pre-interaction discussion/guidance for process recording

By now the learner will have experience of observing her mentor, of note taking, of giving feedback on observations and contributing to the analysis of interactions. In addition she will have had an input into the setting of new targets for the next mentor–patient interaction.

If agreeable to the learner, the next stage would be to plan for an experience – an interaction or activity which she would conduct herself under supervision. (For the purpose of this exercise we will concentrate on interactions only, but the same planning observation and process recording would also apply to activities.) The learner can select the patient herself as he will be one of the group for which her mentor is primary nurse. She will be aware of his treatment goals, and where he is at, in terms of achieving them. As this is the learner's first encounter with this particular patient, or indeed, may be her first encounter with any patient, she will discuss with her mentor: what she considers the aim of the interaction to be; how it will help facilitate the patient in moving towards the attainment of his treatment goals; her objectives for the interaction; why these objectives are important; what theoretical rationale underpins the objectives; what therapeutic interventions she will use; potential problems that may arise and strategies for their possible resolution; and her personal fears and anxieties and how they might interfere with her performance.

However, it is never possible to plan for all eventualities, so issues may arise which have not been discussed. It must also be emphasized that all interactions, whether carried out by learner or mentor, should be part of the overall plan of care for the patient and will therefore complement each other.

The interaction

The learner is responsible for deciding where the interaction takes place, but it should be in a quiet private area away from distraction. If possible, the mentor should join the learner if that is agreeable to her and to the patient. If she does, it is best if she sits slightly to the side – therefore being less intrusive, but sitting where both patient and learner will be able to see her. However, the seating arrangements will depend on the learner's ability and level of competence, and also on the nature of the patient's problems and their severity at that time. Nevertheless, this arrangement does tend to make the interaction more natural-looking and less like a situation where the learner is been judged. This is an important consideration as some patients may feel that they are not getting the best possible care if it is been delivered by a learner nurse.

During the interaction the learner will focus on, and record, the points as agreed in the pre-interaction discussion and already outlined. It must be remembered that some patients may find note-taking intrusive; consequently, it may interfere with the flow of conversation. There is a need for flexibility and creativity on this issue.

Patient interaction is a complex process; therefore the learner will have a number of issues to address – including monitoring her own feelings about how the teaching/learning process went. The mentor may also record what is happening as this is useful for validation during the post-interaction discussion. On termination of the interaction the learner will proceed to write up the process record and then join her mentor for discussion.

(a) **Process recording** Process recording is not an end in itself but only a means to an end (Travelbee, 1979). Therefore, the data recorded will be those which the learner and mentor consider necessary to facilitate the learning and development of both patient and learner.

Reflecting on the interaction, the learner will re-examine her objectives, the interventions used and their appropriateness. She will apply concepts and principles to the data. She must not, however, go beyond the data and read into it what is not there. Here the mentor's observations will be useful and act as a safety net.

Following this evaluation she will identify nursing problems and make tentative plans for the next interaction. She will also make a detailed examination of her thoughts and feelings prior to the interaction and identify any effects which they might have had on the actual interaction. In order to prevent duplication of material, the points raised in the section (items to be included in the process recording) will be addressed as part of the process recording.

(b) **Analysis of the process record** When reflection is completed and the process record written up, each part is then analysed and critically examined. The learner reads each section, beginning with the background information. Gaps in the information are identified and plans made to consult the appropriate individuals or agencies. Each part as outlined in the guidelines is examined in exactly the same manner – with the section on the actual interaction itself getting careful scrutiny. At the analysis stage it is not enough to identify a problem: the learner must plan exactly how she intends to overcome it.

(c) **Synthesis of data** Once the analysis is completed the learner commences synthesis. As already indicated, this is where the analysed data are looked at in their entirety in order to form a whole. It is here that plans for the future are made based on the insights gained from the interpretation and analysis. These plans will consist of new objectives for the next patient interaction and set the cycle in motion again. However, the new plans will not be put into action until the learner has discussed them with her mentor and also examined her reflections and process recordings.

(d) **Post-interaction discussion** First, the learner will report on what she felt about the interaction, working her way through the points identified as being important for the process recording. She will describe the parts she liked best followed by those she liked least. She will state whether or not she was able to interpret the patient's behaviour and give meaning to it. Time will be spent reflecting on the use of the interventions – were they used at the correct time and were they of themselves correct? For example, if she said she used a supportive intervention, was it recognizable and would it fit Heron's definition of such an intervention? What other approaches could have been used? Why were they not? Finally, the learner will decide on the areas which she feels need more work before her next interaction – for example, practise a particular intervention, consult a member of the multidisciplinary team, or consult a textbook or article. In addition she will outline how she feels she helped the patient move forward in treatment, if at all.

The mentor will then say what she felt about the interaction, and will highlight the positive aspects before looking at the areas which require modification. She will decide whether or not the learner was able to develop valid inferences about the meaning of the patient's behaviour, and whether or not she was able to apply appropriate concepts. She will also give her opinion about the interventions used and their appropriateness. Essentially, she will concentrate on the same areas as the learner and provide validation, as and when appropriate.

So far we have discussed how the learner and mentor will look at the data collected, their interpretation and analysis, as well as considering the application of concepts and principles to nursing practice. Learner and mentor must also look at the learner's synthesis, and consider how the student has planned for the next interaction. This will be based on the insights obtained from the interpretation of the data. The mentor will assess the appropriateness of the decisions taken and the objectives set. If she agrees then this forms the beginning of the next learning cycle. During this session the learner has the opportunity to examine theoretical principles in detail and look at how they influence her practice. She will also be given constructive feedback and praise, thus increasing the possibility of maintaining and/or further improving her clinical competence. The importance of relating theory to practice will also be reinforced.

It must be emphasized that process recording can be time-consuming and difficult to use; however, the gains from it are potentially enormous. When the learner has acquired both clinical and recording skills it is possible to modify the number of items included in the process records. Alternatively, it might be agreed that only one to two interactions per week are selected to be looked at in this manner. As part of the learning process the learner needs to produce some form of written documentation of patient interactions, and the more learning potential this documentation has the better. The data from the process records can form the basis of the weekly discussion between tutor, mentor and learner. They can also form part of the assessment process by providing a clear picture of how the learner is developing, both clinically and personally, as well as supplying the student with valuable feedback.

An alternative form of documentation is the use of a daily log book, which of itself is valuable but contains more general information. (It could be used in addition to the process record.) Here the learner would record on a daily basis particular experiences or activities which she found of interest. For example, it might be a completely new experience, or one which she was reliving having done additional preparation, or perhaps a difficult or unpleasant experience. This information would then be used in discussion with her mentor as outlined previously. Whatever form of recording is used it must produce a live working document which is of value to learner, mentor and tutor and ultimately of benefit to the patient.

The above model describes how learners can acquire psychiatric nursing skills in the clinical environment through active participation. This will engender increased commitment and challenge and create an atmosphere where the learner will feel part of the ward team and will want to acquire knowledge and skills so that she can increase her contribution as well as pursuing knowledge for its own sake.

Summary

This chapter has looked at the essential features of psychiatric nursing and how psychiatric nurse learners might be helped to learn in the clinical environment. The characteristics of a good ward-learning climate were considered, and the importance of student-centred learning was emphasized. It was stated that the best way to learn psychiatric nursing skills was through the process of doing, and a model for achieving this was outlined.

References

Alexander, M. F. (1985) *Learning to Nurse: Integrating Theory and Practice*, Churchill Livingstone, Edinburgh.

Altschul, A. T. (1972) *Patient–Nurses Interaction: a study in Acute Psychiatric Wards*, Churchill Livingstone, Edinburgh.

Ausubel, D. P., Novak, D. and Hanesian, H. (1978) *Educational Psychology: a Cognitive View*, 2nd edn, Holt, Rinehart and Winston, New York.

Bandura, A. (1969) *Principles of Behaviour Modification*, Holt, Rinehart and Winston, New York.

Berger, S. M. (1961) Incidental learning through vicarious reinforcement. *Psychol. Rep.*, **9**, 477–91.

Birney, R. C., Burdick, H. and Teevan, R. C. (1969) *Fear of Failure*, Van Nostrand Reinhold, New York.

Burnard, P. (1987) Towards an epistemological basis for experiential learning in nurse education. *J. Adv. Nurs.*, **12**, 189–93.

Burnard, P. (1989) Exploring nurse educators' view of experiential learning: a pilot study. *Nurs. Ed. Today*, **9**, 39–45.

Chambers, M. (1989) Learning psychiatric nursing. Paper presented at the Royal College of Nursing Research Society Conference, Swansea.

Clark, L. (1988) Ideology, tradition and choice: questions psychiatric nurses ask themselves. *Senior Nurse*, **8**, 11–13.

Clinton, M. E. (1981) Training psychiatric nurses: a sociological study of the problems of integrating theory and practice. Unpublished PhD thesis, University of East Anglia.

Cormack, D. (1988) The myths and realities of interpersonal skill use in nursing, in *Interpersonal Skills in Nursing: Research and Applications* (ed. C. Kagan), Croom Helm, London.

Davis, B. D. (1981) Social skills nursing, in *Social Skills and Health* (ed. M. Argyle), Methuen, London.

Dewey, J. (1916) *Democracy and Education*, Free Press, New York.

Fairbanks, J. (1980) Primary nursing: what's so exciting about it? *Nurs. Times*, **10**, 55–7.

Firth, H., McIntee, J. M., McKeown, P. and Brittan, P. (1986) Interpersonal support amongst nurses at work. *J. Adv. Nurs.*, **11**, 273–82.

Fretwell, J. E. (1978) Socialisation of nurses. Teaching and learning in hospital wards. Unpublished PhD thesis, University of Warwick.

Heron, J. (1975) *Six, category intervention analysis. Human potential research project*, University of Surrey, Guildford, Surrey.

Heron, J. (1981) Philosophical basis for a new paradigm, in *Human Inquiry: a Source Book of New Paradigm Research* (eds P. Reason and J. Rowan), John Wiley, Chichester.

Hersey, P. and Blanchard, K. (1977) Management of organizational behaviour, cited in *The Teaching Process: Theory and practice in nursing* (eds H. van Hoozer *et al.*), Appleton-Century-Crofts, Norwalk, CT.

Hyland, M. E., Millard, J. and Parker, S. (1988) How hospital ward members treat learner nurses: an investigation of learners' perceptions in a British hospital. *J. Adv. Nurs.*, **13**, 472–7.

Jaques, D. (1984) *Learning in Groups*, Croom Helm, London.

Jones, W. J. (1981) Self directed learning and student selected goals in nurse education. *J. Adv. Nurs.*, **6**, 59–69.

Kanfer, F. H. (1965) Vicarious human reinforcement. A glimpse into the black box, in *Research in Behaviour Modification* (eds L. Krasner and L. P. Ullman), Holt, Rinehart and Winston, New York.

Knowles, M. (1980) The modern practice of adult education, cited in *The Teacher Practitioner in Nursing Midwifery and Health Visiting* (P. Jarvis and S. Gibson), Croom Helm, London, 1985.

Kolb, D. A. (1971) *On management and the learning process*. Working paper 652–773, Alfred P. Sloan School of Management, Massachusetts. Institute of Technology.

Kolb, D. A. and Fry, D. (1975) Towards an applied theory of experiential learning, in *Theories of Group Processes* (ed. C. L. Cooper), John Wiley, Chichester.

Kreigh, M. and Perko, J. (1979) *Psychiatric and Mental Health Nursing: Commitment to care and concern*. Reston, Virginia.

Lewin, D. and Jacka, K. (1987) *The Clinical Learning of Student Nurses*. NERU Report No. 6, King's College, University of London.

Luft, J. (1970) *Group Processes: an Introduction to Group Dynamics*, Mayfield, Pal Alto, CA.

Marlett, C. A. (1968) Vicarious and direct reinforcement control of verbal behaviour in an interview setting, cited in *Principles of Behaviour Modification* (A. Bandura), Holt, Rinehart and Winston, New York, 1969.

Maslow, A. (1954) *Motivation and Personality*, Harper and Row, New York.

Mayeroff, M. (1971) *On Caring*, Harper and Row, New York.

Mezirow, J. (1981) *A critical theory of adult learning and education in Adult Education 32,* 1, Washington.

McClelland, D. C. (1959) *The Achievement Motive,* Appleton-Century-Croft, New York.

Ogier, M. E. (1982) *An Ideal Sister,* Royal College of Nursing, London.

Orton, H. D. (1979) Ward Learning Climate and Student Nurse Response. Unpublished MPhil thesis, CNAA (available from Royal College of Nursing library, London).

Pearson, J. (1979) Educational Encounters in the Ward. Unpublished MPhil thesis, CNAA (available from Royal College of Nursing library, London).

Peplau, H. (1952) *Interpersonal Relations in Nursing: a Conceptual Frame of Reference for Psychodynamic Nursing,* Putnam, New York.

Peplau, H. (1969) Theory: the professional dimensions, in *Proceedings of the First Nursing Theory Conference* (ed. M. Norris), Department of Nurse Education, University of Kansas.

Reid, N. G. (1985) *Wards in Chancery,* Royal College of Nursing, London.

Reynolds, W. (1982) Patient-centred teaching: a future role for the psychiatric nurse teacher? *J. Adv. Nurs.,* **7,** 469–75.

Rogers, C. (1957) The necessary and sufficient conditions of therapeutic personality change. *J. Consult. Psych.,* **21,** 95–103.

Rogers, C. (1961) *On Becoming a Person,* Houghton Mifflin, Boston.

Rogers, C. (1983) *Freedom to Learn for the 80s,* Merrill, London.

Skinner, B. F. (1953) *Science and Human Behaviour,* Macmillan, New York.

Strang, J. (1982) Psychotherapy by Nurses – some special characteristics. *J. Adv. Nurs.,* **7,** 167–71.

Stuart, G. W. and Sundeen, S. J. (1979) *Principles and Practice of Psychiatric Nursing,* Mosby, St Louis, MO.

Stuart, G. W. and Sundeen, S. J. (1988) *Pocket Nurse Guide to Psychiatric Nursing,* Mosby, St Louis, MO.

Travelbee, J. (1979) *Intervention in Psychiatric Nursing: Process in the One-to-One Relationship.* FA. Davis, Philadelphia.

Uys, L. R. (1980) Towards the development of an operational definition of the concept 'therapeutic use of self'. *Int. J. Nurs. Studies,* **17,** 175–80.

Chapter 21

Research and psychiatric nursing

B. D. DAVIS

Introduction

It is a truism that nursing is a skills-based profession. All branches of nursing have their particular ranges of skills which differentiate them. Some of these skills involve the manipulation of instruments and equipment, often in relation to the human body. Others involve interactions with people, patients/clients, the lay public and other professionals. Yet another group of skills involve cognitive activity, for example, problem solving and planning. Related to these latter skills are the skills of reading, critical analysis and writing. All nurses must be prepared, trained in these skills, with the various types of nursing having different skills profiles. Psychiatric nursing has a skills profile that is weighted towards interpersonal problem solving and planning. Reading, critical analysis and writing skills apply equally to all nurses. Generally speaking, the acquisition of these skills is a function of practice and experience. Most courses leading to a qualification in nursing, at both basic and post-basic levels, are concerned with the provision of experience and opportunities for practice. In particular the most apt experience seems to be that in the clinical setting where, under supervision, the student can develop the relevant skills. Much can also be done in preparation, in learning laboratories.

However, nursing skills, especially those more concerned with interpersonal relationships, problem solving and planning, but also the other more physical skills, have to be practised on people. Those who have practised such skills on people will know that these skills have to be modified and varied in the light of the differences that are always to be found between people. These differences can be most acute when they are behavioural. It is argued here that a professional is one who can effect such modifications and variations on the skills, in the light of a relevant knowledge base.

The importance of a knowledge base

Knowledge is gained from experience. The experience can be personal or vicarious, through conversation with others or through reading or observation. Elsewhere I have discussed the nature of knowledge and the importance of public, scientific knowledge above private knowledge in professional practice (Davis, 1986a). Knowledge becomes public, and scientific when it is tested and validated. The experience and practice from which the knowledge derives is shared with others, compared and evaluated.

When it is necessary to modify a skill or practice, or to vary an approach, then a reference to the public, scientific knowledge base will greatly enhance the likelihood of success in the modification or variation. An understanding of the why's of the situation is most important. This knowledge base is sometimes referred to as theory.

The development of a professional knowledge base

A professional knowledge base is the collected, validated and tested knowledge available for those engaged in the practice of the profession. It is gained from experience. The better the control, evaluation and recording of that experience, the stronger the knowledge base. The control and evaluation of experience is the research process, ensuring that any conclusions drawn from the experience are valid, and reliable. Knowledge gained thus, when collected together and organized in a systematic way, becomes theory. Theory can then explain and predict and thus inform decisions about practice or generate further research questions.

As a practitioner, it is important that not only is one prepared and competent in the range of skills required, but that one is aware of the dynamics of the caring situation. When the evaluation of the practice suggests that the aims are not being achieved, then changes, adjustments or innovations must be introduced as necessary. Having access to a knowledge base resulting from controlled and evaluated experience (research) greatly facilitates this process. Practitioners with any claim to being professional should be supportive of research and utilizers of the knowledge that results from it. That said however, the nursing profession in general and psychiatric nursing in particular as yet does not have a very strong knowledge base outside of that provided by the other disciplines in health care. Nevertheless the situation is changing slowly, and at an increasing rate. More and more research is being done into psychiatric nursing, and the rest of this chapter consists of a review of research reported during the last few years.

It is hoped that this presentation will demonstrate the range and amount of work being done and the developing strength of the professional knowledge base. Where relevant or possible, it is hoped that it will help psychiatric nurses to plan their work and to make descisions about practice. It is also hoped that it will stimulate nurses to undertake further research into as yet unexplored areas, as well as continuing the research currently being undertaken.

The research review

The search

In order to compile this review a search was undertaken of material from the UK, the USA, Canada and Australia – in other words, material in English. The first stage in the process was to search bibliographies and indexes. The following were consulted:

Royal College of Nursing Bibliography
International Nursing Index
Department of Health and Social Security (DHSS) Nursing Research
    Abstracts

From these, 124 research papers covering the period 1983–88 were found. The following journals were consulted:

Australian Journal of Advanced Nursing
Australian Nursing Journal
British Journal of Clinical Psychology
British Journal of Medical Psychology
British Journal of Psychiatry
British Medical Journal
Canadian Nurse
Community Psychiatric Nursing Journal
International Journal of Nursing Studies
Journal of Advanced Nursing
Journal of Emergency Nursing
Journal of Neurosurgical Nursing
Journal of Nursing Education
Journal of Psychosocial Nursing
Nurse Education Today
Nursing Clinics of North America
Nursing Mirror
Nursing Research
Nursing Times
Perspectives in Psychiatric Care
Research in Nursing and Health

This is not an exhaustive list of nursing or related journals, but it reflects the range readily available.

Table 21.1 Categories of research

Theory development and methods		
Theory development	4	
Reviews	2	
Instrumentation	12	
		18
Psychiatric nursing		
General research	30	
CPN	24	
Interpersonal skills	9	
Transcultural	3	
		66
Management		
General research	7	
Job stress	12	
		19
Education		
Basic	9	
Post-basic	12	
		21
	Total	124

Types of research

Table 21.1 shows the types of research included in the total of 124 reports found; four main categories with various sub-categories. The largest category is that of psychiatric nursing (52%), which demonstrates that the main thrust of research is very much practice-related. Community psychiatric nursing comprises a large proportion of this category (36.36%).

The categories of management and education consist of relatively small numbers of reports, at 19 and 21 respectively. However, a large proportion of the former are concerned with the issue of stress in psychiatric nursing and the problems of maintaining staff morale in the face of a variety of stressors.

Table 21.2 shows the professional orientation of the authors of the various research reports. As can be seen, a small but significant proportion of reports have been written by psychologists (13.7%) and seven of those initiated by nurses have had the collaboration of psychologists. Fewer of

Table 21.2   Research by author's profession

Category	Nurses	Psychologists	Psychiatrists	Social workers
Theory/methods	18			
Nursing	20	4	5	1
CPN	23		1	
Interpersonal	7	2		
Transcultural	2		1	
Management	6		1	
Job stress	7	5		
Education, basic	11			
Education, post-basic	4	6		
Totals	98	17	8	1

the reports are by psychiatrists (nearly 6.45%), with seven of the nursing-initiated reports having the collaboration of psychiatrists. One report is by a social worker.

The majority of the reports by psychologists are concerned with education (six reports, 28.57%). A similar number but larger proportion are concerned with job stress (five reports, 41.66%). Two of these are from the USA.

There was some difficulty in the definition of nursing research, particularly when research by other professionals was considered. Generally the research had to be concerned with the practice, management or education of psychiatric nurses. Research into psychometrics, psychopathology, or psychiatry has not been considered unless it applied specifically to the work of nurses. Thus some reports of the development of behavioural assessment forms and of treatment have been included.

As the review of psychiatric nursing research was to be international, Table 21.3 shows the research by country. By far the majority of reports are British, but a substantial minority are from the USA (29.8%). Very few were found from Australia or Canada. This may reflect the inadequacies of the search process, or the state of psychiatric nursing research in those countries. Certainly there is much written about psychiatric nursing in these countries but only very few research papers could be found. It may be that there is much research being undertaken and not being reported in the nursing or related journals.

A major proportion of the reports from the USA concern the development of research or clinical instruments (35.14%) with a similar proportion being concerned with psychiatric nursing. None of the American reports

Table 21.3   Research by country

Category	UK	USA	Australia	Canada
Theory/methods	5	13		
Nursing	17	12		1
CPN	23		1	
Interpersonal	6	3		
Transcultural	2	1		
Management	4	3		
Job stress	7	5		
Education, basic	10		1	
Education, post-basic	10			
Totals	84	37	2	1

are concerned with community psychiatric nursing, however. A significant minority are concerned with job stress (13.5%). Most of the reports from the USA are by nurses.

Generally, work done for master's and doctoral dissertations has not been included here. The emphasis has been on material available for general consumption by the profession. It is not fair to expect practising nurses to obtain theses from university or college libraries. Nurses pursuing academic studies will be able to make such searches. Those who feel aggrieved that their theses have not been included should make the material readily available in journal or similar form (e.g., Royal College of Nursing Research Reports or research collections, such as those by Altschul (1985), Brooking (1986), and Davis (1987)). However, as examples of higher degrees, six studies are mentioned in this chapter, from the categories of research, nursing, management and education. Abstracts of these are available in *Nursing Research Abstracts*.

The review

Theory development and methods

(a) **Theory development** Very few papers have been published in the reviewed journals about psychiatric nursing theory or the development of the professional knowledge base. Those that are included under this heading are from the USA, and two are about the adequacy of the research process used in much (American) psychiatric nursing research. One in particular insists that only quantitative research with adequate statistical analysis to support the findings is acceptable for incorporation into a professional body of knowledge (Jones and Jones, 1987). No acknowledgement is given of the value of qualitative data and inductive forms of theory development.

Baier (1988) discusses some of the many difficulties facing the would-be researcher into the care of the mentally ill. These include ethical problems; the individual nature of the presentation of patients and their problems; and the consequent difficulty in establishing satisfactory treatment outcome variables, and the measurement of these. The question of the adequacy of research designs for suitable levels of control is also discussed in the light of sampling errors and difficulty in achieving consistency in the independent variables. In an accompanying commentary, Babich (1988) argues against too rigorous standards being imposed before research can reach acceptability. Nevertheless these two papers are useful reminders for nurse researchers. Brooker (1984) who considers methodological issues is referred to in more detail in the section Community Psychiatric Nursing.

In the third of these papers, it is argued that psychosocial nursing has come of age regarding the development of professional theory (McBride, 1986). This paper relates to the situation in the USA. However, the author also points out that much of the knowledge gained by psychosocial nurses has been taken up by nurses in other fields as well, and psychosocial nursing seems to be losing its differentiating characteristics. In particular she refers to the research in communications and interpersonal skills. However, it can be argued that a knowledge base for psychiatric nursing can share elements with other areas in nursing. McBride also treats the problem of dealing with both psychiatry and mental health; are they the same? She quotes Sills (1977) as arguing that they are different. McBride concludes by arguing for a continuing programme of research and emphasizes that the chronically mentally ill should be included in the programmes. The research should also emphasize nursing issues rather than psychiatric issues.

(b) Research reviews   There have been two reviews of psychiatric nursing research in the period under review. Brooking (1986) has discussed the quality and value of research undertaken by students of the BSc (Hons) degree in nursing studies at King's College (London). Eight studies are presented and evaluated. The main conclusions are the value of such research in research training and in the development and refinement of research questions, although the issue of the ethics of such research is discussed.

Davis (1986a) has reviewed psychiatric nursing research for the period 1980–84. The volume of research found then and in a previous review (Davis, 1981), it was argued, demonstrated that psychiatric nursing was indeed developing a substantial body of knowledge. However, it was also pointed out that much of the research was descriptive, formulating further

Table 21.4 Instrument development

Nursing diagnosis	
Hinds, P. S.	(1984)
Munns, D. C.	(1985)
Thomas, M. D. *et al.*	(1986)
Bruss, C. R.	(1988)
Mental status questionnaires	
Turner, H. B. *et al.*	(1984)
Foreman, M. D.	(1987)
Patient coping	
Graydon, J. E.	(1984)
Jalowiec, A. *et al.*	(1984)
Good psychiatric nursing	
Shanley, E.	(1985)
Psychiatric nursing patient assessment form	
Tissier, J.	(1986)
Level of cognitive functioning scale	
Dowling, G. A.	(1985)
Evaluation of nursing	
Stanley, B.	(1984)

research questions. In a major discussion the author considers priorities for research in the future, and illustrates the discussion with reference to particular attempts to develop research strategies. The question is raised as to whether research should be theory-generated or practice-generated. A solution is perhaps that there is room for both.

(c) The development of instruments Table 21.4 shows the different types of instrument under development. Two types are concerned specifically with the assessment of nursing needs, nursing diagnosis and patient assessment form. Others contribute to the assessment of patients and the development of nursing care plans; mental status questionnaires, patient coping, and level of cognitive functioning scales. One paper, Stanley (1984), is concerned with the development of a scale to evaluate the implementation of nursing care using goal attainment strategies. The final type of instrument is concerned with the assessment of the characteristics of a good psychiatric nurse.

The second group are of a multidisciplinary nature and offer information for the whole mental health care team. Most of these are for use in general medical situations as well. The coping instruments are concerned with the ability of the patient/client to cope with stress, and in particular the stress of illness and hospitalization. The aim is to obtain evidence indicating the individual level of stress-related support needed for clients.

Foreman's paper is particularly useful as a critical comparative evaluation of a series of mental status questionnaires in the general health care setting but with relevance to that of mental health (Foreman, 1987). Mental status in this context involves sensory and cognitive behaviour.

All of these papers are concerned with the accurate assessment of clients and the relationship of that to the development of more individual plans of care, their implementation and evaluation. Little work has been done yet into the evaluation of care, apart from that of Stanley (1984), who argues for a goal attainment model of evaluation. This issue is also tackled to some extent in the other sections.

Shanley's work is concerned to assess the criteria of effectiveness of mental nurses, and in particular the personality characteristics of those considered by other nurses and by clients to be effective or ineffective (Shanley, 1985). Although only a piloting of the new instrument, the findings indicate that such assessments are possible. Further reports concerned with the measurement of the quality of care are discussed in later sections.

In conclusion to this section it seems that, in the USA in particular, there is a concern to achieve higher, more objective standards in patient assessment in relation to the nursing process. It would be useful if nurses in the UK could take up some of this work and use it, modified as necessary to the British situation, in an attempt to apply the nursing process more effectively.

Psychiatric nursing research

Table 21.5 shows the range of work classified under this heading. As can be seen, five sub-categories are presented, and they will be discussed separately.

(a) **Quality of care**   This seems to have been a relatively recent development in psychiatric nursing research. Many of these papers are by non-nurses, i.e., psychologists and a social worker. The major source of evidence has been patient/client perception of care, using in the main specially developed questionnaires or interviews.

One study that used patient behaviour as evidence for evaluation of nursing intervention was that of Youssef (1983). The author quotes two addresses in her report – one in Egypt and the other in the USA – so that the setting for the research is uncertain, but it has been taken as the USA for the purposes of the classification. One other study used changes in patient behaviour in a quasi-experimental design providing some degree of control of a range of variables (Lavender, 1987a). In an extension of the

Table 21.5 Psychiatric nursing

Quality of care		
Youssef, F. A.	(1983)	
Wright, F. and Briggs, S.	(1986)	
Lavender, A.	(1987a)	
Lavender, A.	(1987b)	
Richards, D. A. and Lambert, P.	(1987)	
Richardson, B. K.	(1987)	
Teasdale, K.	(1987)	
Shields, P. J. *et al.*	(1988)	
Nurse therapists		
Hardin, S. B. and Durham, J. D.	(1985)	
Marks, I. M.	(1985)	
Brooker, C. D. and Brown, M.	(1986)	
Roach, F. and Farley, N.	(1986)	
Tilley, S. and Weighill, V. E.	(1986)	
Group psychotherapy		
Levin, D. *et al.*	(1985)	
Selander, J. M. and Miller, W. C.	(1985)	
Murphy, J. F. and Cannon, D. J.	(1986)	
Nurses' views of psychiatry		
Hussain, M. F. and Varadaraj, R.	(1983)	(Nurses holding power)
Phillips, M. S.	(1983)	(Forensic psychiatry)
Berkowitz, R. and Heinl, P.	(1984)	(Schizophrenia)
Pothier, P. C. *et al.*	(1985)	(Child psychiatry)
Jones, R. G.	(1986)	(Geriatric psychiatry)
Bhattacharyya, A.	(1987)	(General nurses)
Special investigations		
Whiteside, S. E. *et al.*	(1983)	(Patient education re drugs)
Floyd, J. A.	(1984)	(Patient sleep patterns)
Francis, G. *et al.*	(1985)	(Pets as therapy)
Coupar, A. and Conway, A.	(1986)	(Depression)
Gordon, V.	(1986)	(Group therapy for depression in women)
Berrios, G. E. and Sage, G.	(1986)	(Fasting for ECT)
Mullis, M. R. and Byers, P. M.	(1987)	(Social support and suicide)
Walder, C. P. *et al.*	(1987)	(Aerophobia)

same study, Lavender also used staff responses on a model standards questionnaire to monitor the effects of changes (Lavender, 1987b).

The studies in this section utilized the analysis of interview data, patient satisfaction questionnaire surveys, and quasi-experimental and experimental designs. These latter studies where those by Youssef (1983) on education and compliance with medication; Wright and Briggs (1986) on patient and staff attitudes towards structural changes to rehabilitation wards; Lavender (1987a, 1987b), who looked at the effects of changes in rehabilitation wards on patient behaviours and staff and patient attitudes; and Richards and Lambert (1987) on patient satisfaction with nursing process versus traditional care. Generally they managed to achieve quite high levels of control although randomization was limited to one study, the others dealing with convenience samples. All except Richards and Lambert showed significant changes or differences.

Of the surveys, that by Richardson (1987) in the USA had the most structure and offered correlations between patients' views of seclusion-room experience and various demographic and clinical variables as well as with nurses' notes. This study and those by Shield *et al.* (1988) and Teasdale (1987) showed how even such relatively simple studies can provide information offering insights into the care being given and evidence to inform changes in policy.

The existence of these studies demonstrates that the profession is beginning to be sensitive to the evaluation aspect of the nursing process and of professional practice. However there is not much that is generalizable from such small scale, situation-specific studies except perhaps the development of some instruments and the general methodological movement. The studies do show that opportunist or planned changes can be evaluated and that the results may be of value to future practice. However, Shields *et al.* (1988) highlight the problems of getting the results of such research taken up and acted on by the relevant staff.

(b) Nurse therapists Two national surveys inform this section, one in the UK and the other in the USA (Hardin and Durham 1985; Brooker and Brown 1986). Hardin and Durham also included responses from clients of the therapists. Both surveys describe the preparation and work of the therapist with attitudes to those from the therapists. Demographic and professional data were also collected by both studies. The American study also includes evaluations of psychotherapy by the clients, using a specially developed questionnaire based on previous work. Generally the evaluations are positive.

The study of Marks (1985) and that of Roach and Farley (1986) are evaluative in a more structured way, utilizing pre- and post-hoc designs. That of Roach and Farley however concerns the input of one therapist, whereas that of Marks compared the input of the nurse therapist with that of a general practitioner. Both studies utilized a variety of measures and both studies report significant improvement for those patients treated by the nurse therapist. In the case of Marks, more improvement was obtained by the nurse therapist patients than that obtained by those treated by the general practitioner.

Tilley and Weighill (1986), found from a survey of a small group of nurse therapists that they play an active and extended role in the assessment and management of the use of alcohol and sedatives by patients referred to them. Their policies are based on those gained in training and show no sign of development or modification in the light of the literature or experience.

The research in this section would therefore seem to indicate that the nurse therapist has a valuable part to play in the care of the mentally ill, although such nurses may be in need of continuing education.

(c) Group psychotherapy Three studies in this section, all from the USA, evaluate the effects of nurse-managed group psychotherapy. Levin *et al.* (1985) show that alternating leadership has a better outcome than that from the comparison groups with co-leaders and with single leaders. Selander and Miller (1985) show that group work in support of chemotherapy reduced recidivism (in terms of number and length of hospitalizations). Murphy and Cannon (1986) found that improved selection and preparation techniques were associated with reduced drop-out rates from nurse- or social-worker-led group therapy. All three studies indicate that nurse-led group therapy can be effective and that there are techniques for improvement.

(d) Nurses' views of psychiatry The papers in this section report surveys of nurses' views of various aspects of psychiatry. Table 21.5 shows the aspects considered. The data were collected by means of questionnaires, some specially constructed, but others (e.g., Bhattacharyya, 1987) borrowed from other sources. Some were used in an interview setting (e.g., Berkowitz and Heinl, 1984) and others used in a postal survey (e.g., Pothier *et al.*, 1985). Some studies were small-scale single-hospital studies (e.g., Hussain and Varadaraj, 1983), whereas others were national surveys (e.g., Phillips, 1983).

Generally the surveys found positive attitudes to the aspect of psychiatry being investigated – as, for example, surveys by Hussain and Varadaraj (1983), Phillips (1983) in Canada, and Jones (1986). Pothier *et al.* (1985) found great need and under-utilization in child psychiatry, and Berkowitz and Heinl (1984) found differences between the attitudes of nurses working in acute or chronic settings, but also similarities in nurturance and coping strategies. Bhattacharyya (1987) found naive and misinformed attitudes among the general nurses towards psychiatry.

Surveys are an important part of the development of the research process in any discipline. They provide a base-line from which it is possible to generate further questions and the possibility of manipulating variables in order to bring about change, where the evidence suggests that change might be beneficial or facilitate further insights and understanding. The results of the studies presented here all offer the possibility of further work to enhance the body of knowledge behind psychiatric nursing practice.

(e) Special investigations This group of studies consists of a mixed bag which indicate the wide range of research issues now stimulating nurses. A large group consist of evaluations of particular interventions for specific clinical situations. A further one (Coupar and Conway, 1986) explores the experience of being depressed, finding that factors making the patients more depressed varied, depending on whether or not they occurred at home or in hospital, some being more influential at home, others in hospital, and others influential in either setting. (Berrios and Sage, 1986) studied the problem of fast-breaking before ECT, finding that patients who were not married, detained, non-consenting, and disagreed with the use of ECT were more likely to break their fast. A third study (Floyd, 1984) looked at the relationship between patients' morning and eveningness and rest-activity schedules in a hospital in the USA, finding that there was disruption of the patients' sleep patterns as a result of hospital schedules, whatever the individual's morning or eveningness.

The evaluation studies looked at a wide range of interventions as indicated in Table 21.5. They all report positive outcomes for the particular intervention, and make recommendations concerning the application of the results to practice. Three of the studies were undertaken in the USA, one is a comparative study between the USA and the UK (Gordon, 1986) and one was undertaken in the UK (Walder *et al.*, 1987).

These studies indicate that nurses are attempting the kind of change and manipulation of variables suggested at the end of the previous section on surveys. Coupled with the findings from the group therapy and nurse therapist sections, these findings indicate a fair degree of success in experimental and quasi-experimental investigations into general psychiatric nursing.

Community psychiatric nursing

As can be seen in Table 21.6, a wide range of studies have been undertaken under this heading, including six special investigations which do not fall into any other section. Two of the remaining sections are evaluations of community psychiatric nursing, and three are concerned with various groups' perceptions of community psychiatric nursing.

(a) Evaluations of community psychiatric nursing services The evaluation studies are led by a discussion of problems associated with such research (Brooker, 1984) in the context of a proposed evaluation study. Highlighting weaknesses in the internal validity of the proposed design the author argues for continuing rigour in research design so that

Table 21.6 Community psychiatric nursing

Evaluation of community psychiatric nursing	
Brooker, C. D.	(1984)
Brooker, C. D. and Simmons, S. M.	(1985)
Brooker, C. D.	(1987)
Senicle, L.	(1987)
Pollock, L.	(1988a)
Pollock, L.	(1988b)
Carers perceptions	
Simmons, S. M.	(1984)
Pollock, L.	(1986)
Adams, T.	(1987)
GP's perceptions	
Hendon, J.	(1984)
Godin, P. and Wilson, I.	(1986)
White, E. G.	(1986)
Conhye, A.	(1987)
Base location of community psychiatric nurses	
Friend, W.	(1984)
Dyke, R.	(1984)
Skidmore, D.	(1986)
Lay public perceptions	
Foster, J. *et al.*	(1986)
Barnett, C.	(1987)
Special investigations	
Dawe, A.-M.	(1983)
Thomas, W.	(1984)
Hugo, M. *et al.*	(1985)
Rushforth, D.	(1986)
Storer, D. *et al.*	(1987)
Wetherill, J. *et al.*	(1987)

only the highest standards should obtain and thus ensure the credibility of the professional knowledge base. (This study could have appeared in the section, theory development and methods, but it was felt that it would have greater impact alongside similar studies.)

The other evaluation studies involve comparisons between different CPN services to demonstrate the development and quality of the services being offered (e.g., Brooker and Simmons, 1985; Brooker, 1987). Both studies provide information which demonstrates the importance of systematic evaluation for the management and delivery of effective services.

In her paper, Senicle (1987) argues for the importance of including costs and benefits in any evaluation of services and offers a model for such an exercise. Pollock uses qualitative data from interviews to evaluate the work of community psychiatric nurses, and finds that there is poor definition of their tasks and priorities, inadequate preparation for the role, and insufficient levels of authoritative supervision (Pollock, 1988a p. 5), the nurses having constantly to seek to legitimize their work and...juggle resources (Pollock, 1988b, p. 537) in order to provide individual care to their clients.

(b) Base-location of the CPN Two papers are concerned with the base-location of the CPN. Dyke (1984) found that referrals to CPNs were facilitated when they were based in the primary health-care setting, and when the primary health-care team were aware of the role that might be played by the CPN. Both Skidmore (1986) and Friend (1984) in a thesis, found no differences between the intervention styles of hospital-based and primary-health-care-based CPNs. However, they did find that hospital/institutional approaches tended to be used; they argue for more specialized preparation for the role. Skidmore's study, although reported later, was in fact undertaken before that of Dyke, and we may be seeing improvements as a result of changes in the preparation of CPNs in the differences found by Dyke.

The papers concerned with perceptions of the community psychiatric nursing service are also evaluative in much the same way as that of Pollock (1988b). However, they are classified separately here to allow a clearer presentation of these various views from other groups: carers, GPs and the lay public (not involved in caring for a mentally ill person).

(c) Carers' perceptions The views of carers have been explored by Simmons for her thesis (1984), Pollock (1986) and Adams (1987). Simmons found that the experiences of carers differed depending on the degree of involvement and relationship to the mentally ill person. Duty to care and attitudes to community care also influenced the burden of being a carer. Pollock found that CPNs were seen as being easy to talk to and valued in a crisis. However, they often felt that they did not receive all the help they needed in particular situations. Simmons used a guided interview for data collection, and Pollock used a special idiographic method, based on repertory grid technique, and the PQRST technique (Shapiro, 1961). In a small-scale study, using diaries and interviews with carers of sufferers from Alzheimer's disease, Adams found that the patient's problems became family problems and advocates a family-centred approach to care.

(d) GPs perceptions The studies exploring the perception of GPs find generally that there are many different kinds of perception, and of relationships between them and the CPN. Most GPs who had had extensive dealings with CPNs generally trusted them and their recommendations (e.g.,

Hendon, 1984) although Hendon found that they tended to prefer a psychiatrist to back these up. Godin and Wilson (1986), however, found that many GPs were not well informed about the service that could be provided. This finding was supported by that of Conhye (1987). White (1986) found that the situation was more complex than one of lack of experience or information. Models of psychopathology, FPC management strategies, and nurse/doctor power relations influenced the nature of the referral policies, and were a function of individual relationships.

(e) Lay public perceptions   Attitudes of the public in one town were explored by Barnett (1987) who found generally a positive perception of those questioned, to community day care for the mentally ill. Foster, Beck and Wright (1986) studied the attitudes of children in one grammar school to mental illness generally and to its presence in the community. They found a high level of accurate knowledge in the thoughtful replies given. The children expressed themselves in a sensitive and compassionate way, although worries were expressed about the presence of a group home near to their own home, possible violence being given as the main reason.

(f) Individual investigations   The final section under community psychiatric nursing concerns more individual investigations. Dawe (1983) studied the factors influencing the size and type of case-load carried by CPNs based at one hospital. A high proportion of re-opened cases was found and also a high proportion of hospital re-admissions, indicating that the support required by the patients in the community was not being provided. The author argues for increased support services including a higher ratio of CPNs to clients. In a small-scale study however, Thomas (1984) makes a strong case for the value of depot drugs in community psychiatry.

Hugo *et al.* (1985) in an Australian study argue for the value of screening instruments to facilitate the care of the elderly in the community. Although they acknowledge limitations to the study, the authors claim to have successfully discriminated among levels of psychiatric need in the elderly attending a non-psychiatric community day centre. However, there was a tendency for those with a probable psychiatric problem to inhibit their emotional responses to the questionnaires. A case is made for a role for the CPN in helping such people to acknowledge and express their feelings more easily.

In a small-scale, single-hospital study a case is made for a CPN service to be involved in the A and E department by Storer *et al.* (1987), while Rushforth (1986) in his thesis was concerned to demonstrate the role of the CPN in the management of self-poisoning cases. The study is also concerned with assessing the use of the problem-oriented nursing record system. However, in a study of CPN involvement in the care of patients

Table 21.7   Interpersonal relationships and skills

Patient–nurse interactions	
Marshall, P. D.	(1985)
Scadden, J. G.	(1985)
Sugden, J.	(1985)
Teaching social skills to patients	
George, P. and Dudley, M.	(1986)
Whetstone, W. R.	(1986)
Non-verbal communication	
Marlow, H. A. and Marcotte, A.	(1984)
Welt, S. R.	(1984)
Smith, B. J. and Cantrell, P. J.	(1988)
Relationships between patients	
Harries, C., Frois, M. and Healey, J.	(1984)

suffering from alcoholism, Wetherill, Kelly and Hore (1987) were unable to find a significant effect from the CPN input.

Interpersonal relationship and skills

The studies classified under this heading fall into four sections as shown in Table 21.7.

(a) Nurse–patient interaction   This section is led by a study continuing the work into nurses' perceptions of patients as reviewed by Kelly and May (1982) and Davis (1984d). Using a visual analogue scale, and a questionnaire in a relatively small-scale study, Marshall (1985) found that nurses did discriminate between patients in terms of enjoying caring for them or not. Scadden's (1985) thesis describes the monitoring by tape recorder of nurse–patient interactions in order to identify the styles of interaction used and from these to identify ideal types. The thesis discusses the value of this research and suggestions made for further research. The work of Sugden (1985) demonstrates, however, the influence of the social and physical environment on relationships and therapy in ward settings. The author argues for the role of nurses in monitoring the efficiency of the therapeutic environment.

(b) Teaching social skills to patients   Poor social skills seem to be a major part of the difficulty in the rehabilitation of long-term mentally ill people. George and Dudley (1986) describe in their paper a group-approach involving problem-solving to the development of verbal skills in rehabilitation, and Whetstone (1986), in a small-scale study in Canada, describes the use of social dramatics. Using an experimental design and videotape feedback, he demonstrated significant improvement in social competence, but not for social interest, neatness or irritability. There was no change in psychotic or depressive states. Both of these studies suggest that further work in this area might be well rewarded.

(c) **Non-verbal communication** Marlow and Marcotte (1984), in the USA, describe a programme designed to improve non-verbal decoding in the long-term mentally ill, claiming that it did achieve its goals, was positively received, and was considered worthwhile by the clients. However, this paper was subjected to a critical evaluation by Welt (1984), who argued that the presentation of the study was inadequate in that no data were offered to support the conclusions, and also that the theoretical assumptions of the study could be challenged. This critique was published in the same issue of the same journal as an insert to the main paper and seems to offer a useful aid to the clinical practitioner attempting to utilize research findings.

Smith and Cantrell (1988), also in the USA, use an experimental design to study the effect of distance (social or intimate) and verbal input (personal or impersonal questions) on measures of stress in psychotic patients. They found that the more personal the question, the more the increase in anxiety, whatever the level of distance, whereas distance only aroused anxiety if associated with verbal intrusion.

(d) **Relationships between patients** In an interesting study, Harries, Frois and Healey (1984) investigated factors influencing the relationships developed between long-stay psychiatric residents. In particular they report the usefulness of multidimensional scaling as a method of studying this phenomenon. They found that the residents were willing to cooperate in the study and that the technique did provide maps which demonstrated meaningful dimensions to the inter-patient relationships. The implications for the management of long-stay residents are discussed.

Transcultural psychiatric nursing

The area of transcultural nursing is one that, although very obvious in practise, has had relatively little attention from researchers, particularly in the UK. This is surprising in such a multicultural country, although the USA and Canada have begun to develop a body of knowledge and of education in the field. For this review three papers have been found (see Table 21.8).

The use of special instruments to assess cultural diversity in attitudes and perceptions of aspects of health care in general, and in psychiatry in

Table 21.8 Transcultural psychiatric nursing

Brink, P. J.	(1984)
Davis, B. D.	(1986b)
London, M.	(1986)

particular, is an area of interest, and Brink's (1984) paper is an example of the few attempts to evaluate them. The value orientations tool described and evaluated in relation to the Annang people in Nigeria in this paper seems to offer a valid and reliable form for investigating cultural diversity. Arguing for further assessment of the tool in the USA with larger sample sizes and different ethnic groups, the author, a noted researcher and writer in this aspect of nursing, emphasizes the importance of increasing the rigour with which assessments and judgments are made in the transcultural setting.

Davis (1986b) has reviewed much of the research and educational developments in this area and makes recommendations for the incorporation of multicultural strands in basic and post-basic nurse education. He argues that such developments could be built on social and interpersonal skills courses, or that they should incorporate an interpersonal skills foundation, with an emphasis on empathy skills.

London, a psychiatrist, has reviewed research into the incidence and nature of mental illness among immigrant minorities in the UK (London, 1986). He argues that earlier recognition and treatment of psychiatric disorder is needed and that health care personnel require special preparation in order to be able effectively to assess for and provide the care needed, and, perhaps, to re-examine the psychiatric concepts that inform current practice in this cultural framework.

Management

A relatively small number of papers are classified under this heading, which is surprising in the context of the number of papers reviewed (see Table 21.9). One would have expected a much greater interest in the management issues involved in the transfer of patients from hospital settings to the community, the management issues of delivering community-based services, and the management of small centres in relation to the wider geographical context. However, the next section, job stress, does demonstrate a strong interest in this one aspect of nursing.

(a) **Planned change: innovation** Two papers inform this section: Bevvino *et al.* (1984) from the USA, and Lemmer (1986) in the UK. The former describes and evaluates the introduction of a psychosocial rehabilitation

Table 21.9 Management

Planned change: innovation	
Bevvino, C. A. *et al.*	(1984)
Lemmer, W.	(1986)
Ward/unit management	
Rix, G.	(1983)
Wake, P.	(1986)
Berry, M. and Freeman, M.	(1987)
Garritson, S. H.	(1988)
Assessing establishment needs	
Pardue, S. F. and Dick, C. T.	(1986)

programme. This focuses primarily on the patients' successful adjustment and return to the community. The programme is not concerned with custody issues, or with socialization into an institutional role; rather it is concerned with developing coping strategies, a new sense of self, involved in a self-directed programme rather than the recipient of treatment. It is claimed that the change has produced significant financial savings with improved patient outcomes, such as employment gained, development of interpersonal relationships outside the institution, and more adaptive behaviour. This paper seems to describe a process that is also being attempted in this country.

The project described by Lemmer (1986) is one such study. The paper describes an action research project involving a preliminary assessment of the work of trained and untrained staff on five wards for the care of the elderly mentally ill, followed by feedback to the staff in terms of the strengths and many weaknesses found, via management and educational input. The major change was from custodial, task-centred nursing to in-dividualized problem-orientated care. The second assessment demon-strated the changes achieved and the value of the group work involved in bringing them about.

The value of action research as a way of bringing about innovation and change is one that could be applied much more frequently in nursing in general and psychiatric nursing in particular. The collaborative cycle of innovation and evaluation brings a research-based approach to the man-agement of services and care that adds to the professional knowledge base in a way that integrates theory and practice.

(b) Ward/unit management Studies of management at ward or unit level have tackled a variety of issues. Rix (1983) was concerned with the management of patients' time in an adolescent unit, and found that the girls had become bored and apathetic. Feedback to staff from the study has led to more constructive activities being developed. Wake (1984) also was concerned about the management of wards and in particular the deployment of charge nurses. From a national survey he found that many hospitals were trying to break from the traditional model of a two-charge nurse system to a single leader with overall responsibility, as was the case in the home hospital of the researcher. He discusses the perceived advantages and disadvantages of the change.

Berry and Freeman (1987) report a survey of attitudes to working in a secure unit. Many problems and disadvantages were identified but many positive points were made also. This study is not a nursing study, being undertaken by a clinical psychologist and an occupational therapist and dealing with the multidisciplinary nature of the units. Nevertheless, it has many implications for nursing management.

The paper by Garritson (1988) is of interest in that it discusses the ethical implications of nursing decisions in the management of psychiatric nursing care. It considers the kind of factors influencing the decisions made by nurses and relates these to basic ethical principles of beneficence, autonomy and distributive justice. The paper discusses some of the management implications of the dilemmas highlighted by the study in a series of illustrative vignettes.

(c) **Assessing establishment needs** The one paper in this section describes the development and piloting of a new instrument for the assessment of the nursing need of patients as a method for determining staffing needs. In particular the instrument tries to move away from the physical orientation of previous examples and to incorporate more of the psychosocial health care needs. The results of extensive piloting and evaluation of the instrument indicates its reliability and validity as a management tool although the authors acknowledge that staff will need special perparation in achieving accurate assessment using it.

Job stress

Table 21.10 shows that three sections were identified under this classification, each with a fair number of studies. The first group were concerned with the identification of stressors.

(a) **Stressors** Of the four papers in this section, that by Dawkins *et al.* (1985) in the USA is the earliest. It uses the Holmes and Rahe technique (Holmes and Rahe, 1967) in the development of a psychiatric nurses' occupational stress scale to aid the identification of job stresses. This consists of 78 items, which the researchers have grouped into six categories, listed here in order of number of high stress items: administrative

Table 21.10 Job stress

Stressors	
Dawkins, J. E. *et al.*	(1985)
Trygstad, L. N.	(1986)
Jones, J. G. *et al.*	(1987)
Larson, D. G.	(1987)
Violence	
Casseem, M.	(1984)
Hodgkinson, P. *et al.*	(1984)
Rix, G.	(1987)
Dawson, J. *et al.*	(1988)
Burnout/staff morale	
Cronin-Stubbs, D. and Brophy, E. B.	(1985)
McCarthy, P.	(1985)
Reed, M. T.	(1986)
Jones, R. G.	(1988)

issues, resources, staff conflicts, scheduling issues, negative patient char-acteristics and staff performance. The top ten stressors in the study of nurses in one hospital were all in relation to organizational issues, and the highest rated stressor was not being notified of changes before they occur. Negative patient characteristics were rated as relatively unstressful. The authors acknowledge that the instrument needs testing in other set-tings and may require further modification. These findings are supported by those of Trygstad (1986), also in the USA, and Jones *et al.* (1987) in the UK. Trygstad used a grounded theory approach, whereas Jones *et al.* used structured interviews with a specially developed questionnaire. Trygstad found that staff and staff relations were the greatest stressor and yet other staff were the greatest resource in coping with job stress, after self.

In another study from the USA, Larson (1987) describes a survey of emotional experiences related to job stress, also using an experiential, ethnographic approach. Nine categories of stressor were identified (includ-ing 'other'), the most frequently occurring being emotional and physical distancing, feelings of inadequacy and of anger or frustration.

These four studies are most important in breaking through the barriers of stress in psychiatric nursing and provide a most useful baseline for the study of staff morale and burnout.

(b) Burnout Few studies were found that looked at factors which might improve staff morale or decrease the incidence or occurrence of burnout. However, two of the studies presented under this section do just that. The first, from the USA, by Cronin-Stubbs and Brophy (1985), looked at the influence of social support. Interpersonal relationships were reported as the most frequent source of stress by four groups of nurses (psychiatry, OR nurses, intensive care, medicine). The psychiatric nurses experienced less support than did the nurses and intensive care nurses.

In another small-scale study in the UK, and using another, specially developed questionnaire, Jones (1988) demonstrated that nurses working in a high-stimulation environment achieved higher morale scores than did those in a ward with a traditional approach. Because of the design of the study with control and experimental wards, the author claims that it was the high level of stimulation that caused the higher morale scores. McCarthy (1985) using the SBS-HP, as had Cronin-Stubbs and Brophy, found it difficult to demonstrate differences in levels of burnout between nurses working in different clinical areas in psychiatry. He did find, however, that younger nurses scored higher than older ones (29–59), and argues that this is related to different expectations in the two groups.

This is obviously an area where much more research is required to confirm the identification of stressors and their measurement at an individual level, as well as to strategies in management and preparation which may confound or reduce their impact.

Finally in this section, a paper is presented which reports a descriptive study of chemically dependent nurses. Reed (1986) draws on research in the USA, and in particular the state of Georgia, where her work was undertaken, using a specially developed interview schedule with nurses who were attending for therapy for drug dependence. The results of the survey indicate that high achievers, more frequently in critical care settings, and those experiencing high levels of stress were more at risk. Education and early diagnosis and treatment were seen by the sufferers as being most important, coupled with the belief that there is help and hope. A copy of the interview schedule is published with the report.

(c) Violence Although not appearing high on the lists of stressors in studies reported above, there is evidence that some staff feel inadequate in the face of patient assaults, and that they are more likely to consider changing jobs, as well as taking more short-term absence to cope with stress (e.g., Lanza (1983) quoted in Rix (1987)).

Two studies here report on the number and nature of violent incidents in single-hospital studies. Casseem (1984) found reports of 152 incidents during a four-month period, more being committed by females, and some of them being self-directed. Forty-seven incidents involved nurses. Problems were identified in the reporting system, and recommendations were made to improve this. Hodgkinson *et al.* (1984) argue that there is no evidence that psychiatric patients are more violent than members of the general population. In a survey of the incidents over a four-year period a dramatic annual increase in the incidence was found, although most incidents do not lead to serious injury. Again, females committed more assaults, with the age group 20 to 29 being associated with more incidents for both sexes. No attempt was made in the study to enumerate possible causes, although a variety of correlates was found.

During a ten-month period, Rix (1987) found 293 incidents reported. In an attempt to relate these to short-term sickness absence he found no evidence to support the hypothesis. Dawson *et al.* (1988) in the USA describe and evaluate a peer support programme for staff victims of patient assaults. The programme utilizes a buddy system where a pair of victims help each other until an assault support team member can be contacted. Staff generally evaluated the programme positively and there was evidence that staff turnover was reduced although the design does not allow causal relations to be identified.

Education

A substantial group of papers has been classified under this heading, and divided into two major sub-groups: basic education and post-basic education. However, one report has been separated from these groups: that of Leiba (1984) which is an historical review of the development of psychiatric nursing with particular reference to education, written as a thesis for a higher degree. The author acknowledges that this research is only the early stages of what is hoped to be a more systematic study.

Basic Education
This category has been divided into four sections.

(a) **Student nurse attrition**   In the first paper James *et al.* (1983), in an Australian study, attempted to identify psychological tests predictive of success as measured by clinical appraisal, examination and employment recommendation in a short conversion course for enrolled nurses to become registered mental nurses. Although not concerned strictly with wastage during training, this study found that there was a low attrition rate from this kind of course, and also that there was no predictive ability shown by any of the tests, confirming findings from other studies with non-psychiatric nurses as well as with psychiatric nurses.

Davis (1984a, 1984b) reports findings from a small-scale study of wastage during psychiatric nurse training, and relates this to poor staff relationships, particularly between junior and senior staff. Findings included the following: an age group difference in attitudes to treatment in one psychiatric hospital; a difference in attitudes between teaching and senior nursing staff; that anxiety levels correlated with attitude scores; and that student attitudes could change over time, particularly if influenced by relevant informational input. The author discusses the importance of the attitudinal

Table 21.11   Education

History		
Leiba, P. A.	(1984)	
Basic education		
Student nurse attrition		
James, J. et al.	(1983)	
Davis, B. D.	(1984a)	
Davis, B. D.	(1984b)	
Student nurse socialization		
Davis, B. D.	(1984c)	
Davis, B. D.	(1986c)	
Teaching interpersonal skills		
Reynolds, W. and Cormack, D.	(1985)	
Reynolds, W.	(1987)	
Sankar, S.	(1987)	
Reynolds, W. and Presly, A. S.	(1988)	
Psychiatric content of BSc/RGN courses		
Muir-Cochrane, E.	(1986)	
Post-basic education		
Evaluation		
Milne, D.	(1984a)	
Milne, D.	(1984b)	
Milne, D.	(1985a)	
Milne, D.	(1985b)	
Milne, D. et al.	(1985)	
Gournay, K.	(1986)	
Chambers, M.	(1988)	
Milne, D. and Whyke, T.	(1988)	
Needs		
Kennedy, J.	(1986)	(Alcoholism)
Robinson, S.	(1988)	(Violence)

climate within hospitals and with respect to staff morale as well as attrition. These findings reflect those of Sugden (1985) and the studies on stressors above.

(b) Student nurse socialization   In two separate studies, Davis (1984c, 1986c) reports on the process of becoming a psychiatric nurse. In the first, data from interviews with students were subject to content analysis. In this paper the author discusses in some detail the problems of collecting such qualitative data and analysing it in an unbiased way to maintain academic rigour. The ward experience and the ward staff were seen as important influences, but the school and tutors were seen as not achieving their potential. Job satisfaction was related to patient care. In the second study, the socialization process was studied in more detail, using repertory grid technique and personal construct theory. Problems were identified, as were resources, as well as the quality of the relationships with various significant others, supporting and amplifying the earlier findings.

(c) **Teaching interpersonal skills** The papers in this section relate to those in the psychiatric nursing section above but have been placed here because they are specific to basic nurse education. In a series of reports, a project to develop a new approach to the teaching of such skills is described and evaluated (Reynolds and Cormack, 1985; Reynolds, 1987; Reynolds and Presly, 1988). The main emphasis was on the development of empathy. Reynolds explored and evaluated the literature and interviewed nurse teachers with regard to their understanding of the concept and practice of empathy and their consequent teaching. Reynolds and Presly found that state empathy was unstable and therefore a possible target for teachers. Also, major differences were found in the teaching strategies of the teachers in three schools of nursing. Reynolds and Cormack evaluated a trial clinical teaching programme for teaching group dynamics. They demonstrated the value of teachers as practitioners in influencing the development of skills in learners.

In a small-scale study, Sankar (1987) described and evaluated an attempt to put into practice the implications of the 1982 syllabus for psychiatric nurse education, using Peplau's model, and with particular reference to the teaching of interpersonal skills. He found that the learners' experiences in the clinical setting were not supportive of the integration of theory and practice.

(d) **Psychiatric content of BSc/RGN courses** In a review of such courses, Muir-Cochrane (1986) has found great differences between the content of different degree courses and between degree courses and conventional ones. An argument is made for the evaluation of these courses and for the development of nationally agreed standards regarding the educational requirements for student psychiatric nurses.

Post-Basic Education

(a) **Evaluation** Milne (1984a, 1984b, 1985a, 1985b) and Milne *et al.* (1985), report an extensive programme of research involving the establishment and evaluation of post-basic courses in behaviour therapy. The evaluations led to the development of an approach based on behavioural ecology, where the unexpected consequences (positive and negative) of interventions can be considered and included in the evaluation. The papers are important in terms of their description of the educational input and teaching strategies of the course and also for their development of course evaluation.

A survey of nurses' attitudes to post-basic education was undertaken by Gournay (1986). He reviews the problems of measuring attitudes and some specific instruments before describing the results of his own survey. Differences in attitudes were found between nurses undertaking different post-basic courses, and it was also found that nurse therapist trainees changed the most during their courses. The author calls for more behavioural validation of attitude studies.

Chambers (1988) describes an illuminative evaluation approach, involving interviews with participants: students and teachers; group discussions; a course evaluation questionnaire; classroom and clinical observations; and student assessment. Generally the evaluations were positive although weaknesses were identified which could be modified for adjustment of the educational process.

Finally in this section, Milne and Whyke (1988) describe the development and assessment of formative and summative evaluation measures for a short course of training (ENB 953). The results indicate that the measures are valid and reliable but showed that the course itself required revision. There are links between the findings of this study and that of Shanley discussed above under Instrument Development.

(b) Needs The two papers in this section are concerned with exploring the continuing educational needs of psychiatric nurses with respect to two specialist areas. Kennedy (1986) has looked at the area of alcoholism. Using a specially designed questionnaire, a national survey of nurses working in alcohol rehabilitation establishments was undertaken, and a high return rate was achieved. The majority of respondents wanted further training and identified psychotherapy and behaviour therapy as the main areas of interest. Very few had attended ENB 620 courses, however. In another survey, Robinson (1988) studied some aspects of the role and education of the nurse regarding violent behaviour by mentally ill patients. The methods used include document analysis, interviewing and non-participant observation.

Conclusion

Psychiatric nursing research is becoming established, on the evidence of the preceding review. However, apart from a few areas, it is still in its infancy, as can be seen by the nature of the research questions being asked and the methods being used to investigate them. As has been pointed out on a previous occasion (Davis, 1986a), there is a hierarchy to the process of research and before major additions can be made to the knowledge base and thus to practice, research must climb that hierarchy (see Clark and Hockey, 1979).

The relationship between research, knowledge-base (theory), and practice is a very complex one. That between research and the development of theory has been discussed earlier, but the relationship between research (via theory) and practice is one that can usefully be explored here.

In a few areas there would seem to be a reasonable body of knowledge that could be the basis of research utilization projects or programmes of planned change. These include student nurse socialization, where recent national developments under UKCC 2000 may allow such research to be implemented as part of new educational strategies. Another area is that of job stress and burnout where the insights gained by the research so far should be enough to form the basis of efforts to change the situation. There is now a substantial amount of material concerning the work and preparation of CPNs which could form the basis of new approaches to education for, and management of, this service. The importance of interpersonal skills in psychiatric nursing and insights into the dynamics of the training of these in relation to nurse–patient relationships would suggest that the time is ripe for major changes to be made to management strategies so that these are optimized at ward/unit level as well as at a more individual level in hospital and community situations.

As was pointed out under that heading, there does seem to be little evidence of a research-based approach to management. Examples of monitored programmes of innovation and change are few in the literature. Two only were found for inclusion in this review, although there are earlier examples in the literature. One would like to see senior managers investing in programmes of research replication and utilization, whereby researchers are employed to monitor and evaluate planned change in respect of particular research issues such as those mentioned here.

Programmes like this could utilize strategies pioneered by the CURN project in the USA (Horsley, 1983), or that advocated by Rothman (1980). In the UK some pioneering work has been undertaken by workers such as Towell and Harries (1979), Harries (1982), and Lemmer (1986). Brighton Polytechnic in the UK has established a nursing research unit in association with local health authorities, particularly Brighton and Eastbourne where a programme of research utilization (including psychiatry) has already been initiated and is being developed as one of the major thrusts of the unit. A privately endowed unit, the Foundation of Nursing Studies has also been established recently in London with a similar remit. It is to be hoped that these enterprises will stimulate similar developments in other areas and include psychiatric nursing research in their plans.

Nurses with a preparation in research (for example, with higher research degrees) and now in positions of management and policy making should be using those positions to undertake this kind of innovative exercise, utilizing research in relation to the nursing demands in their service. Those in academic positions should be establishing relationships with local senior nurse managers in order to facilitate the same.

These innovations and collaborative exercises may indeed be underway in different parts of the country. The unfortunate thing is that, if they are, no one else knows about them. They remain private, adding to the local, private body of knowledge, but not adding to the general scientific body of knowledge where others can draw on them, incorporating findings or techniques into their own developments.

We now have a resource of research into psychiatric nursing reaching back for at least 35 years, much of it of high calibre, and yet in many cases we are repeatedly confirming situations warranting change without taking further the research process leading to the evaluation of changes in policy. We have had many changes in policy, local and national, without much reference to research and without attempts to scientifically evaluate those changes. It is time to acknowledge the importance of a scientific knowledge base of nursing practice, to education for it and to the management of it. Nursing is not just skills; it is the intelligent, informed use of those skills, and that means both doing and using research at all levels in the profession.

References

Adams, T. (1987) How does it feel to be a caregiver? *Commun. Psych. Nurs. J.*, 11–17.

Altschul, A. T. (1985) *Psychiatric Nursing*, Churchill Livingstone, Edinburgh.

Babich, K. (1988) Obstacles in research: another point of view. *J. Psychosoc. Nurs.*, **26**, 30–1.

Baier, M. (1988) Why research doesn't yield treatment. *J. Psychsoc. Nurs.*, **26**, 29–33.

Barnett, C. (1987) What will the neighbours say? *Nurs. Times*, **83**, 31–2.

Berkowitz, R. and Heinl, P. (1984) The management of schizophrenic patients: the nurses' view. *J. Adv. Nurs.*, **9**, 23–33.

Berrios, G. E. and Sage, G. (1986) Patients who break their fast before ECT. *Brit. J. Psych.*, **149**, 294–5.

Berry, M. and Freeman, M. (1987) Staffing in secure units. *Nurs. Times*, **83**, 38–9.

Bevvino, C. A., Burns, B., Lewis, M. H. and Allen, J. K. (1984) Planned change: an innovative nursing rehabilitation model. *Perspect. Psych. Care*, **22**, 149–58.

Bhattacharyya, A. (1987) Nurses' attitudes to psychiatry in a general hospital. *Brit. J. Psych.*, **151**, 418.

Brink, P. J. (1984) Value orientations as an assessment tool in cultural diversity. *Nurs. Res.*, **33**, 198–203.

Brooker, C. G. (1984) Some problems associated with the measurement of community psychiatric nurse intervention. *J. Adv. Nurs.*, **9**, 165–74.

Brooker, C. G. (1987) An investigation into the factors influencing variation in the growth of community psychiatric nursing services. *J. Adv. Nurs.*, **12**, 367–75.

Brooker, C. G. and Brown, M. (1986) National follow-up survey of practising nurse therapists, in *Psychiatric Nursing Research* (ed. J. Brooking), Wiley, Chichester.

Brooker, C. G. and Simmons, S. M. (1985) A study to compare two models of community psychiatric nursing care delivery. *J. Adv. Nurs.*, **10**, 217–23.

Brooking, J. (1986) Undergraduate research in psychiatric nursing, in *Psychiatric Nursing Research* (ed. J. Brooking), Wiley, Chichester.

Bruss, C. R. (1988) Nursing diagnosis of hopelessness. *J. Psychosoc. Nurs. Mental Health Serv.*, **26**, 28–31.

Casseem, M. (1984) Violence on the wards. *Nurs. Mirror*, **158**, 14–16.

Chambers, M. (1988) Curriculum evaluation: an approach towards appraising a post-basic psychiatric course. *J. Adv. Nurs.*, **13**, 330–40.

Clark, J. M. and Hockey, L. (1979) *Research for Nursing*, H M and M, Aylesbury.

Conhye, A. (1987) Hidden assets. *Nurs. Times*, **83**, 49–50.

Coupar, A. and Conway, A. (1986) Hospital admission for depression. *J. Adv. Nurs.*, **11**, 697–704.

Cronin-Stubbs, D. and Brophy, E. B. (1985) Burnout: can social support save the psych nurse? *J. Psychosoc. Nurs. Mental Health Serv.*, **27**, 8–13.

Davis, B. D. (1981) Trends in psychiatric nursing research. Occasional paper, *Nurs. Times*, **77**, 73–6.

Davis, B. D. (1984a) Student nurse wastage and attitudes to treatment. *Nurs. Ed. Today*, **4**, 89–91.

Davis, B. D. (1984b) Student nurses' attitudes: their modification and associations. *Nurs. Ed. Today*, **4**, 117–20.

Davis, B. D. (1984c) Interviews with student nurses about their training. *Nurs. Ed. Today*, **4**, 136–40.

Davis, B. D. (1984d) What is the nurse's perception of the patient? In *Understanding Nurses* (ed. S. Skevington) Wiley, Chichester.

Davis, B. D. (1986a) A review of recent research in psychiatric nursing. In *Psychiatric Nursing Research* (ed. J. Brooking), Wiley, Chichester.

Davis, B. D. (1986b) Culture and psychiatric nursing. In *Transcultural Psychiatry* (ed. J. Cox), Croom Helm, Beckenham, Kent.

Davis, B. D. (1986c) The strain of training. In *Psychiatric Nursing Research* (ed. J. Brooking), Wiley, Chichester.

Davis, B. D. (1987) *Nursing Education: Research and Developments*, Croom Helm, Beckenham, Kent.

Dawe, A-M. (1983) The nursing needs of the mentally ill in the community. *Commun. Psych. Nurs. J.*, **3**, 38–41.

Dawkins, J. E., Depp, F. C. and Selzer, N. E. (1985) Occupational stress in a public mental hospital. *J. Psychosoc. Nurs. Mental Health Serv.*, **23**, 8–15.

Dawson, J., Johnston, M., Kehiayan, N. *et al.* (1988) Responses to patient assault. *J. Psychosoc. Nurs. Mental Health Serv.*, **26**, 8–15.

Dowling, G. A. (1985) Levels of cognitive functioning. *J. Neurosurg., Nurs.*, **17**, 129–34.

Dyke, R. (1984) CPN's and primary health care team attachment. Occasional paper, *Nurs. Times*, **80**, 55–7.

Floyd, J. A. (1984) Interaction between personal sleep–wake rhythms and psychiatric hospital rest–activity schedule. *Nurs. Res.*, **33**, 255–9.

Foreman, M. D. (1987) Reliability and validity of mental status questionnaires in elderly hospitalized patients. *Nurs. Res.*, **36**, 216–20.

Foster, J., Beck, J. and Wright, D. (1986) A child's view. *Nurs. Times*, **82**, 38–9.

Francis, G., Turner, J. T. and Johnson, S. B. (1985) Domestic animal visitation as therapy with adult home residents. *Int. J. Nurs. Studies*, **22**, 201–6.

Friend, W. (1984) An appraisal of the effectiveness of CPN's. Unpublished MPhil thesis, Manchester Polytechnic.

Garritson, S. H. (1988) Making patterns. *J. Psychosoc. Nurs. Mental Health Serv.*, **26**, 22–9.

George, P. and Dudley, M. (1986) Problem solving skills training for chronic psychiatric patients. *Commun. Psych. Nurs. J.*, **6**, 8–12.

Godin, P. and Wilson, I. (1986) Selling skills. *Nurs. Times Commun. Outlk.*, **5**, 27–8.

Gordon, V. (1986) Treatment of depressed women by nurses in Britain and the USA, in *Psychiatric Nursing Research* (ed. J. Brooking), Wiley, Chichester.

Gournay, K. (1986) A pilot study of nurses' attitudes with relation to post-basic training, in *Psychiatric Nursing Research* (ed. J. Brooking), Wiley, Chichester.

Graydon, J. E. (1984) Measuring patient coping. *Nurs. Pap.*, **16**, 3–12.

Hardin, S. B. and Durham, J. D. (1985) First rate: exploring the structure, process and effectiveness of nurse psychotherapy. *J. Psychosoc. Nurs. Mental Health Serv.*, **23**, 8–15.

Harries, C. (1982) Establishing order in a hospital hostel for the long term mentally ill. Unpublished MSc thesis, Guildford, University of Surrey.

Harries, C., Frois, M. and Healey, J. (1984) The hidden society: the practical use of multi-dimensional scaling to illuminate the pattern of relationships between long-stay psychiatric residents. *J. Adv. Nurs.*, **9**, 619–25.

Hendon, J. (1984) Liaising with the community. Psychiatry forum, *Nurs. Mirror*, **158**, vii–viii.

Hinds, P. S. (1984) Inducing a definition of hope through the use of grounded theory methodology. *J. Adv. Nurs.*, **9**, 357–62.

Hodgkinson, P., Hillis, T., and Russell, D. (1984) Assaults on staff in a psychiatric hospital. *Nurs. Times*, **80**, 44–6.

Holmes, T. H. and Rahe, R. H. (1967) The social readjustment rating scale. *J. Psychosom. Res.*, **11**, 213–8.

Horsley, J. A. (1983) *Using Research to Improve Nursing Practice: CURN Project*, Grune and Stratton, New York.

Hugo, M., Goldney, R., Skinner, E. *et al.* (1985) Using screening instruments in community psychiatric nursing for the elderly. *Aust. J. Adv. Nurs.*, **2**, 13–17.

Hussian, M. F. and Varadaraj, R. (1983) Responses to holding power. *Nurs. Times*, **79**, 44–5

Jaloweic, A., Murphy, S. P. and Powers, M. J. (1984) Psychometric assessment of the Jaloweic Coping Scale. *Nurs. Res.*, **33**, 157–61.

James, J., Goldney, R. and Spence, N. (1983) Psychological tests as predictors of success in psychiatric nurse education. *Aus. J. Adv. Nurs.*, **1**, 44–8.

Jones, R. G. (1986) Extended study to evaluate nurses' attitudes to geriatric psychiatry, in *Psychiatric Nursing Research* (ed. J. Brooking), Wiley, Chichester.

Jones, R. G. (1988) Experimental study to evaluate nursing staff morale in a high stimulation psychiatry setting. *J. Adv. Nurs.*, **13**, 352–7.

Jones, S. L. (1987) Detecting statistically significant differences. *J. Psychosoc. Nurs. Mental Health Serv.*, **25**, 38–42.

Jones, S. and Jones, R. (1987) Detecting statistically significant differences in psychiatric nursing research. *J. Psychosoc. Nurs.*, **25**, 38–45.

Jones, J. G., Janman, K., Payne, R. L. and Rick, J. T. (1987) Some determinants of stress in psychiatric nurses. *Int. J. Nurs. Studies*, **24**, 129–44.

Kelly, M. P. and May, D. (1982) Good and bad patients: a review of the literature and theoretical critique. *J. Adv. Nurs.*, **7**, 147–56.

Kennedy, J. (1986) The previous training and present training needs of nurses in charge of alcohol treatment units and community alcohol teams. *J. Adv. Nurs.*, **11**, 283–8.

Lanza, M. L. (1983) The reactions of nursing staff to physical assault by a patient. *Hosp. Commun. Psych.*, **34**, 44–7.

Larson, D. G. (1987) Helper secrets: internal stressors in nursing. *J. Psychosoc. Nurs. Mental Health Serv.*, **25**, 20–7.

Lavender, A. (1987a) Improving the quality of care on psychiatric hospital rehabilitation wards. *Brit. J. Psych.*, **150**, 476–81.

Lavender, A. (1987b) The effects of nurses changing from uniforms to everyday clothes on a psychiatric rehabilitation ward. *Brit. J. Med. Psychol.*, **60**, 189–99.

Leiba, P. A. (1984) Changes in the concept and practice of mental nursing with special reference to training. Unpublished MSc thesis, University of London.

Lemmer, W. (1986) The management of change: an evaluation of work upon five psychogeriatric wards of a London psychiatric hospital, West Lambeth Health Authority.

Levin, D., Diamond, R. and Goldstein, S. (1985) A study of alternating leadership for group psychotherapy in an aftercare clinic. *Perspect. Psych. Care*, **23**, 33–8.

London, M. (1986) Mental illness among immigrant minorities in the United Kingdom. *Brit. J. Psych.*, **149**, 265–73.

Marks, I. M. (1985) Psychiatric nurse therapists in primary care. Royal College of Nursing Research Report.

Marlow, H. A. and Marcotte, A. (1984) Client skills: non-verbal decoding. *J. Psychsoc. Nurs. Mental Health Serv.*, **22**, 9–15.

Marshall, P. D. (1985) Nursing patients – an enjoyable task? *J. Adv. Nurs.*, **10**, 429–34.

McBride, A. B. (1986) Theory and research: present issues and future perspectives of psychosocial nursing. *J. Psychosoc. Nurs. Mental Health Serv.*, **24**, 29–32.

McCarthy, P. (1985) Burnout in psychiatric nursing. *J. Adv. Nurs.*, **10**, 305–10.

Milne, D. (1984a) The development and evaluation of a structured learning format: introduction to behaviour therapy for psychiatric nurses. *Brit. J. Clin. Psychol.*, **23**, 175–85.

Milne, D. (1984b) Improving the social validity and implementation of behaviour therapy training for psychiatric nurses using a patient-centred learning format. *Brit. J. Psychol.*, **23**, 313–4.

Milne, D. (1985a) An observational evaluation of the effects of nurse training in behaviour therapy on unstructured ward activities and interactions. *Brit. J. Clin. Psychol.*, **24**, 149–58.

Milne, D. (1985b) 'The more things change the more they stay the same': factors affecting the implementation of the nursing process. *J. Adv. Nurs.*, **10**, 39–45.

Milne, D. and Whyke, T. (1988) New measures for the formative and summative evaluation of a post-basic psychiatric nurse education course. *J. Adv. Nurs.*, **13**, 79–86.

Milne, D. Burdett, C. and Conway, P. (1985) Review and replication of a 'core-course' in behaviour therapy for nurses. *J. Adv. Nurs.*, **10**, 137–48.

Muir-Cochrane, E. (1986) An examination of the psychiatric nursing component of degree/RGN courses in Britain, in *Psychiatric Nursing Research* (ed. J. Brooking), Wiley, Chichester.

Mullis, M. R. and Byers, P. M. (1987) Social support in suicidal patients. *J. Psychosoc. Nurs. Mental Health Serv.*, **25**, 16–19.

Munns, D. C. (1985) A validation of the defining characteristics of the nursing diagnosis of potential for violence. *Nurs. Clin. N. Amer.*, **20**, 711–72.

Murphy, J. F. and Cannon, D. J. (1986) Avoiding early drop-outs; patient selection and preparation techniques. *J. Psychosoc. Nurs. Mental Health Serv.*, **24**, 21–6.

Pardue, S. F. and Dick, C. T. (1986) Patient classification: illness acuity and nursing care needs. *J. Psychosoc. Nurs. Mental Health Serv.*, **24**, 23–30.

Phillips, M. S. (1983) Forensic psychiatry: nurses' attitudes revealed. *Dimens. Health Care*, **5**, 41–3.

Pollock, L. (1986) An evaluation study of community psychiatric nursing employing the personal questionnaire rapid scaling technique. *Commun. Psych., Nurs.*

J., **11**, 11–21.

Pollock, L. (1988a) The future work of community psychiatric nursing. *Commun. Psych. Nurs. J*, **5**, 5–13.

Pollock, L. (1988b) The work of the community psychiatric nurse. *J. Adv. Nurs.*, **13**, 537–45.

Pothier, P. C., Norbeck, J. S. and Laliberte, M. (1985) Child psychiatric services: the gap between need and utilisation. *J. Psychosoc. Nurs. Mental Health Serv.*, **23**, 18–23.

Reed, M. T. (1986) Descriptive study of chemically dependent nurses, in *Psychiatric Nursing Research* (ed. J. Brooking), Wiley, Chichester.

Reynolds, W. (1987) Empathy: we know what we mean, but what do we teach? *Nurs. Ed. Today*, **7**, 265–9.

Reynolds, W. and Cormack, D. F. S. (1985) Clinical teaching of group dynamics: an evaluation of a clinical teaching programme. *Nurs. Ed. Today*, **5**, 101–8.

Reynolds, W. and Presly, A. S. (1988) A study of empathy in student nurses. *Nurs. Ed. Today*, **8**, 123–30.

Richards, D. A. and Lambert, P. (1987) The nursing process: the effect on patients' satisfaction with nursing care. *J. Adv. Nurs.*, **12**, 559–62.

Richardson, B. K. (1987) Psychiatric in-patients' perceptions of the seclusion-room experience. *Nurs. Res.*, **36**, 234–8.

Rix, G. (1983) Time on their hands. *Nurs. Mirror*, **156**, 24–6.

Rix, G. (1987) Staff sickness and its relationships to violent incidents on a regional secure psychiatric unit. *J. Adv. Nurs.*, **12**, 223–8.

Roach, F. and Farley, N. (1986) The behavioural management of neurosis by the psychiatric nurse therapist, in *Psychiatric Nursing Research* (ed. J. Brooking), Wiley, Chichester.

Robinson, S. (1988) A study of some aspects of the role and education of the nurse in relation to the prevention and management of violent behaviour by mentally ill patients. Nursing Education Research Unit, Kings' College, London.

Rothman, J. (1980) *Using Research in Organisations: A Guide to Successful Application*, Sage, Beverley Hills.

Rushforth, D. (1986) An evaluation of the management of deliberate self-poisoning within a health authority, using the community psychiatric nurse as an agent of change. Unpublished MPhil thesis, Manchester Polytechnic.

Sankar, S. (1987) Teaching psychiatric nursing: curriculum development for the 1982 syllabus, in *Nursing Education: Research and Development* (ed. B. D. Davis), Croom Helm, Beckenham, Kent.

Scadden, J. G. (1985) An ideal typical approach to the study of nurse–patient interactions in psychiatric settings. Unpublished MSc thesis, Guildford, University of Surrey.

Selander, J. M. and Miller, W. C. (1985) Prolixin group: a recidivism rate study using mirror image controls. *J. Psychosoc. Nurs. Mental Health Serv.*, **23**, 16–20.

Sencicle, L. (1987) Assessing the objectives for an economic evaluation of community psychiatric nursing care. *Commun. Psych. Nurs. J.*, **3**, 18–21.

Shanley, E. (1985) A study of the relationship between the characteristics of mental nurses and the perception of others of mental nurses in acute admission wards. Unpublished PhD thesis, University of Edinburgh.

Shapiro, M. B. (1961) A method of measuring psychological changes specific to the individual psychiatric patient. *Brit. J. Med. Psychol.*, **134**, 151–5.

Shields, P. J., Morrison, P. and Hart, D. (1988) Consumer satisfaction on a psychiatric ward. *J. Adv. Nurs.*, **13**, 396–400.

Sills, G. M. (1977) Research in the field of psychiatric nursing. *Nurs. Res.*, **26**, 206–10.

Simmons, S. M. (1984) Family burden: what does it mean to the carers? Unpublished MSc thesis, Guildford, University of Surrey.

Skidmore, D. (1986) The effectiveness of community psychiatric nursing teams and base-locations, in *Psychiatric Nursing Research* (ed. J. Brooking), Wiley, Chichester.

Smith, B. J. and Cantrell, P. J. (1988) Distance in nurse–patient encounters. *J. Psychosoc. Nurs. Mental Health Serv.*, **26**, 22–6.

Stanley, B. (1984) Evaluation of treatment goals: the use of goal attainment scaling. *J. Adv. Nurs.* **9**, 351–6.

Storer, D., Whitworth, R., Salkovskis, P. and Atha, C. (1987) Community psychiatric nursing intervention in an accident and emergency department: a clinical pilot study. *J. Adv. Nurs.*, **12**, 215–22.

Sugden, J. (1985) The psychiatric treatment setting: some general considerations, in *Psychiatric Nursing* (ed. A. T. Altschul), Churchill Livingstone, Edinburgh.

Teasdale, K. (1987) Stigma and psychiatric day care. *J. Adv. Nurs.*, **12**, 339–46.

Thomas, W. (1984) Depot drugs in community psychiatry. *Nurs. Times*, **80**, 43–6.

Thomas, M. D., Sanger, E. S. and Whitney, J. D. (1986) Nursing diagnosis of depression: clinical identification on an inpatient unit. *J. Psychosoc. Nurs. Mental Health Serv.*, **24**, 6–12.

Tilley, S. and Weighill, V. E. (1986) How nurse therapists assess and contribute to the management of alcohol and sedative use among anxious patients. *J. Adv. Nurs.*, **11**, 499–503.

Tissier, J. (1986) The development of a psychiatric nursing assessment form, in *Psychiatric Nursing Research* (ed. J. Brooking), Wiley, Chichester.

Towell, D. and Harries, C. (1979) *Innovation in Patient Care*, Croom Helm, Beckenham, Kent.

Trygstad, L. N. (1986) Stress and coping in psychiatric nursing. *J. Psychosoc. Nurs. Mental Health Serv.*, **24**, 23–7.

Turner, H. B., Kreutzer, J. S., Lent, B. and Brockett, C. A. (1984) Developing a brief neuropsychological mental status exam: a pilot study. *J. Neurosurg. Nurs.*, **16**, 257–61.

Wake, P. (1986) Shifting the system. *Nurs. Times*, **82**, 34–5.

Walder, C. P., McCracken, J. S., Herbert, M. *et al.* (1987) Psychological intervention in civilian flying phobia: evaluation and three year follow-up. *Brit. J. Psych.*, **151**, 494–8.

Welt, S. R. (1984) Can training do the job?: another view on 'non-verbal decoding'. *J. Psychosoc. Nurs. Mental Health Serv.*, **22**, 12–13.

Wetherill, J., Kelly, T. and Hore, B. (1987) The role of the community psychiatric nurse in improving treatment compliance in alcoholics. *J. Adv. Nurs.*, **12**, 707–11.

Whetstone, W. R. (1986) Social dramatics: social skills development for the chronically mentally ill. *J. Adv. Nurs.*, **11**, 67–74.

White, E. G. (1986) Factors influencing general practitioners to refer patients to community psychiatric nurses, *Psychiatric Nursing Research* (ed. J. Brooking), Wiley, Chichester.

Whiteside, S. E., Harris, A. and Whiteside, H. D. (1983) Patient education. *J. Psychosoc. Nurs. Mental Health Serv.*, **21**, 17–21.

Wright, F. and Briggs, S. (1986) Great expectations? *Nurs. Times*, **80**, 38–40.

Youssef, F. A. (1983) Compliance with therapeutic regimes: a follow-up study for patients with affective disorders. *J. Adv. Nurs.*, **8**, 513–7.

Index